The Essential Guide to Coding in Otolaryngology

Coding, Billing, and Practice Management

The Essential Guide to Coding in Otolaryngology

Coding, Billing, and Practice Management

Seth M. Brown, MD, MBA
Kimberly J. Pollock, RN, MBA, CPC, CMDP
Michael Setzen, MD
Abtin Tabaee, MD

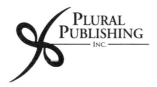

PLURAL PUBLISHING INC.

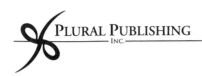

5521 Ruffin Road
San Diego, CA 92123
e-mail: info@pluralpublishing.com
Website: http://www.pluralpublishing.com

Typeset in 11/13 Palatino by Flanagan's Publishing Service, Inc.
Printed in the United States of America by McNaughton & Gunn, Inc.

NOTICE TO THE READER
Care has been taken to confirm the accuracy of the indications, procedures, codes and diagnoses presented in this book and to ensure that they conform to the practices of the general medical and health services communities. It is recommended that International Classification of Diseases (ICD), Current Procedural Terminology (CPT®) and best practice guidelines are followed at all times. All procedures performed must be done for the proper indications. However, the authors, editors and publisher are not responsible for errors or omissions or for any consequences from application of the information in this book and make no warranty, expressed or implied, with respect to the currency, completeness, or accuracy of the contents of the publication. Application of this information in a particular situation remains the professional responsibility of the practitioner. Because standards of practice and usage change, it is the responsibility of the practitioner to keep abreast of revised recommendations and procedures. It is recommended that the practitioner reviews updated CPT, ICD and practice guidelines as published by the American Medical Association, the Centers for Medicare and Medicaid Services and the American Academy of Otolaryngology-Head and Neck Surgery, amongst others. A coding professional should be consulted when necessary to confirm that the services are coded properly.

CPT copyright 2015 American Medical Association. All rights reserved. Fee schedules, relative value units, conversion factors and/or related components are not assigned by the AMA, are not part of CPT, and the AMA is not recommending their use. The AMA does not directly or indirectly practice medicine or dispense medical services. The AMA assumes no liability for data contained or not contained herein. CPT is a registered trademark of the American Medical Association.

Library of Congress Cataloging-in-Publication Data

Names: Brown, Seth M., editor. | Pollock, Kimberly J., editor. | Setzen,
    Michael, editor. | Tabaee, Abtin, editor.
Title: The essential guide to coding in otolaryngology : coding, billing, and
    practice management / [edited by] Seth M. Brown, Kimberly J. Pollock,
    Michael Setzen, Abtin Tabaee.
Description: San Diego, CA : Plural Publishing, [2016] | Includes
    bibliographical references and index.
Identifiers: LCCN 2015046756| ISBN 9781597566162 (alk. paper) | ISBN
    1597566160 (alk. paper)
Subjects: | MESH: Otolaryngology--organization & administration | Clinical
    Coding--methods | Practice Management, Medical--economics
Classification: LCC RF56 | NLM WV 100 | DDC 617.5/10068--dc23
LC record available at http://lccn.loc.gov/2015046756

Contents

Introduction

The goal of this book is to provide a readable, yet searchable coding text. Unlike most coding books, which are often reference texts and written entirely by coding professionals, the ultimate goal was to create an otolaryngology coding book geared for physicians with significant physician input in the content. To make this project possible, the authors are a combination of leaders in otolaryngology, physicians with an interest in coding, and leading coding and practice management professionals in otolaryngology.

This book will appeal to all practicing otolaryngologists, residents, fellows, physician extenders, and coding professionals. It is basic enough for a resident to read and learn, yet detailed enough to appeal to the most advanced practitioner and coder and use as a reference text. The goal is not to be the exhaustive reference source, but to be a guide to use to assist in correct coding initiatives. The reader should use this in addition to standard American Medical Association (AMA) coding sources that are the gold standard. Although every effort has been made to be as accurate as possible, many of the clinical coding chapters are written by practicing physicians without formal coding education. When in doubt, consult your coding professional, the American Academy of Otolaryngology-Head and Neck Surgery, or the AMA.

This book is designed in 3 sections. The first provides a framework to coding and is designed to be read as a text. It includes chapters written by practice management and coding experts in the field and covers the fundamentals of coding, including billing strategies, dealing with appealing denials, *International Classification of Diseases, Tenth Revision, Clinical Modification* (ICD-10-CM), and the use of modifiers. The next 2 sections are divided by subspecialty focus area and type of service, office vs surgery. Although this causes some overlap, it allows one to either read an entire chapter on an area of interest or use this as a reference. The authors of these chapters are practicing providers, thus incorporating real-life experiences in these 2 sections. Pertinent references and resources are included in the text for the reader; however, it is important to note that some references may require login to the American Academy of Otolaryngology-Head and Neck to access the reference.

The ideal of incorporating different authors does limit standardization of this text; however, we feel strongly that this allows the text to have a true subspecialty focus and incorporate the ideas of multiple experts in the field. We have also included *International Classification of Diseases, Ninth Revision, Clinical Modification* (ICD-9-CM) codes in addition to ICD-10-CM codes. During production, ICD-9-CM was still in use, and it is our belief that for this edition leaving ICD-9-CM in place along with ICD-10-CM will provide a smoother transition to our physicians and health care providers.

Preface

Physicians spend years training for their careers in medicine through medical school, residency, and fellowship; however, little formal training has traditionally been provided in coding, business, and practice management for physicians during this path. These topics are critical for financial success in practice. This leads to common, often preventable errors and inefficiencies. The potential negative impact of improper coding is huge, including underpayment, overpayment, noncompliance with government guidelines, audits, and financial and sometimes even criminal penalties. There is also a paucity of available quality resources out there geared toward practicing physicians.

As a result, all of the editors have spent significant time independently and often together, educating peers, residents, fellows, and other coding professionals. This book is a compilation of our ideas, teaching, and teamwork to provide a text that is specifically geared to practicing otolaryngologists but in depth enough for coding professionals to find useful. Enlisting the help of some of not only the most recognizable names in otolaryngology and otolaryngology coding and practice management, but also physicians with a genuine interest in coding made this book a reality. We feel confident you will find this book useful in your practice endeavors now and in the future.

Acknowledgments

We would like to acknowledge all of the outstanding contributors to this book who took time out of their busy clinical and professional practices to make this book a reality.

Contributors

Debra Abel, AuD
Arch Health Partners
Poway, California
Chapter 17

Amit D. Bhrany, MD
Assistant Professor
Department of Otolaryngology-Head and Neck
    Surgery
University of Washington
Seattle, Washington
Chapter 18

R. Cheyenne Brinson, MBA, CPA
Consultant and Speaker
KarenZupko & Associates, Inc.
Chicago, Illinois
Chapter 6

Seth M. Brown, MD, MBA, FACS
Connecticut Sinus Institute
ProHealth Physicians
Assistant Clinical Professor
Department of Surgery
Division of Otolaryngology Head and Neck
    Surgery
University of Connecticut School of Medicine
Farmington, Connecticut
Chief of Service - Otolaryngology
St. Francis Hospital and Medical Center
Hartford, Connecticut
Chapters 12 and 23

Manderly A. Cohen, MS, CCC-SLP
Director of Voice and Swallowing
Michael Setzen Otolaryngology, PC
Great Neck, New York
Chapter 15

Marc A. Cohen, MD, MPH
Assistant Professor
Department of Otolaryngology
Weill Cornell Medical College
New York Presbyterian Hospital
New York, New York
Chapter 19

John P. Dahl, MD, PhD, MBA
Fellow Pediatric Otolaryngology
Seattle Children's Hospital
Department of Otolaryngology-Head and Neck
    Surgery
University of Washington
Seattle, Washington
Chapter 20

Rebecca E. Fraioli, MD
Assistant Professor
Department of Otolaryngology
Montefiore Medical Center
Albert Einstein College of Medicine
Bronx, New York
Chapter 27

Neal D. Futran, MD, DMD
Professor and Chair
Director of Head and Neck Surgery
Department of Otolaryngology-Head and Neck
    Surgery
University of Washington
Seattle, Washington
Chapter 29

Babak Givi, MD, FACS
Assistant Professor
Department of Otolaryngology-Head and Neck
    Surgery
New York University
New York, New York
Chapter 29

Andrew M. Hinson, MD
Otolaryngology-Head and Neck Surgery
University of Arkansas for Medical Sciences
Little Rock, Arkansas
Chapter 28

Patricia S. Hofstra, Esq
Partner
Duane Morris LLP
Chicago, Illinois
Chapter 7

John W. Ingle, MD
Assistant Professor
Director, University of Rochester Voice Center
Department of Otolaryngology
Rochester, New York
Chapter 14

Adam S. Jacobson, MD
Associate Professor
Department of Otolaryngology-Head and Neck
  Surgery
NYU Langone Medical Center
Laura and Isaac Perlmutter Cancer Center
New York, New York
Chapter 29

Mary Lally, MS, CAE
Deputy CEO IAC
Ellicott City, MD
Chapter 22

Jivianne T. Lee, MD
Co-Director, Orange County Sinus Institute,
  SCPMG
Clinical Assistant Professor
Department of Otolaryngology-Head and Neck
  Surgery
David Geffen School of Medicine
University of California, Los Angeles
Los Angeles, California
Chapter 24

Fred Y. Lin, MD
Icahn School of Medicine at Mount Sinai
Assistant Professor
Director, Mount Sinai Sleep Surgery Center
Department of Otolaryngology-Head and Neck
  Surgery
New York, New York
Chapter 33

Natalie Loops, CPC-A
Practice Management Programs Manager
KarenZupko & Associates, Inc.
Chicago, Illinois
Chapter 1

Michelle M. Mesley-Netoskie, CPC
Senior Billing Analyst

Albany ENY and Allergy Services, PC
Albany, New York
Chapters 13 and 22

Elinor Hart Murárová, JD
Associate
Duane Morris LLP
Chicago, Illinois
Chapter 7

Jason G. Newman, MD, FACS
Associate Professor
Department of Otorhinolaryngology-Head and
  Neck Surgery
Perelman School of Medicine
University of Pennsylvania
Philadelphia, Pennsylvania
Chapter 31

Betsy Nicoletti, MS, CPC
Medical Practice Consulting, LLC
Speaker, Educator, Author
Springfield, Vermont
Chapters 9 and 10

Bert W. O'Malley, Jr., MD
Professor and Chairman
Department of Otorhinolaryngology -Head and
  Neck Surgery
University of Pennsylvania Health System
Philadelphia, Pennsylvania
Chapter 31

Sanjay R. Parikh, MD, FACS
Professor
Department of Otolaryngology-Head and Neck
  Surgery
University of Washington
Seattle Children's Hospital
Seattle, Washington
Chapter 20

Anit T. Patel, MD, MBA, FACS
Otolaryngologist
Plymouth ENT
Medical Director
South Shore Sleep Diagnostics
Plymouth, Massachusetts
Chapter 21

Kimberley J. Pollock, RN, MBA, CPC, CMDP
Consultant
KarenZupko & Associates, Inc.
Chicago, Illinois
Chapters 9, 10, and 11

Teri Romano, RN, MBA
Consultant
KarenZupko & Associates, Inc.
Chicago, Illinois
Chapter 2

Clark A. Rosen, MD, FACS
Professor of Otolaryngology
University of Pittsburgh School of Medicine
Director
University of Pittsburgh Voice Center
Pittsburgh, Pennsylvania
Chapter 14

Babak Sadoughi, MD, FACS
Assistant Professor of Otolaryngology
The Sean Parker Institute for the Voice
Department of Otolaryngology-Head and Neck
   Surgery
Weill Cornell Medical College
New York Presbyterian Hospital
New York, New York
Chapter 25

Gavin Setzen, MD, FACS, FAAOA
Clinical Associate Professor of Otolaryngology
Albany Medical College
Chief of ENT Surgery
St. Peter's Hospital
Albany, New York
Chapters 13 and 22

Michael Setzen, MD
Clinical Associate Professor of Otolaryngology
New York University School of Medicine
Adjunct Clinical Assistant Professor of
   Otolaryngology
Weill Cornell University College of Medicine
Section Chief of Rhinology
North Shore University Hospital
Great Neck, New York
Chapter 15

Jack A. Shohet, MD
President
Shohet Ear Associates Medical Group, Inc.
Clinical Professor
University of California, Irvine
Department of Otolaryngology-Head and Neck
   Surgery
Irvine, California
Chapter 30

Lawrence M. Simon, MD, FAAP, FACS
Pediatric and General Otolaryngologist
Hebert Medical Group
Clinical Assistant Professor
Department of Otolaryngology-Head and Neck
   Surgery
Louisiana State University Health Sciences
   Center
New Orleans, Louisiana
Chapters 4 and 32

Margaret A. Skurka, MS, RHIA, CCS, FAHIMA
Professor
College of Health and Human Services
Chair
Department of Health Information
   Management
Indiana University Northwest
Gary, Indiana
Chapter 3

Brendan C. Stack, Jr., MD, FACS, FACE
Professor
Otolaryngology-Head and Neck Surgery
University of Arkansas for Medical Sciences
Little Rock, Arkansas
Chapter 28

Lucian Sulica, MD
Sean Parker Professor of Otolaryngology
Director, Sean Parker Institute for the Voice
Department of Otolaryngology-Head and Neck
   Surgery
Weill Cornell Medical College
New York, New York
Chapter 25

Charles A. Syms III, MD, MBA
President, Ear Medical Group
Clinical Professor of Otolaryngology-Head and
	Neck Surgery
University of Texas Health Science Center at San
	Antonio
San Antonio, Texas
Chapter 26

Abtin Tabaee, MD
Associate Professor
Department of Otolaryngology-Head and Neck
	Surgery
Weill Cornell Medical College
New York, New York
Chapter 19

Belachew Tessema, MD, FACS
Connecticut Sinus Institute
ProHealth Physicians
Assistant Clinical Professor
University of Connecticut School of Medicine
Department of Surgery
Division of Otolaryngology Head and Neck
	Surgery
Farmington, Connecticut
Chapter 30

Christopher R. Thompson, MD
Chief Resident
Department of Otolaryngology-Head and Neck
	Surgery
University of Texas Health Science Center
San Antonio, Texas
Chapter 26

Cheryl Toth, MBA
Consultant and Trainer
KarenZupko & Associates, Inc.
Chicago, Illinois
Chapter 5

Richard W. Waguespack, MD, FACS
Clinical Professor
Department of Otolaryngology-Head and Neck
	Surgery
University of Alabama at Birmingham
Section Chief, Otolaryngology
Birmingham VA Medical Center
Birmingham, Alabama
Chapter 4

Gregory S. Weinstein, MD
Professor and Vice Chair
Director, Division of Head and Neck Surgery
Co-Director, The Center for Head and Neck
	Cancer
Department of Otorhinolaryngology-Head and
	Neck Surgery
The University of Pennsylvania
Perelman School of Medicine
Philadelphia, Pennsylvania
Chapter 31

Sarah Wiskerchen, MBA
Consultant and Speaker
KarenZupko & Associates, Inc.
Chicago, Illinois
Chapter 8

Benjamin J. Wycherly, MD
Assistant Clinical Professor
Division of Otolaryngology
Department of Surgery
University of Connecticut
Farmington, Connecticut
Chapter 16

Karen A. Zupko
President
KarenZupko & Associates, Inc.
Chicago, Illinois
Chapter 5

I would like to dedicate this book to my mentors in medicine, health care and life: Dr. Marvin Fried, Dr. Vijay Anand and my parents Dr. David and Barbara Brown. I would like to thank my partners, Drs. Belachew Tessema and Ben Wycherly, for their friendship, companionship, and support with this project. Finally, and most importantly, I would like to thank my family, Betsy, Ella, and Tessa who put up with me on a daily basis and make life more enjoyable.

—SB

This book is dedicated to my wife, Elsa, for her support and love in all of our moments together. I would also like to thank Vijay Anand and Mark Persky for their mentorship throughout my career. Finally, I would like to convey my sincere gratitude to the co-editors and authors of this book for their dedication, hard work, and expertise.

—AT

A special thanks to my wife Sheryl for her never-ending support throughout my entire professional career and without whom I could not have been successful.

—MS

Dedicated to the memory of my mentor in consulting, Debra Dorf, who introduced me to the world of coding and taught me that accurate coding is not only ethical but helps both the physician and patient. Thank you to my colleagues at KarenZupko & Associates, Inc. for the excellent chapters. Sincerest appreciation to my co-authors for their patience with me and the invaluable professional dialogue we had while reviewing chapters. Finally, my heartfelt gratitude to Arthur for his endless support and love throughout this book process and always.

—KP

SECTION I

Basics of Coding and Billing

CHAPTER 1

Essentials of Coding

Natalie Loops

There are few complex entities in the world that can be summed up in 5 digits. Medical coding does this with a *Current Procedural Terminology* (CPT®) code. Would 99205, in any other system, be able to tell you as much as it does in CPT? Creating a system that strives to describe a complex procedure or diagnosis with just a few digits is a very enterprising task. Not surprisingly, the coding process has been an evolution leading to reams of information, multiple exceptions, and revisions. The information presented in this book has been curated to present you with just the essentials, making otolaryngology coding simple and straightforward.

Starting with the basics, the three main sets of codes used are the *International Classification of Diseases, Ninth Revision, Clinical Modification* (ICD-9-CM) as well as *International Classification of Diseases, Tenth Revision, Clinical Modification* (ICD-10-CM), which is published by the World Health Organization (WHO); the *Current Procedural Terminology (CPT) Manual*, which is published by the American Medical Association (AMA); and the Healthcare Common Procedure Coding System, Level II (HCPCS Level II), which is released by the Centers for Medicare and Medicaid (CMS). These code sets come out with updates annually. Make sure you have the most recent versions of these texts. The new books are not just sales gimmicks. There are actual changes made to these codes, which are very important and affect the coding and reimbursement process. Practitioners are required to follow the AMA's CPT coding guidelines. However, payers such as Medicare may have their own payment or reimbursement

rules. It is important not to confuse the two—coding versus reimbursement.

If you are here reading this text it is evident that you think coding is important, but do you know the multitude of reasons why? Perhaps the most obvious reason is that correct coding can significantly increase the amount you are reimbursed for your efforts. As if that is not motivating enough, correct medical coding also decreases your practice's risk for an audit and thus minimizes the chance you will experience a payment take-back. Having a thorough knowledge of coding, billing, and practice management will also allow you to lead an efficient and high-functioning practice.

In 2002 the Improper Payments Information Act was signed into law. The act requires federal agencies to review programs they administer, estimate improper payments, and improve the steps they have been taking to bring back to the government the money that was given erroneously. The report for 2013 estimates that $9.5 billion of improper payments were allocated due to no documentation, insufficient documentation, medical necessity, incorrect coding, or "other".[1] This report and the subsequent call to action has led to some very aggressive Recovery Audit Contractors (RAC). A RAC is an entity hired by the Centers for Medicare and Medicaid Services (CMS) to recoup as much as possible of the $9.5 billion. The RAC is paid a percentage of the amount of money regained, which is extremely motivating for the RAC. According to CMS, "In Fiscal Year (FY) 2013, Recovery Auditors collectively identified and corrected 1,532,249 claims for improper payments, which resulted in $3.75 billion in improper payments being corrected."[2] So if the prospect of receiving accurate payment is not incentive enough to learn to code correctly, perhaps keeping the RAC out of your practice is.

Still not convinced that coding is imperative? Here is another reason it should be done correctly; it helps others. Medical codes assist public health officials in tracking diseases and procedures to plan for resource allocation in the future. The codes provided are used by a multitude of others who are working to make health care run more smoothly. For example, the WHO did not just publish the ICD-9-CM codes and say, "that's it, we're done." The WHO regularly tracks this epidemiological data and uses it to focus new research on the progress of diseases in order to better understand and treat them, while also teaching others to prevent future illness. Coding trends are also utilized to negotiate funds for public education on topics that range from hand washing to tobacco use. Last, medical management uses trends in these data to make sure you have the right supplies when you need them. In summation, correct coding helps you be reimbursed to the fullest extent without concerns of an audit or a take-back of funds, it aids research and assists epidemiologists, and it provides trend data to administrators providing for the allocation of future funds and supplies.

Right now you are thinking, "Wow medical coding is important"! So, who is the best person to code? Typically the provider does the coding himself or herself or a medical coder provides this service based on the documentation. If a medical coder is the chosen route, it is important that the provider be involved in the correct reporting of services since his or her name will be on each claim that is submitted. Coding is a complex subject and the provider should want to make sure that the coding reflects the documentation, is in accordance with the most recent changes, and correctly reflects the work performed. Therefore, if the coding is delegated from the provider to the coder, it is crucial to be sure the coder is capable, accurate, properly educated, comfortable enough to query the provider when there are questions, and up to date on all the changes continually released. Ideally the coder should be certified, though there are many very capable and knowledgeable coders

who are not. The coder should have access to tools that enhance coding accuracy, as well as ongoing education about current diagnosis and procedure code changes.

The two most recognized certifying bodies for medical coding are the AAPC (formerly American Academy of Professional Coders) and the American Health Information Management Association (AHIMA). Each of these organizations issues a variety of certificates acknowledging medical coding proficiency. The two that are the most common for physician-based settings are the Certified Professional Coder (CPC) certification from AAPC and the Certified Coding Specialist-Physician-Based (CCS-P) certification from AHIMA. Passing these respective board exams to receive these certifications requires demonstrative and detailed knowledge of CPT, ICD-9-cm/icd-10-cm, and HCPCS Level II coding systems.

If you are unsure of a coder's abilities, this can be discerned by asking him or her a few questions. A certified coder should have a robust working knowledge of important topics such as those of Medicare's global surgical periods. In case you are unfamiliar with this term, certain procedure codes have a postoperative global period that is also known as "postop global days." This means that the Medicare reimbursement for that CPT code includes all necessary services that are normally performed for that procedure after the surgery. A global period applies for all settings including the doctor's office and the hospital and ranges from zero for a procedure such as an endoscopy (eg, 31231) to 90 days for a surgery like a septoplasty (30520). Some services that are included in the global surgical package for a CPT code are the preop visit after the decision for surgery has been made, removal of sutures, and management of postoperative pain. Billing of any of these reasonable situations to the patient's payer when he or she is in a global period is considered unbundling. You will see the terms *global surgical package* and *global period* used throughout this book. Remember, this is a Medicare payment rule because the CPT definition of "typical follow up care" is vague and subjective. To find out what a procedure code's global period is, one can head to National Medicare Physician Fee Schedule Database on the CMS website.[3]

For most otolaryngologists, the vast majority of service codes selected are evaluation and management (E/M) CPT codes. Thus, it is imperative that these services are coded correctly. An important concept to understand is how to choose the appropriate coding level for the visit. In most cases, the complexity of the patient's situation and in turn the difficulty of the medical decision making is the decisive component determining the level of the office visit. CMS defines medical decision making as follows:

The complexity of establishing a diagnosis and/or selecting a management option, which is determined by considering the following factors:

- The number of possible diagnoses and/or the number of management options that must be considered
- The amount and/or complexity of medical records, diagnostic tests, and/or other information that must be obtained, reviewed, and analyzed
- The risk of significant complications, morbidity, and/or mortality as well as comorbidities associated with the patient's presenting problem(s), the diagnostic procedure(s), and/or the possible management options[4]

These factors are somewhat subjective, and many medical coders do not have a clinical background. Therefore, this is another reason the medical coder/provider relationship must have open lines of communication. In order to accurately code the service provided, the coder must feel comfortable querying the provider when the complexity of the patient's visit is unclear in the documentation.

The information contained in this book is based on the coding guidelines specified in the CPT, ICD-9-CM/ICD-10-CM, and HCPCS Level II coding books and from information released by these same sources. Occasionally payer rules are contrary to the CPT guidelines stated. In these situations, it is important to understand the payer's rules in order to receive accurate reimbursement, but deference should be made to the CPT rules.

Similar to the need for accuracy in medical diagnosis and treatment, accurate information is essential in the world of medical coding. If you are looking for further information, refer to the AMA's CPT Assistant as well as "CPT Changes: An Insider's View" publications, CMS' National Correct Coding Initiative (CCI) Policy Manual, and individual payer's websites. The CPT Assistant is a monthly publication released by the same organization that wrote the CPT book. Here they provide more detailed information than the format the printed book can allow. This makes the CPT Assistant a superb tool to reference when appealing denials. The CMS' National Correct Coding Initiative (CCI) Policy Manual is released quarterly, and its sole purpose is to provide accurate payments on Part B claims. Finally, when in doubt head to the payer's website. Payers such as Blue Cross and Blue Shield and CMS have an abundance of information on coding as well as the medical necessity they deem appropriate. These are all tools that our professional coder colleagues utilize on a regular basis, and communication with them is of the utmost importance to remain accurate and up to date.

References

1. Centers for Medicare & Medicaid Services. Comprehensive Error Rate Testing (CERT). http://www.cms.gov/Research-Statistics-Data-and-Systems/Monitoring-Programs/Medicare-FFS-Compliance-Programs/CERT/Downloads/CERT-101-07-2013.pdf. Accessed November 23, 2014.
2. Centers for Medicare and Medicaid Services. Recovery auditing in Medicare for fiscal year 2013. http://www.cms.gov/Research-Statistics-Data-and-Systems/Monitoring-Programs/Medicare-FFS-Compliance-Programs/Recovery-Audit-Program/Downloads/FY-2013-Report-To-Congress.pdf. Accessed November 23, 2014.
3. Centers for Medicare and Medicaid Services. Medicare physician fee schedule. http://www.cms.gov/apps/physician-fee-schedule/overview.aspx. Accessed November 23, 2014.
4. Centers for Medicare and Medicaid Services. Evaluation and management services guide. http://www.cms.gov/Outreach-and-Education/Medicare-Learning-Network-MLN/MLNProducts/downloads/eval_mgmt_serv_guide-ICN006764.pdf. Accessed November 23, 2014.

CHAPTER 2

Navigating the CPT® Book

Teri Romano

What is CPT?

Current Procedural Terminology (CPT®) is a comprehensive compilation of descriptive terms and identifying codes that are used to report services provided by physicians and other health care professionals. The intent of CPT codes is to provide a uniform, nationwide nomenclature that can be used to accurately describe medical, surgical, and diagnostic services.

First developed in 1966, CPT codes describe what a physician does during a patient encounter. In 2000, CPT codes were designated by the Department of Health and Human Services as the national coding standard, and as such, all financial and administrative health care transactions require the use of the CPT code set. The current version is *Current Procedural Terminology* (CPT) 2015, fourth edition.

Simply stated, CPT codes describe physician work and are the basis for reporting of services. Payment from governmental and private entities is calculated based on these nationally utilized codes. Otolaryngologists should understand how these codes are developed and used if their services are to be reported accurately.

The American Medical Association (AMA) owns and is responsible for maintaining the CPT codes and overseeing code development and revision. New, revised, and deleted CPT codes are officially introduced each year and become effective on January 1 of the upcoming year. The AMA publishes an annual CPT book (referred to as a *CPT Manual*) listing all CPT codes that are effective for that year including new, revised, and deleted codes. This publication is typically available in early fall of the prior year, giving users of the codes approximately 2 months to incorporate the use of any new codes that impact their specialty. The CPT code set is published as both electronic data files and a book. Physicians should purchase a current data file or book each year (the Professional Edition is recommended) to ensure the use of current and accurate CPT codes.

The CPT Development Process

The CPT code development is an ongoing process managed by the AMA. Over 80 medical societies, representing all specialties, have representatives on what is known as the *AMA CPT Advisory Committee* and provide input to code development. This committee evaluates proposed new codes as well as the revision of existing codes. A new CPT code may be proposed by a physician, a medical society, a medical device company, or anyone with an interest in the establishment of a new code. The CPT Advisory Committee (not just the relevant specialty groups) evaluates all new or revised codes and, if approved, these become part of the CPT code set.

7

The *CPT Manual*: Content and Format

Content

The *CPT Manual* includes the following main chapters:

Introduction

Illustrated Anatomical and Procedural Review

Evaluation and Management (E/M) Services

Anesthesia

Surgery

Radiology

Pathology and Laboratory

Medicine

Category II codes

Category III codes

Appendices

Codes for otolaryngologists and their staff will primarily come from the E/M section (office and inpatient visits), the surgery section (eg, sinus, head, and neck surgery), as well as from the radiology (eg, in-office sinus computed tomography [CT]) and medicine sections (eg, audiology testing, allergy). However, codes used by otolaryngologists can come from any of the above sections. CPT codes are not specialty specific. Any specialty may use any CPT code if it accurately describes the work performed.

Code Format

There are three types of CPT codes: Category I, II, and III. A description of each type of CPT code is found in Table 2–1. Category I and III codes, those used most commonly by otolaryngologists, are defined below.

Category I CPT Codes

Category I CPT codes, the bulk of the CPT codes used, are identified with a 5-digit numerical code.

A Category I code designates that a procedure is Food and Drug Administration (FDA) approved, consistent with current medical practice, and performed frequently by many physicians in the United States. Each Category I CPT code includes a brief description of the specific procedure or service. For example,

30100 Biopsy, intranasal

Many codes will have a base code and one or more indented codes that describe a related but different procedure. For example,

31254 Nasal/sinus endoscopy, surgical; with ethmoidectomy, partial (anterior)

31255 with ethmoidectomy, total (anterior and posterior)

In the above case, the root description is "nasal/sinus endoscopy, surgical." The semicolon indicates the end of the base or root description. The wording following the semicolon further describes the procedure. In the related codes (in this example 31255), everything after the semicolon is replaced by the descriptors of the second, related code. For example, the full procedure represented by code 31255, is read as follows:

31255 Nasal/sinus endoscopy, surgical; with ethmoidectomy, total (anterior and posterior)

Category III CPT Codes

Some new procedures or new technologies do not meet the description or intent of an existing Category I code. In this case, the AMA may decide to develop a Category III code. Category III codes, often referred to as "T" codes, are 4-digit codes followed by the letter T. The procedures and devices described by a Category III code may not yet be FDA approved, are not yet performed routinely across the country, or are not yet supported by the peer-reviewed, published data. Because most Category III codes are not assigned a fee by Medicare, payers determine whether to provide reimbursement for a Category III code. Practices should always obtain preauthorization prior to performing a procedure or placing a device that

Table 2–1. Types of CPT Codes

Code	Description

Category I CPT Codes	• These are 5-digit numerical codes. The majority of CPT codes are Category I codes.
	• They designate procedures and services performed frequently by many physicians and other qualified health care professionals in the United States.
	• All devices and drugs used to perform the procedure are Food and Drug Administration (FDA) approved.
	• The procedure is consistent with current medical practice.
	
	Stand-alone Category I codes are 5-digit codes for procedures that may be performed as sole or primary procedures.
	
	    Example: **30520** Septoplasty or submucous resection, with or without cartilage scoring, contouring or replacement with graft
	
	Add-on Category I codes are also 5-digit numerical codes but are preceded by the + symbol. Add-on codes are always performed in addition to a stand-alone or primary procedure. These primary procedures may be referred to as "parent" codes. Add-on codes describe additional intraoperative work performed. These codes are not subject to the multiple procedure reduction and should be reimbursed full fee.
	
	    Example: **+60512** Parathyroid autotransplantation (List separately in addition to code for primary procedure)

Category II Codes	• These are optional supplemental tracking codes for performance measurement—4-digit codes followed by letter F. • Intended to facilitate data collection by coding certain services and/or test results that are agreed upon as contributing to positive health outcomes and quality patient care. • The use of these codes is optional. Example: 4000F – Tobacco use cessation intervention, counseling
Category III Codes	• These are emerging technology codes—often referred to as "T" codes. They are 4-digit codes followed by the letter T. • These are codes for new technology—not yet FDA approved, not done routinely across the country, or not supported by the published data. • The purpose of this category of codes is to facilitate data collection and assessment of new services and procedures. These codes are intended to be used for data collection purposes to substantiate widespread usage or during the FDA approval process. • Codes may remain as Category III codes for up to 5 years while their use is being evaluated. At that time, they are either retired or upgraded to Category I codes. • They are updated twice a year, in January and July, by the AMA. Example: 0210T Speech audiometry threshold, automated

is reported with a Category III code. An example of a Category III code in otolaryngology is as follows:

    0208T Pure tone audiometry (threshold), automated; air only

The majority of procedures and services performed by otolaryngologists will be reported with Category I codes. However, each year all new and revised codes, especially those classified as Category I or Category III, should be carefully reviewed for potential relevance to otolaryngology practice.

Key Sections for Otolaryngologists

Evaluation and Management (E/M) Codes (99201-99499)

Evaluation and Management codes referred to as E/M codes, are codes used to describe office (new, established, or consultation), inpatient (admission, consultation, followup, and discharge) hospital observation (same day, subsequent days, discharge), emergency room, nursing home, hospice, and other nonprocedural patient encounters. Subsequent chapters will provide a more detailed description of these codes and their appropriate use by otolaryngologists.

Surgical Codes (10021-69990)

Surgical procedures comprise the largest section of the *CPT Manual*. The introduction of the surgical section describes general surgical guidelines, including the services considered to be inherent to a surgical procedure. The remaining sections organize procedure codes by organ system, body area, or procedure:

- General
- Integumentary system
- Musculoskeletal system
- Respiratory system
- Circulatory system
- Cardiovascular system
- Hemic and lymphatic systems
- Mediastinum and diaphragm
- Digestive system
- Urinary system
- Male genital system
- Reproductive system procedures
- Intersex surgery
- Female genital system
- Maternity care and delivery
- Endocrine system
- Nervous system
- Eye and ocular adenexa
- Auditory system
- Operating microscope

Otolaryngologists will find many of their surgical procedure codes, both open and endoscopic, in the respiratory section, codes 30000-31899. This section includes nose and sinus procedures as well as procedures on the larynx and trachea. In addition, auditory system procedures, codes 69000-69979, will be part of an otolaryngologist's commonly used codes. These codes include surgical procedures of the ear.

Otolaryngologists who perform surgery with other surgeons, typically performing the head and neck approach and resection portion of procedure, will use codes from different sections of CPT (eg, the nervous system for skull base surgery or digestive system for oral cavity procedures).

CPT codes are not restricted by specialty, so an otolaryngologist may use CPT codes from any section of the surgical chapter if it is appropriate for the procedure performed.

Radiology Codes (70010-79999)

The Radiology section of the *CPT Manual* includes most diagnostic and guidance imaging, the exception being noninvasive diagnostic ultrasound, which is part of the Medicine chapter. Diagnostic imaging, including plain-film x-rays of the head and neck, computed tomography (CT), computed tomographic angiography (CTA), magnetic resonance imaging (MRI), and magnetic resonance angiography (MRA) are located in this chapter.

As with other CPT codes, these codes are not solely used by radiologists and may be reported by otolaryngologists if the work performed meets the description and intent of the code.

Pathology and Laboratory (80047-89398)

Otolaryngologists who perform in-office allergy or other blood testing will use codes from this section of the *CPT Manual*.

Medicine and Therapy Codes (90281-99607)

The section includes a wide range of medicine codes: testing, therapy, immunizations, and more. For an otolaryngologist, this section includes codes 92502-92700, and covers otorhinolaryngologic testing such as vestibular function, audiologic function, and other evaluation and therapeutic services (eg, cochlear ear implant analysis).

Additional codes used by ear, nose, and throat providers (ENTs) are in the Allergy and Clinical Immunology section (95004-95199) and Sleep Medicine Testing area (95782-95811).

Modifiers

Appendix A of the *CPT Manual* includes a description of modifiers used in CPT coding. Modifiers are 2-digit codes that are appended to a 5-digit CPT code to describe a specific circumstance that alters (modifies) the intent of that code. Modifiers provide a short-cut means for providers to communicate this circumstance to payers and hopefully facilitate appropriate reimbursement for this altered situation. Modifiers will be more thoroughly described in Chapter 11.

Clinical Examples

An important but often overlooked section of the *CPT Manual* is Appendix C (Clinical Examples). In this section CPT provides clinical examples for each of the E/M codes mentioned previously. The examples are specialty specific and describe a typical patient encounter and how that encounter would be accurately reported. Subsequent chapters in this book provide additional information on E/M coding and documentation.

CPT Code Symbols

CPT uses a variety of symbols to provide additional information about codes. These are described as follows:

- • This designates a CPT code that was newly developed for this calendar year.

- Δ This designates a CPT code that was revised for this calendar year. The 5-digit code is the same, but the text description is different.

- + This designates an add-on code. An add-on code describes additional intraoperative work and is always reported with a parent code, also referred to as a stand-alone or primary code.

- ∅ This designates a code that is exempt from use of the 51 modifier. If two stand-alone

surgical procedures are reported as performed at the same operative session, the lower valued of the two (in terms of payment value) is generally subject to a reduction in payment. This symbol indicates that a CPT code is not subject to this reduction (eg, is exempt from a payment reduction). More information on the use of 51 modifier can be found in Chapter 11, "Demystifying Modifiers."

⊙ This designates a code that includes moderate sedation in its code description. For these codes, moderate sedation, if used, is included in the primary procedure and is not separately reported/coded.

\# This designates a code that is out of order in the *CPT Manual*. If it is impossible to place a new code directly below related codes (because the numerical sequence is already full), the new code is placed out of order. This symbol alerts the user to this out-of-sequence listing of codes.

Using Unlisted CPT Codes

Not every procedure or service performed by physicians has an existing CPT code. Recognizing this, CPT provides a number of unlisted codes to be used in reporting these procedures. If a code does not exist that specifically describes what the physician did, he or she must use an unlisted code. It is incorrect coding to select a code that just resembles the procedure performed.

Unlisted codes can be found in each major surgical section as well as other CPT chapters. For example,

31299 Unlisted procedure, accessory sinuses

42999 Unlisted procedure, pharynx, adenoids, or tonsils

92700 Unlisted otorhinolaryngological service or procedure

More can be found about how to select and report an unlisted code under "Basics of Surgical Coding" (Chapter 23).

Supplementing CPT: AMA Resources

In the *CPT Manual*, each code provides a brief description of a specific procedure. Some descriptions provide fairly detailed information about the procedure, but others leave room for interpretation by the user. To facilitate accurate use of CPT codes, it is advisable to invest in supplemental resources that clarify or expand on information provided in the *CPT Manual*. These resources should be considered "must haves" in a physician's arsenal of coding tools.

CPT Assistant

AMA publishes a monthly newsletter entitled *CPT Assistant*. In this publication, CPT provides expanded information on one or more codes or series of codes, typically recently established or revised codes. In addition, a section with coding questions and answers in several specialty areas provides expanded information that can greatly facilitate coding education and correct code usage.

If an edition of *CPT Assistant* published additional information on a particular code, this is indicated directly under the CPT code, as shown by the example below. This reference directs the user to refer to *CPT Assistant*, August 2012, page 13, for additional information about code 30630:

30630   Repair nasal septal perforations

CPT Assistant Aug 12:13

The primary purpose and benefit of the *CPT Assistant* is to enhance coding knowledge, but practices may also find this resource helpful in appealing denials. If a code or a code combination is inappropriately denied by a payer, a confirmation of coding accuracy by this official AMA publication can be useful in defending an appeal.

The *CPT Assistant* is available as a monthly publication, and past issues (1990–present) are available in electronic format through AMA.

Clinical Examples in Radiology

Similar *to CPT Assistant, Clinical Examples in Radiology* is a quarterly newsletter, also available in both hard copy and archived electronic formats. An example is shown below:

70540   Magnetic resonance (eg, proton) imaging, orbit, face, and/or neck; without contrast material(s)

Clinical Examples in Radiology Spring 05:3, Summer 07:7, Summer 13:9

CPT Changes: An Insider's View

In addition to the annual *CPT Manual*, AMA publishes a separate book, *CPT Changes: An Insider's View*, each year. This resource provides description of each new and revised CPT code for that year. It includes clinical examples for each new CPT code, providing valuable information regarding the intent of the code and what clinical activities are considered part of the CPT code. In the CPT manual, a notation of the code's inclusion in an edition of *CPT Changes* is indicated directly under the code as shown below:

30117   Excision or destruction (eg, laser), intranasal lesion; internal approach

CPT Changes: An Insider's View 2002

Conclusion

The *CPT Manual* is the official source for reporting services and procedures provided by physicians and other qualified heath care professionals. An otolaryngologist and his or her staff should be able to navigate this essential resource and supplement it as necessary to ensure accurate coding and, as a result, optimal reimbursement.

CHAPTER 3

Transition to ICD-10-CM

Margaret A. Skurka

Introduction

International Classification of Diseases, Tenth Revision, Clinical Modification (ICD-10-CM) was developed for use in the United States under the leadership of the National Center for Health Statistics and is owned and published by the World Health Organization. With 21 chapters and approximately 69,000 codes, it replaces and significantly expands Volumes 1 and 2 of *International Classification of Diseases, Ninth Revision, Clinical Modification* (ICD-9-CM) diagnosis codes.

Why the Shift to ICD-10-CM?

ICD-9-CM has been in use since 1979 in the United States. Its classification's numeric constrain does not allow for expansion of codes resulting in codes being grouped in general, nondescriptive and inadequate categories. ICD-10-CM expansion of codes allows for more precise coding of clinical diagnoses including emerging diseases and technology, current medical knowledge, and available treatment options. Other countries in the world including Canada, Australia, and most of Europe have been using their countries' versions of ICD-10 since 2000.

One of the primary goals of the ICD-10-CM structure is to better capture accurate clinical data and, thereby, improve patient outcomes. In ICD-10-CM, there is increased detail regarding the severity of conditions and more linear connection between diagnosis and treatment. Proper documentation to support the correct diagnostic code is key to successful coding in ICD-10-CM.

Key Points for Otolaryngology

Most Pertinent Chapters for Otolaryngology

- Chapter 2. Neoplasms
- Chapter 8. Diseases of the Ear and Mastoid Process
- Chapter 10. Diseases of the Respiratory System
- Chapter 11. Diseases of the Digestive System
- Chapter 12. Diseases of the Skin and Subcutaneous Tissue
- Chapter 18. Symptoms, Signs and Abnormal Clinical, and Laboratory Findings, Not Elsewhere Classified
- Chapter 19. Injury, Poisoning and Certain Other Consequences of External Causes

What Stays the Same

1. The Alphabetic index (Volume II) is an alphabetical list of diseases and injuries. This index

13

contains the Neoplasm Table, the Table of Drugs and Chemicals, and the Index to External Cause of Injuries. There is no hypertension table in ICD-10-CM as there is in ICD-9-CM.
2. The Tabular list (Volume I) is an alphanumerical list of codes divided into chapters based on condition and/or body system.
3. The Coding Conventions (the Rules of the Road) are similar including instructional notes (eg, code also, code first, use additional code), punctuation marks, relational terms (eg, and/or), cross-reference notes (eg, see, see also), and abbreviations.

What Is Different

1. ICD-10-CM codes are alphanumeric and from 3 to 7 characters long.
   a. All the letters of the alphabet are used with the exception of "U."
   b. Alpha characters are not case sensitive.
2. Certain chapters have been reorganized.
   a. Some conditions have been reassigned to a more appropriate chapter. For example, Streptococcal tonsillitis was in the Infectious and Parasitic Diseases chapter in ICD-9-CM, but is now in the Respiratory chapter in ICD-10-CM.
3. Certain descriptive titles have changed. For example, 381.10, Chronic serous otitis media, simple or unspecified in ICD-9-CM has become H65.20, Chronic serous otitis media, unspecified ear in ICD-10-CM.
4. New chapters were created specifically for eye and ear diseases. Diseases and conditions of the sense organs have been separated from the nervous system diseases and conditions and now have their own chapters: Chapter 7, Diseases of the Eye and Adnexa, and Chapter 8, Diseases of the Ear and Mastoid Process.
5. Injury codes are now grouped by specific site (eg, nose, ear, throat), then by type of injury (eg, fracture, open wound). In ICD-9-CM injuries were grouped first by type of injury then anatomic location.
6. Some postoperative complications have been moved to specific body system chapters. Examples include:

a. Category H95 Intraoperative and postprocedural complications and disorder of ear and mastoid process, not elsewhere classified
b. H95.41 Postprocedural hemorrhage and hematoma of ear and mastoid process following a procedure on the ear and mastoid process
7. A dash (-) at the end of an index entry indicates that an additional character(s) is required to be a valid code. For example,
   a. H83.3- Noise effects on inner ear
   b. H83.3X1 Noise effects on *right* inner ear.
8. The code structure is very different in ICD-10-CM as all codes start with a letter followed by a number. The remaining 3 to 7 characters may be alpha or numeric. A graphic depicting the code structure of ICD-9-CM to ICD-10-CM is shown in Figure 3–1.
9. Seventh character: Some codes require a seventh character to be a complete, valid code.
   a. Pertinent codes for ENT that require a seventh character mainly fall into injury categories including fractures, foreign bodies, and open wounds.
   b. When seeing this √ 7th notation, the applicable seventh character options will be at the code category level (the first 3 characters) and must be appended to report a valid code.
   c. The seventh character extensions are not the same for all code categories. Some code categories have 3 options while others have 6 options for the seventh character extension.
   d. To accomplish correct 7th character placement, an "X" placeholder is used in the empty character spaces. For example, the appropriate seventh character is to be added to each code from category T16:
   A—Initial encounter
   D—Subsequent encounter
   S—Sequela
   Yet ICD-10-CM provides only the first 4 characters of the code and the instructions to √ x 7th for T16.1 Foreign body in right ear.
      i. Incorrect code assignment. T16.1A
      ii. Correct code assignment: T16.1XXA

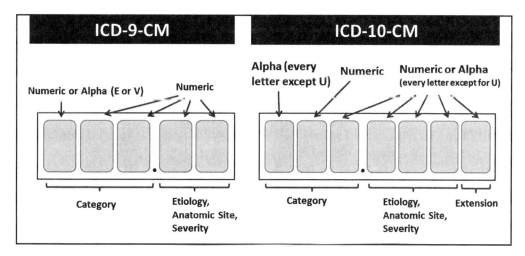

Figure 3–1. Code Structure. Used with permission from KarenZupko & Associates, Inc.

e. The seventh character extension detail is as follows:

A—Initial: This extension is used when the patient is receiving active treatment for the condition. *Examples of active treatment are surgical treatment, emergency department encounter, and evaluation and continuing treatment by the same or a different physician.*

D—Subsequent: Used for encounters after the patient has received active treatments and is now in the healing phase receiving routine care for the condition. Examples include cast change or removal, an x-ray to check healing status of fracture, removal of external or internal fixation, device medication adjustment, other aftercare, and follow-up visits following treatment of the injury or condition.

S—Sequela: Used as an extension to the active injury code, to indicate that a condition is the result of a previous injury. Examples include scar formation resulting from a burn, deviated septum due to a nasal fracture, and infertility due to tubal occlusion from old tuberculosis. The code for the current condition is also used. For example, a scar resulting from a previous laceration is a "late effect" or "sequela" of the laceration. Late effect codes are not used in ICD, but rather the condition itself and then the original injury code with the extension of "S."

1. L91.0 Hypertrophic scar
2. S01.411S Laceration without foreign body of right cheek and temporomandibular area, sequel

10. The "X" placeholder: The "X" placeholder is also used with certain codes to allow for future code expansion as in the example below:
   a. H66.3X3 Other chronic suppurative otitis media, bilateral ear

11. Excludes Notes: Two types of notes are used, each with a different definition, but both indicate that codes excluded from each other are independent of each other. In ICD-9-CM, there was only one type of Excludes note.
   a. Excludes 1: Means "NOT CODED HERE"
      i. The code excluded should never be used at the same time as the code above the Excludes 1 note.
      ii. Used when two conditions cannot occur together.

      J36 Peritonsillar abscess
      Excludes 1   acute tonsillitis (J03.-)
                   chronic tonsillitis (J35.0)
                   retropharyngeal abscess (J39.0)
                   tonsillitis NOS (J03.9-)

   b. Excludes 2: Means "NOT INCLUDED HERE"
      i. The condition excluded is not part of the condition represented by the code,

but the patient may have both conditions at the same time.

ii. It is acceptable to use both the code and the excluded code together, when both conditions exist at the same time.

K11.7 Disturbances of salivary secretion
Excludes 2   dry mouth NOS (R68.2)

R07.0 Pain in throat
Excludes 2   dysphagia (R13.1-)
                      pain in neck (M54.2)

12. Some conditions do not have "in diseases classified elsewhere" in the title, instead the same instructional notes appear at the etiology and the manifestation to help guide the user for correct sequencing. See Table 3–1.

13. Acute and chronic conditions: When the same condition is described as both acute and chronic, and separate entries exist in the Alphabetic Index, at the same indentation level, both codes are assigned, with the code for the acute condition sequenced first.

14. Laterality: Laterality is a prominent concept in ICD-10-CM particularly for otolaryngologists with regard to the ear diagnosis codes. Some blocks, particularly the ear codes, provide specificity for right, left, or bilateral conditions. If a condition is specified as bilateral and a bilateral code does not exist, assign separate codes for the left side and the right side. If the side is not documented in the medical record, the coder should query the provider rather than use the code for "unspecified" site. Interestingly, the sinusitis codes (J01.-, J32.-) do not have specific codes for right, left, or bilateral conditions.

Most Significant Chapters for Otolaryngologists

Chapter 2: Neoplasms

An instructional note appears at the beginning of Chapter 2 of the ICD-10-CM book that includes the following:

All neoplasms are classified in this chapter whether they are functionally active or not. Ch. 2 classifies neoplasms primarily by site, with broad groupings for behavior, malignant, in situ, benign, etc. A primary malignant neoplasm that overlaps two or more contiguous sites should be classified to the subcategory/code .8 (overlapping lesion), unless the combination is specifically indexed elsewhere. For multiple neoplasms of the same site that are not contiguous, codes for each site should be assigned.

Many code categories direct the user to add additional codes to identify alcohol abuse/dependence and/or tobacco use/dependence.

Example: C02 Malignant neoplasm of other and unspecified parts of tongue

Use additional code to identify:

alcohol abuse and dependence (F10.-)

history of tobacco use (Z87.891)

tobacco dependence (F17.-)

tobacco use (Z72.0)

This chapter contains the following blocks of codes of major relevance to ENT:

Table 3–1. Examples of "Use Additional Code" and "Code First" Guidelines

"Use Additional Code"	"Code First"
H65 Nonsuppurative otitis media	**H72 Perforation of tympanic membrane**
Use additional code for any associated perforated tympanic membrane (H72.-)	Code first any associated otitis media: (H65.-, H66.1-, H66.2-, H66.3-, H66.4-, H66.9-, H67-)

C00-C14   Malignant neoplasms of lip, oral cavity and pharynx

C15-C26   Malignant neoplasms of digestive organs

C30-C39   Malignant neoplasms of respiratory organs

Chapter 8: Diseases of the Ear and Mastoid Process

Pertinent code blocks include:

H60-H62: Disease of external ear

H65-H75: Diseases of middle ear and mastoid

H80-H83: Disease of inner ear

H90-H94: Other disorders of ear

H95: Intraoperative and postprocedural complications and disorders of ear and mastoid process, not elsewhere classified

Chapter 8 is a new chapter in ICD-10-CM. The 5 code blocks listed above are divided in such a way as to make it easier to identify the types of conditions that would occur in the ear. Block 5 contains codes for intraoperative and postprocedural complications. Rather than being scattered throughout other code categories, these codes are grouped together at the end of the chapter.

An instructional note appears at the beginning of this chapter instructing the coder to use an external cause code following the code for the ear condition, if applicable, to identify the cause of the ear condition. Most conditions in this chapter have codes to indicate if the condition is in the right, left, or bilateral ears.

Example:

H60.311   Diffuse otitis externa, **unspecified** ear

H60.312   Diffuse otitis externa, **right** ear

H60.313   Diffuse otitis externa, **left** ear

H60.319   Diffuse otitis externa, **bilateral**

H61.121   Hematoma of pinna, **right** ear

H61.122   Hematoma of pinna, **left** ear

H61.123   Hematoma of pinna, **bilateral**

H61.129   Hematoma of pinna, **unspecified** ear

In some categories, notes have been added indicating that any underlying disease should be coded first.

Example:

H62.4   Otitis externa in other diseases classified elsewhere

Code first underlying disease, such as:

erysipelas (A46)

impetigo (L01.0)

Chapter 10: Diseases of the Respiratory System

Pertinent code blocks include:

J00-J06: Acute upper respiratory infections

J30-J39: Other diseases of upper respiratory tract

J40-J47: Chronic lower respiratory diseases

J95: Intraoperative and postprocedural complications and disorders of respiratory system, not elsewhere classified

The following guideline appears at the beginning of Chapter 10:

Note: When a respiratory condition is described as occurring in more than one site and is not specifically indexed, it should be classified to the lower anatomic site (eg, tracheobronchitis to bronchitis in J40).

Another instructional note appears at the beginning of Chapter 10, and also at the category level, which instructs the coder to use an additional code where applicable to identify:

exposure to environmental tobacco smoke (Z77.22)

exposure to tobacco smoke in the perinatal period (P96.81)

history of tobacco use (Z87.891)

occupational exposure to environmental tobacco smoke (Z57.31)

tobacco dependence (F17.-)

tobacco use (Z72.0)

Smoking information does not need to be in any particular section of the medical record (eg, History of Present Illness, Social History). If documented, the additional code to identify any smoking exposure, use, or dependence can be added. Some codes have been expanded to include notes indicating an additional code should be assigned or an associated condition should be sequenced first:

- Use an additional code to identify the infectious agent:

   J01 Acute Sinusitis: Use additional code (B95-B97) to identify infectious agent.
- Use an additional code to identify the virus.
- Code first any associated lung abscess.
- Code first the underlying disease:

   J99 Respiratory disorders in diseases classified elsewhere
- Code first the underlying disease, such as
   amyloidosis (E85.-)
   ankylosing spondylitis (M45)
   congenital syphilis (A50.5)
   cryoglobulinemia (D89.1)
   early congenital syphilis (A50.0)
   schistosomiasis (B65.0-B65.
- Use an additional code to identify other conditions such as tobacco use or exposure.
- Change. Acute Sinusitis (J01.) In ICD-9-CM each sinus that was infected

was coded separately unless all were infected (eg, 461.8 for acute pansinusitis). However, in ICD-10-CM when 2 or 3 sinuses are documented as infected, the "other acute recurrent sinusitis" code, J01.81, is used rather than coding each sinus separately. The same is true for the Chronic Sinusitis codes (J32.-).

Chapter 11: Diseases of the Digestive System

Pertinent code blocks include

K00-K14: Disease of oral cavity and salivary glands

K20-K31: Disease of esophagus, stomach and duodenum

Most codes in this chapter are classified in a similar way to ICD-9-CM. Most of the categories contain the instructional note to identify any tobacco exposure. Many combination codes and exclusion notes appear in this chapter. Categories have been restructured to group together that are related in some way.

Example: Gastro-Esophageal Reflux Disease (GERD) (K21)

   EXCLUDES 1   newborn esophageal reflux (P78.83)

   K21.0 Gastro-esophageal reflux disease with esophagitis

      Reflux esophagitis

   Classified under esophagitis codes in ICD-9-CM (530.11)

      K21.9 Gastro-esophageal reflux disease *without esophagitis*

         Esophageal reflux NOS

   Classified under "other specified" disorders of esophagus in ICD-9-CM (530.81)

Many of the codes in this category have 1:1 mapping from ICD-9-CM to ICD-10-CM. See Table 3–2.

Table 3–2. ICD-9-CM to ICD-10-CM Mappings for Common Salivary Gland Conditions

ICD-9-CM	ICD-10-CM
527.0 Atrophy of salivary gland	K11.0 Atrophy of salivary gland
527.1 Hypertrophy of salivary gland	K11.1 Hypertrophy of salivary gland
527.3 Abscess of salivary gland	K11.3 Abscess of salivary gland
527.4 Fistula of salivary gland	K11.4 Fistula of salivary gland
527.5 Sialolithiasis	K11.5 Sialolithiasis
527.6 Mucocele of salivary gland	K11.6 Mucocele of salivary gland
527.7 Disturbance of salivary secretion	K11.7 Disturbance of salivary secretion

Chapter 12: Diseases of the Skin and Subcutaneous Tissue

Pertinent code blocks include:

L00-L08: Infections of the skin and subcutaneous tissue

L55-L59: Radiation-related disorders of the skin and subcutaneous tissue

L60-L75: Disorders of skin appendages

L76: Intraoperative and postprocedural complications of skin and subcutaneous tissue

L80-L99: Other disorders of the skin and subcutaneous tissue

Categories in Chapter 12 bring together groups of diseases that are, in some way, related to each other. Many instructional and excludes notes in this chapter.

Example: L02 Cutaneous abscess, furuncle and carbuncle

Use additional code to identify organism (B95-B96)

L02.0 Cutaneous abscess, furuncle and carbuncle of face

Excludes 2   abscess of ear, external (H60.0)

abscess of eyelid (H00.0)

abscess of head [any part, except face] (L02.8)

abscess of lacrimal gland (H04.0)

abscess of lacrimal passages (H04.3)

abscess of mouth (K12.2)

abscess of nose (J34.0)

abscess of orbit (H05.0)

submandibular abscess (K12.2)

Chapter 18: Symptoms, Signs, and Abnormal Clinical and Laboratory Findings

Pertinent code blocks include:

R00-R09: Symptoms and signs involving the circulatory and respiratory system

R10-R19: Symptoms and signs involving the digestive system and abdomen

R20-R23: Symptoms and signs involving the skin and subcutaneous tissue

R47-R49: Symptoms and signs involving speech and voice

R50-R69: General symptoms and signs

R70-R79: Abnormal findings on examination of blood, without diagnosis

R90-R94: Abnormal findings on diagnostic imaging and in function studies, without diagnosis

Chapter 18 contains codes for conditions that are associated with more than one disease process or for conditions that are of an unknown etiology. Codes from this chapter should only be used as a primary diagnosis when a more definitive diagnosis has not been established or confirmed by the provider. Codes from this chapter may be reported as an *additional* diagnosis when the sign or symptom is not routinely associated with the primary definitive diagnosis. The primary definitive diagnosis should be sequenced first, followed by the code(s) for the sign(s)/symptom(s). Codes that are routinely associated with a disease process should not be reported separately.

Chapter 19: Injury, Poisoning, and Certain Other Consequences of External Causes

Pertinent code blocks include:

S00-S09: Injuries to the head

S10-S19: Injuries to the neck

T15-T19: Effects of foreign body entering through natural orifice

T80-T88: Complications of surgical and medical care, not elsewhere classified

Chapter 19 has been reorganized compared to ICD-9-CM. Injuries are now arranged first by body region, beginning with the head and ending with the ankle and foot, and then by type of injury.

Example: S00-S09 Injuries to the head

S00 Superficial injury of head

S01 Open wound of head

This chapter uses the S-section for coding different types of injuries related to single anatomic regions and the T-section to code injuries to unspecified body regions, as well as poisonings and certain other consequences of external causes:

S11.011A   Laceration without foreign body of larynx, initial encounter

T17.320A   Food in larynx causing asphyxiation, initial encounter

The following instructional notes appear at the beginning of Chapter 19 and apply to the entire chapter:

Note: Use secondary code(s) from Chapter 20, External causes of morbidity, to indicate cause of injury. Codes within the T section that include the external cause do not require an additional external cause code. **Use an additional** code to identify any retained foreign body, if applicable (Z18.-).

Another major change is the addition of a seventh character extension to most of the codes. The seventh character must always be in the seventh character field. When a code is less than 6 characters, an "X" must be used to fill the empty character positions so the seventh character can be maintained in the 7th position:

Example: T16 Foreign body in ear

Includes: foreign body in auditory canal

The appropriate seventh character is to be added to each code from category T16

A—Initial encounter

D—Subsequent encounter

S—Sequela

Invalid code   T16.1D Foreign body in right ear, subsequent encounter

Valid code   T16.1XXD Foreign body in right ear, subsequent encounter

Seventh characters for fractures have different values and have been expanded as follows:

A—Initial encounter for closed fracture

B—Initial encounter for open fracture

D—Subsequent encounter for fracture with routine healing

G—Subsequent encounter for fracture with delayed healing

K—Subsequent encounter for fracture with nonunion

S—Sequela

Fractures not documented as open or closed are coded to "closed" according to ICD-10-CM guidelines. There are no official definitions of "routine" "delayed" or "nonunion"; therefore, the provider's documentation should specifically use these terms.

Conclusion

ICD-10-CM is a detailed and expanded coding system that will positively impact otolaryngology coding. Most codes have a higher level of specificity, many codes will have laterality, and detailed coding will more accurately describe the acuity of the patient seen by the otolaryngologist. The coding is not difficult, but rather more comprehensive and more detailed. The otolaryngologist need only be specific in the documented diagnosis(es) and accurate coding will follow. The system should be embraced as it is a positive and necessary change to what we have been doing since 1979. Welcome ICD-10-CM.

Acknowledgments: A thank you goes out to Patricia Cervantes Johnson, RHIT at Indiana University Northwest, for her invaluable aid in compiling the material in this chapter.

CHAPTER 4

Health Policy

Richard W. Waguespack and Lawrence M. Simon

Introduction

There are many facets involved with health policy, mainly, in our context, dealing with payment and reimbursement for physician and provider services. This begins by reporting a medical service with *Current Procedural Terminology* (CPT®) coding to a payer and ends with a payment (often shared by the patient and covering entity and rarely what was submitted by the provider) or a denial. There are many steps in this process that we will explore in this chapter.

Introduction to Coding and Reimbursement

Establishing diagnostic and procedural codes and allocating a value to a given physician service is a complex process. For diagnoses, the endpoint is the creation of an *International Classification of Diseases, Ninth Revision, Clinical Modification* (ICD-9-CM) or *International Classification of Diseases, Tenth Revision, Clinical Modification* (ICD-10-CM) code; the latter code set implemented on October 1, 2015. Procedural and physician work reporting begins with the creation of a CPT code and then proceeds to the assignment of Relative Value Units (RVUs), which determine payment in most instances. Although procedures may be reported in the *International Classification of Diseases* (ICD) system (hospitals generally do so), using the *Pro-*

cedure Coding System (PCS), physicians virtually always report them with CPT codes.

ICD-9-CM

The *International Classification of Diseases* system was first devised by the World Health Organization (WHO) in 1900 to aid in the statistical reporting of mortality. The current iteration used in the United States is the 9th revision—ICD-9-CM. These codes contain up to 5 characters and may be either numeric or alphanumeric. They are used to specify a certain disease, condition, or symptom. There are approximately 14,000 diagnosis codes in ICD-9-CM, and familiarity with them is important because all billable patient encounters, ordered tests, and medications must be associated with a diagnosis code. *International Classification of Diseases, Ninth Revision, Procedure Coding System* (ICD-9-PCS), for the procedural coding system, is not used by physicians for professional billing but is used by facilities for coding of procedures.

ICD-10-CM

The 10th revision of the codes (ICD-10) was finalized in 1992 and implemented in 1999 in Europe. The clinical modification (CM) used in the United States provides for codes that are alphanumeric and far more specific than ICD-9-CM codes. Consequently, there are many more ICD-10-CM codes than ICD-9-CM codes, with approximately 70,000 diagnostic codes at last count. All entities covered by the Health Insurance Portability and Accountability Act (HIPAA) were mandated to switch to ICD-10-CM in the United States on October 1, 2015; however, non– HIPAA covered entities, such as Worker's Compensation, are not required to switch and may still require ICD-9-CM codes after this deadline.

CPT

The AMA first developed and published CPT in 1966 in conjunction with the initiation of Medicare. CPT codes are a system of numerical identifiers used for reporting medical services and procedures. They represent the most widely used and accepted system for communicating with both public and private health insurance programs and are the property of the American Medical Association (AMA). By statute (HIPAA), physician and similar provider services use the CPT system.

The code set is maintained by the AMA CPT Editorial Panel (Panel), composed of a number of physicians, nonphysician members of the Health Care Professionals Advisory Committee (HCPAC), and one each nominated from the Blue Cross Blue Shield Association, the Health Insurance Association of America, the Centers for Medicare and Medicaid Services (CMS), and the American Hospital Association. The Panel is advised by, and code changes are often proposed by, the CPT Advisory Committee that has representatives from specialty societies. All societies that have a seat at the AMA House of Delegates are eligible to have a seat on the CPT Advisory Committee. Otolaryngology has one Advisor each from the American Academy of Otolaryngology-Head and Neck Surgery (AAO-HNS; plus an Advisor Alternate), the Triological Society, the American Academy of Otolaryngic Allergy and Foundation (AAOA) and the American Academy of Facial Plastic and Reconstructive Surgery (AAFPRS).

Code Change Proposals (CCPs) are formal requests to the Panel for additions, deletions, and other changes to the code-set and may come from individuals, industry, specialty, and medical societies. There is a formal process of submission,

comment, and finally a presentation to the Panel at one of its three annual meetings. CPT codes are divided into Category I, II, and III. Category I codes are used most often for reporting, whereas Category III are designed for new technology services and have a 5-year life, unless renewed. Category II codes are a set of supplemental tracking codes that can be used for performance measurement. More information about CPT, including specifics about criteria for Category I, II, and III codes and the process for proposing code changes, can be found on the AMA CPT website (http://www .ama-assn.org/ama/pub/physician-resources/ solutions-managing-your-practice/coding-billing-insurance/cpt.page).

The AAO-HNS has a formal process for dealing with code changes and engages other relevant societies, both within otolaryngology as well as outside the specialty, to assure all germane possible input.

Once the CPT Editorial Panel assigns a code for a procedure/service, the code may be used for billing. However, the existence of a code does not guarantee payment. Payment is determined by the insurance company (eg, Medicare). CPT policy is explicit in that services that are not well described by an existing CPT code should not be reported with an approximate CPT code but rather with an applicable unlisted code. Occasionally, services are reported with Healthcare Common Procedure Coding System, Level II (HCPCS Level II) codes, such as G or S codes, but this is payer dependent.

Relative Value Units

During the early phases of Medicare, payment was based on a system of "customary, prevailing, and reasonable" (CPR) fees, typically referred to as "usual, reasonable, and customary" (UCR). It was recognized that there was wide variation in the amount that Medicare paid for similar services due to this system. By the mid-1980s, physicians' dissatisfaction with CPR-based payment resulted in several government overhauls of the system. One of these overhauls was the landmark Harvard Resource-Based Relative Value Scale (RBRVS) study, which was authored in 1985 by Bill Hsiao and Peter Braun.

The intent of the Harvard study was to scale all services and procedures relative to each other. As a standard, the repair of an inguinal hernia was rated at 100. All other services and procedures were then assigned "relative values" according to their work in comparison to this standard (inguinal hernia). As such, in the RBRVS system, payments are determined by the "resource cost" of a particular service. This cost is derived from three components: physician work, practice expense, and professional liability insurance. Payments are calculated by multiplying the combined cost (relative value) of the service by a conversion factor—a monetary amount that is determined by Centers for Medicare and Medicaid Services (CMS), or by a commercial carrier that utilizes the RBRVS system. For example, a carrier that reimburses at 120% of Medicare means that its conversion factor is 20% above the CMS value for that year. This system allows for payments to be adjusted for geographical differences in resource cost using a separate multiplier called the geographic practice cost index (GPCI).

Prior to April 1, 2015, the CMS conversion factor was determined by the sustainable growth rate (SGR) formula, which was designed to prevent overspending by statutorily mandating that Medicare spending per beneficiary may not increase at a rate that exceeds growth in the gross domestic product (GDP). After extensive advocacy efforts by numerous medical organizations, including the American Academy of Otolaryngology-Head and Neck Surgery, this formula has now been repealed and replaced by the Medicare Access and Children's Health Insurance Program (CHIP) Reauthorization Act of 2015 (MACRA). This legislation is designed to provide physicians with stable, predictable Medicare payments while facilitating the transition to alternative payment models (APMs). The law calls for annual updates (increases) of 0.5% annually beginning July 1, 2015, and extending through December 31, 2019. By July 1, 2019, the Medicare Payment Advisory Commission (MedPAC) must present recommendations to Congress regarding future updates. Currently, these are set at 0% for 2019 to 2025 and then increase again to 0.75% annually for those participating in eligible APMs and 0.25% annu-

ally for all other providers. The law also consolidates all current reporting systems (physician quality reporting system, value-based modifier, and meaningful use) into the Merit-Based Incentive Payment System (MIPS). Rules have yet to be established regarding the implementation of MIPS, but one key difference from the current system is that penalties to lower performers are no longer required to offset bonus payments. Instead, providers will be assessed against an established threshold level, above which all providers become exempt from penalties and eligible for bonuses. Moreover, no one has to receive a penalty in order for another provider to receive a bonus. Funds will also be available to help small practices implement MIPS, and there are strong incentives for providers to participate in APMs (such as Accountable Care Organizations [ACOs] and medical homes). There are many other provisions within this law, and as of the writing of this chapter, many aspects still need to be clarified and possibly addressed through future advocacy efforts.

The physician work component of the RBRVS accounted (in 2013) for about 51% of the total relative value for most codes. The initial physician work relative values were based on the results of the Harvard studies but are now based on surveys of practitioners. The factors used to determine physician work include the time it takes to perform the service, the technical skill and physical effort, the required mental effort in judgment, and stress due to the potential risk to the patient. The physician work RVUs may be reviewed as frequently as every year to account for changes in medical practice and for budgetary considerations, but if there is a compelling reason to review a code and its related family, re-survey and possibly revision by the CPT Editorial Panel may be performed.

The practice expense component of the RBRVS accounted (in 2013) for about 45% of the total relative value for each code. There are typically two different classifications of practice expense (PE) RVU. A "facility" RVU is assigned if the procedure is performed in a facility setting (eg, hospital inpatient, hospital outpatient, ambulatory surgery center), and a "nonfacility" RVU is assigned if the procedure is performed in a doctor's office or similar location. Determinations of PE are now resource based and differ based on the site of service (facility or nonfacility). The third component of the RBRVS is professional liability or malpractice insurance. It only accounted for 4.3% of the total value of most codes in 2013.

Relative values are assigned for nearly all Category I CPT codes, but not Category III codes, by the AMA Relative Value Scale Update Committee (RUC).

Traditionally, surgical procedures have been designated to have 0-, 10-, or 90-day global periods by CMS. Under this system, all routine pre-, intra-, and postoperative care was considered part of the CPT code. In appropriate circumstances, modifiers can be used to provide reimbursement for services provided during the global period. One CMS proposal that is gaining momentum is to remove the associated evaluation and management (E/M) values currently embedded in the base CPT code and assign all surgical procedures with a 0-day global period. This would radically change RVUs for surgical procedure codes and likely create inconsistent valuations. Also unanswered at this time are the timetable and adoption policies by commercial carriers if CMS eliminates the 10- and 90-day postoperative global period concept. Other changes of this magnitude (eg, CMS's nonreimbursement for consultation codes in 2010) have often been adopted by private payers.

The RUC

The 31-member American Medical Association's Specialty Society Relative Value Scale Update Committee (RUC) was formed in November 1991 to provide RVU recommendation to CMS for new or revised CPT codes. As a committee of the AMA and national medical specialty societies, it recommends updates to the physician work and PE components of the Medicare physician fee schedule. The RUC represents the entire medical profession, with 21 of its 31 members appointed by major national medical specialty societies. Many observers feel the RUC is increasingly oriented toward primary care with a trend for valuations reflecting this impression.

The RUC values new and revised CPT Category I codes, generally by survey. When codes come before the RUC, specialty societies have the option of surveying, commenting, or not commenting. The AAO-HNS has a robust process for responding to RUC queries (including working with other specialty societies) and has a defined member on the RUC as well as a designated RUC Advisor and Alternate. More information is available on the AMA RUC website (http://www.ama-assn.org/ama/pub/physician-resources/solutions-managing-your-practice/coding-billing-insurance/medicare/the-resource-based-relative-value-scale.page).

To pass through the RUC successfully, a two-thirds majority must vote affirmatively for a relative value number. When a new code is presented at the RUC, both the physician work and the PE are determined. Practice expense is determined by the Practice Expense Subcommittee.

Once a code has successfully been passed through the RUC, it is referred to CMS for final approval. At the present time, CMS's acceptance of RUC values is in the mid-90% range. Once these values have been accepted by CMS, they are published in the *Federal Register*, and a 60-day period of discussion will follow. Once the 60-day open period has closed, CMS makes its final decision, and thus the new code and its relative value will be established for Medicare payments.

Because CMS operates on a fixed dollar budget, with only increments for increasing the number of Medicare patients, RVU and code payment assignment is a budget neutral process. As such, the payment authorized is not necessarily what the procedure is worth but is heavily influenced by what Medicare can afford to pay for that procedure or service. No new money comes into the system when a new code is authorized unless that code involves new technology. Examples of procedures that might qualify under this exception include those with recent Food and Drug Administration (FDA) approval, those that use new/novel technology to perform an existing service, and those migrating from Category III to Category I classification. Thus, with the exception of new technology, the typical way CMS funds will be allocated to a new code is by decreasing the money given to existing codes (usually within the same general category). Additionally, many, if not most, third-party payers have adopted the RBRVS system as the cornerstone of their payment policies. However, they do not generally adhere to Medicare payer policy in its entirety, for example, not reimbursing some services deemed "experimental or investigational" or rigorously using its National Correct Coding Initiative (NCCI) edits. Many private payers have more strict code edits and/or more robust medical necessity guidelines than does Medicare.

Coding Edits

Coding edits refer to reimbursement logic and rules used by payers, most commonly when multiple codes are reported together. There are other rules to prevent overpayments, for example, age and gender (eg, to prevent reimbursement for tonsillectomy over age 12, CPT code 42821, when performed on a 4-year-old). The most widespread set of code edits is National Correct Coding Initiative (NCCI—often referred to as CCI), which is maintained by CMS. It is often adopted, at least in part, by other carriers, especially if they use the RBRVS payment methodology. The NCCI edits also define which modifiers may be used, when appropriate, to override the edits. A common example of this is when performing a limited ethmoidectomy (31254) on one side and total (31255) on the other. The edits can be found at the CMS website (http://www.cms.gov/Medicare/Cod ing/NationalCorrectCodInitEd/NCCI-Coding-Edits.html).

Individual payers may develop their own internal code edits.

Payer Policy

This term refers to policies that commercial or governmental payers use to define how they will pay for services. There is no mandate that a carrier must reimburse for a service that has a CPT code or has been valued by Medicare. This is especially true for new technologies. Payers are increasingly using published literature and levels of evidence (or their interpretation of lack thereof) to state that a service is "experimental or investigational." Payers generally may deny reimbursing for ser-

vices that are not a covered service (eg, cosmetic), not medically necessary (providing a service that the payer and presumably most clinicians would not feel is medically indicated), or experimental or investigational. Clinicians must realize that this is an insurance determination. Many payers have criteria used to determine this status, and providers and societies should craft their arguments to prove, based on the strongest levels of evidence, why a contested service satisfies the payer's own criteria. Simply declaring a service is not experimental/investigational by a physician or society generally has no standing with payers. Societies providing position statements with the highest levels of evidence have the greatest likelihood of changing adverse payer policies.

New technology represents a challenge in that there must be a balance struck between paying for unproven, often very expensive new procedures and devices, and the introduction of innovative new technology that truly improves patient care. This is one of the reasons CPT Category III codes are available. The AAO-HNS has a New Technology Pathway to help it determine how to develop its internal policies and positions on innovations within the specialty. More information on this pathway can be found on the AAO-HNS website (http://www.entnet.org/sites/default/files/uploads/PracticeManagement/Reimburse ment/_files/AAOHNS-NewTechnologyPathway Requests_PoliciesandProcedures.pdf).

Blue Cross and Blue Shield companies are independent entities and generally develop their own payer policies that may or may not be in alignment with the Blue Cross Blue Shield Association. Generally, their policies are on their respective websites and proposed changes open for a comment period. Medicaid agencies' policies are typically developed at the state level. Medicare policies are based on local coverage determinations (LCDs) and national coverage determinations (NCDs). There are more LCDs, and these are defined by the local Medicare contractor; thus, changes in these must be approached locally. The AAO-HNS is frequently asked to review such policies and engages its committee structure and other specialty leadership to respond.

Depending on the issue, coalitions of individuals and their state and local medical and specialty societies with involvement of similar national organizations are generally needed to inform and affect payer policies. Clearly national medical and specialty societies must be engaged with issues of that scope (eg, CMS- or congressionally-driven issues). The AAO-HNS (with its Health Policy Department and Board of Governors) is very involved on behalf of otolaryngology, and it almost always works with specialty-related societies to form policy.

The Affordable Care Act

In March 2010, Congress passed the Patient Protection and Affordable Care Act (often referred to as the ACA or "Obamacare") in an effort to decrease the number of Americans who did not have any form of health insurance. The three basic premises behind the bill were the following: (1) mandate that all individuals carry some form of health insurance or face a penalty; (2) expand Medicaid to all patients with an income below 133% of the Federal Poverty Level (FPL—$31,720.50 for a family of 4 in 2014); and (3) offer federal subsidies for the purchase of insurance to all patients with an income at or below 400% of the FPL ($95,400 for a family of 4 in 2014). Subsidized policies are offered through a Health Insurance Exchange Marketplace. Exchange Marketplaces are currently run by either a state or the federal government, or a combination of both. Their basic premise is to group individual patients into one common risk pool in order to allow each individual Exchange customer to benefit from the power of group purchasing. Patients with incomes below 100% of the FPL ($23,850 for a family of 4 in 2014) were excluded from eligibility for subsidies due to the assumption that they would be covered by Medicaid. As a result of the Supreme Court decision to exempt states from the Medicaid requirement, patients with incomes below 100% of the FPL who live in states that did not expand Medicaid are faced with both the unavailability of Medicaid and the inability to receive federal subsidies to purchase insurance.

Parts of the ACA deal with development of alternative payment models (eg, ACOs and value-

based payment programs). Private payers are also engaged in similar efforts to deal with burgeoning health care costs; however, many of these efforts are early in their development and further discussion is beyond the scope of this chapter. As of this writing, there are still legal challenges to parts of the legislation, and some in Congress are trying to repeal all or parts of the ACA.

Resources

- American Medical Association. Coding with CPT® for proper reimbursement. http://www.ama-assn.org/ama/pub/physician-resources/solutions-managing-your-practice/coding-billing-insurance/cpt.page.
- American Medical Association CPT Network. http://www.ama-assn.org/ama/pub/physician-resources/solutions-managing-your-practice/coding-billing-insurance/cpt/cpt-network.page.
- American Medical Association. The RVS Update Committee. http://www.ama-assn.org/ama/pub/physician-resources/solutions-managing-your-practice/coding-billing-insurance/medicare/the-resource-based-relative-value-scale/the-rvs-update-committee.page.
- American Medical Association. The Medicare physician payment schedule. http://www.ama-assn.org/ama/pub/physician-resources/solutions-managing-your-practice/coding-billing-insurance/medicare/the-medicare-physician-payment-schedule.page.
- Centers for Medicare and Medicaid Services. Physician fee schedule. https://www.cms.gov/PhysicianFeeSched/PFSRVF/list.asp.
- American Medical Association. RBRVS: Resource-Based Relative Value Scale. 2014 RVS Update Process. http://www.ama-assn.org/go/rbrvs. Published 2013.
- The Henry J. Kaiser Family Foundation. http://kff.org/health-reform/.

CHAPTER 5

Successful Strategies in Billing

Cheryl Toth and Karen A. Zupko

"Don't worry, you don't need to pay anything today. We'll bill you after insurance pays."

For decades, this has been the basic billing strategy for most practices. A reactive versus proactive approach that has allowed patients to receive services, treatments, and tests in the office and leave without paying anything except a co-pay. In many practices, even the co-pay is not consistently collected at the time of the visit. After the patient leaves your office, staff posts the visit and any other service charges and sends out a claim, crossing their fingers that the front desk has entered the handwritten data from the patient's registration form accurately.

Best case, the practice receives payer reimbursement in 4 to 6 weeks, and the patient is billed his or her portion by snail mail, with a request to pay within 30 days. In other words, *best case*, the practice is not fully paid until 8 to 10 weeks after rendering a service.

With deductibles skyrocketing and reimbursements flat, today's modern otolaryngology practice must do better. The good news is there are many ways to gain billing process efficiency and improve cash flow. New technologies improve data gathering and provide transparency into patient benefit plans and financial responsibilities. Payers offer more details than ever online, if only staff know where to look. And hiring capable, experienced staff and supplying them with knowledge tools and ongoing education is de rigueur over filling empty seats with warm bodies.

The following 5 strategies improve the success of billing and collections and they represent a significantly different approach than the "we'll bill you after insurance pays" mantra of the past. Tactics for implementing each strategy are included in this chapter.

1. Know the Rules. Billing is a detailed business, with reams of rules—from payer reimbursement guidelines and payment schedules to Medicare transmittals and code changes. Most of this information is readily available but requires time and effort to locate, collect, organize, maintain, and update. If you do not assign someone the job of paying attention, you will see a rise in claim rejections and receivables.

For example, vital to successful billing is knowing how payers want claims submitted. There is no industry standard, so your staff must know the rules for each individual payer. One client had a stream of Medicare denials for bilateral, maxillary sinus procedures. A quick look at the Explanation of Benefits (EOB) forms indicated that staff was submitting code 31256 on two lines, with modifier 50. But Medicare's rule is to submit code 31256 on one line, with modifier 50. If staff had taken the time to learn the Medicare rule for claims with bilateral procedures, the claims would have been paid without incident. Instead, they unnecessarily spent many hours putting the denied claims through Medicare's appeal process.

2. Focus on the Front End. Billing has "front-end" and "back-end" processes. Contrary to what you may think, the most common billing

29

mistakes do not actually happen in the billing office. Most of them happen on the "front end" of the process, by the staff that schedules appointments, registers patients, and checks out patients in the office. Modern practices understand that front-end processes must be fine-tuned and nearly pitch perfect if the goal is timely and effective reimbursement. In modern practices, front desk staff is held accountable for accurate registration, eligibility, benefits, and referral verification, and point-of-service collections or payment plan setup. This is a big shift in mindset.

3. Adopt Payment Technologies. Batch eligibility verification, online cost estimators, electronic remittance advice, and recurring payment solutions are a few examples of technologies that improve billing process efficiency and speed payments. These technologies are inexpensive and put powerful data in the hands of practice staff, enabling them to do the billing better and smarter. Yet, it is surprising how many practices are slow to adopt them. In many practices, overcoming inertia is essential in order to gain the benefits of these tools.

4. Optimize the Billing Team. An optimized billing team has the right type of people doing the right things at the right time. The team's primary tasks include sending out claims, processing payments, following up on denials, analyzing accounts receivable and denial patterns, and ensuring coding practices are appropriately followed. Unfortunately, we find many billing teams spend too much time mopping up easy-to-avoid messes that were created before a claim was ever transmitted, on the front end of the billing process. Modern practices shift their mindset to the critical role that front desk staff has in the billing and collections process and holds them accountable so that the billing team can focus on the complexities of denial management and ensure a robust revenue cycle that keeps cash flowing.

5. Empower and Educate Staff. Billing rules and payment technologies are constantly changing. "Saving money" by denying your

staff billing education and training will cost the practice dearly in rejected claims and unpaid patient bills. Regular team attendance at payer webinars, ENT-specific workshops and online courses are vital to your practice's ability to bill and get paid properly. Empowering staff with information such as a new coding book every year and subscriptions to trade publications, as well as access to online billing information, are also essential to the financial health of the practice.

Strategy 1: Know the Rules

Even 5 years ago, obtaining payer rules and guidelines required that staff make lots of phone calls and wait on hold. This has changed significantly. Today, virtually every payer provides most if not all of their coding and claim submission guidelines, as well as provider manuals and reimbursement policies, online. Below is a list of the critical information a practice needs in order to accurately submit claims and understand how to follow up when not paid:

- Which plans are performing prospective audits for levels 4 and 5 evaluation and management (E/M) codes?
- How do we bill bilateral surgery? On one line or two?
- How must we bill for turbinate procedures?
- Where can we download the latest copy of the payment schedule for otolaryngology?
- What is the claim filing limitation?
- How do we appeal a denied claim?
- What are the guidelines for billing for a nonphysician provider? Does the payer allow a nonphysician provider to be credentialed as a provider, or do we bill incident-to?
- What are the rules for global surgery?
- Which otolaryngology procedures require prior authorization? What is the process?
- How do we verify eligibility? What phone number? Which website address?

- Where do we go online to check claims status?

Start with Medicare, which publishes everything you need to know about submitting claims, billing, coding guidelines, how to bill for nonphysician providers, National Correct Coding Initiative (NCCI) edits, and much more at https://www.cms.gov. Each year in the fall, Medicare publishes the full payment schedule that will be implemented the following calendar year. That is available on this site as well, as are lots of e-newsletters and webinars on key topics and upcoming changes. Make sure staff sign up for all relevant e-newsletters and attend every pertinent webinar. In one practice we work with, the administrator requires a representative from the nonphysician provider team, front desk, and physician team to attend.

Next gather policies and information from your Medicare Administrative Contractor (MAC). The MAC is the organization that pays or denies your Medicare claims, your practice must know the details of how to appeal denials and request redeterminations when a claim has been rejected that you think should not have been. MACs generally follow Medicare rules, but not always. Your staff must know the rules and the deviations.

Then, conduct similar fact-finding missions at the websites of commercial payers and Medicaid. Provide everyone on your team account access to these sites. Like Medicare, commercial payers offer e-newsletters, webinars, and ongoing, online training to keep physician offices up to date. If you divide your billing staff by payer account, have each account manager be responsible for distributing new information across the practice. Be vigilant and keep up with policy changes.

To keep data organized and easier to maintain, create a folder structure on your computer network so that all staff has access to the information, even if they are not directly responsible for managing it. Encourage knowledge transfer across the team by dividing responsibilities for obtaining updates, then sharing with the group. In one model, the office staff visit the websites of payers they manage once a month, as well as read e-newsletters and attend webinars. The staff then distill what they learn and present it in bimonthly staff meetings, thereby keeping everyone up to date.

Finally, there is one rule that Medicare and all payers agree on these days: the rule about professional courtesy. The old philosophy of professional courtesy—physicians seeing or treating other health care professionals and their families for free—has for the most part gone the way of the paper chart. In an environment of shrinking reimbursement, many otolaryngologists instead donate their time to patients who have demonstrated financial hardship or are uninsured. This care is typically written off as charity care so it can be tracked and evaluated annually.

The other method of professional courtesy, whereby a physician accepts what insurance pays and does not balance bill the patient or collect a co-pay, is a payer contract violation that practices must avoid. Nearly every managed care contract we reviewed—and certainly Medicare—states that practices are obligated to collect the patient's responsibility. Actuarially speaking, the payer's reimbursement plus the patient's portion is the full cost of the procedure, and practices must attempt to collect all of it. The patient's complete financial responsibility could include deductible, visit co-pay, coinsurance, and noncovered services fees.

Strategy 2: Focus on the Front End

Front-end billing processes are those that happen prior to the patient's first visit, or prior to surgery. *Front-end billing processes are where the majority of billing mistakes are made.* They represent the root causes of the majority of claim denials or lack of patient payment. These include the following:

- The patient did not have a referral on the date of service.
- The patient was not eligible on the date of service.
- Prior authorization was not obtained.
- The patient's plan does not include the service as a benefit. (The staff should have reviewed this with the patient and collected up front.)

- The patient has an unmet deductible/coinsurance. (The staff should have collected prior to the visit.)
- The patient's co-pay was not collected.

Table 5–1 indicates the most common front-end and back-end processes and who performs them. Commonly, employees on the "front end" are responsible for completing competing tasks. For example, the interruptive nature of answering phones and checking in/out patients makes data collection accuracy challenging.

Why are so many mistakes made on the front end? Often it's because of these cultural norms:

1. Front desk staff do not understand that they are part of the billing process.
2. Rejected claims and unpaid patient bills are perceived as the billing office's fault, so front desk staff are not held accountable.
3. Front desk staff are not given the tools or the training necessary to do their job well.
4. The front desk is perceived as an entry-level job so it is filled with inexperienced, untrained individuals who are typically the lowest paid in the practice.
5. The surgery scheduling process does not include a request for presurgical deposits.

Here is the best piece of billing advice we can give your practice: *The most critical people on the billing team are sitting at the front desk, on your appointment scheduling team, and in the Surgery Coordinator's office.* These employees are on the front lines. They gather information from patients. They have eyeball-to-eyeball contact with patients and therefore have the best chance at collecting money at the point of service. Modern practices change the old front desk and surgery scheduling culture to one that is proactive, using tactics such as these:

1. Start the billing process on the first phone call. The new patient appointment call is the most overlooked opportunity in the billing process. Provide staff with the customer service and revenue cycle training to handle this call right. Structure tasks so that staff does not rush new patients off the phone after making the first appointment, and they can collect more information than name, date of birth, and telephone number. In this call, staff must proactively cover key points such as

- "Please bring your tests/scans and referral—or we may reschedule you."
- "We'll collect your co-pay prior to being seen, and the coinsurance and any unmet deductible for the services and tests you receive in our office. We accept Visa/MC, Discover, or check."
- "If you are a candidate for surgery, our Surgery Coordinator will calculate your financial responsibility based on your insurance coverage, and ask for a deposit to secure a surgery date."
- "We offer payment plans and patient financing to those who need a little

Table 5–1. Common Front-End and Back-End Billing Processes

Front-End Processes	Back-End Processes
• Schedule appointment and preregister patient	• Submit claim/send patient statement
• Verify insurance and manage referrals	• Correct front-end edits and resubmit
• Check-in/verify demographic data	• Process and analyze payments
• Conduct patient encounter—code and document (provider)	• Manage denials/resubmit
• Coordinate tests/procedure	• Follow up with payer and patient on overdue receivables
• Check-out and collect at point of service	

extra time paying their bill." This is especially helpful for audiology and hearing aid patients.

- And finally, "we have you all set to see Dr. Wonderful at [DATE] [TIME]. We have reserved this time especially for you. If you must cancel or reschedule your appointment, please call us within 24 hours of your scheduled time, or you may be billed. Our no-show policy is . . . [EXPLAIN POLICY].

As the demand for appointment slots increases, in competitive geographic locations, practices are beginning to charge patients who fail to show up or cancel their appointment within 24 hours of the scheduled time. Medicare and other payers have issued statements supporting these practices, as long as the charge is reasonable. We find that $25 to $30 is a typical fee range for surgical practices that have a policy to charge no-show patients. This fee is billed to the patient, not the insurance company. In-demand physicians who take a credit card number to guarantee an appointment inform patients that their credit card may be billed if they fail to cancel or reschedule within 24 hours.

In addition to communicating your no-show policy, the front desk staff must have deep knowledge of the practice's patient payment policies in order to do an effective job of describing them to patients. Make sure you have clarified these policies in writing so that they can properly explain the rules to patients. Figure 5–1 provides an overview of what should be covered in the policy.

Setting expectations such as these on the first phone call improves overall collections and effectively communicates the patient's financial expectations. Patients appreciate knowing what they owe, and how they can settle their bill. According to a 2009 survey by McKinsey & Company, 74% of patients said they were willing and able to pay out-of-pocket expenses less than or equal to $1000 and 62% were willing to pay medical bills greater than or equal to $1000. Provide options and clear information, and collections will improve.

An effective patient payment policy includes these components, which are reinforced by phone on the first appointment call as well as by staff in the office.

- Patient responsibility in the billing process – for instance, that they arrive with a referral, if required by their plan

- Methods of payment you accept

- What you will collect in the office – copay, coinsurance, unmet deductible

- Explanation of presurgical deposit and what is expected to schedule surgery

- Description of your payment plan options

- Description of patient financing, if you offer this

- Options for patients who are uninsured or who have a financial hardship

- No show policy for patients who fail to show up or cancel within 24 hours of their appointment time

Figure 5–1. Key Components of a Patient Payment Policy.

2. Preregister new patients. Preregistration means obtaining complete patient demographic and insurance information and entering it into the computer system prior to the first visit. We have advocated this for decades and today it is more important than ever to your practice's billing health. Complete and timely information is essential for ensuring the practice verifies eligibility and benefits, knowing what the practice can collect from the patient in the office, and understanding referral or precertification requirements before a visit, test, or surgery.

Patient portals, which allow patients to go online and register themselves, are the most effective way to preregister because the data are automatically entered into your practice management system (PMS). Other options include calling the patient and preregistering by phone, or e-mailing the forms to new patients in advance. You could also ask your website administrator to create an online form for patients to complete, so that registration information is transmitted to the office for data entry into the billing system prior to patient arrival.

3. Verify insurance eligibility and benefits, for new *and* established patients. It amazes us how many practices skip this critical billing step. Or, that verify it for new patients but not for established patients, only to find that the established patient is no longer eligible for the plan on record, which results in a rejected claim.

Before the Internet, eligibility verification took a lot of staff time on the phone. Today, many PMS and electronic health record (EHR) systems can be scheduled to "batch" and perform these checks automatically, 48 to 72 hours prior to the patient's appointment. The system produces a report that indicates which patients are eligible and which are not. If done several days in advance of the patient's appointment, staff can call ineligible patients and explain that they will be responsible for paying for the visit. Front desk staff can also use the report to collect from ineligible patients or give them the option of rescheduling. If your system does not have this "batch eligibility" feature, nearly all payers provide eligibility verification features on their websites.

4. Obtain managed care referrals for all new patients. Depending on the size of the practice, referrals management can be performed at the time of appointment scheduling, or can be a separate process. If a patient arrives for a non-urgent issue without a referral, obtain it before the patient is seen or reschedule the patient. If you do not, your reimbursement for that visit is at risk.

5. Precertify tests and scans. Payers frequently have contracts with separate radiologic diagnostic testing facilities and will not reimburse the practice if tests are not done in an approved facility. Always precertify any diagnostic testing, or at least contact the payer to inquire whether precertification is required. Typical tests that require precertification include magnetic resonance imaging (MRI) and computed tomography (CT) scans, some audiology diagnostic testing, allergy testing, and certain lab tests. In rare cases, the payer may even require precertification for plain films. Since many patients will require further diagnostic testing and therapeutic procedures after being seen in the office, obtain precertification prior to the patient's arrival.

6. Verify patient identity, demographics, and insurance at check-in. The front desk staff plays a vital role here by validating the patient's identity and any previously obtained insurance information. This is critical for both new and established patients. Yet, this step is frequently overlooked due to the fact that the check-in staff is often overwhelmed with phone calls, chart preparation, appointment scheduling, and check-in tasks. Like the first phone call, take the importance of check-in tasks seriously. Set up your team for success by minimizing multitasking and allowing them to focus on verification tasks.

7. Implement point-of-service collections. As patient responsibilities continue to rise, there is more to collect from patients than ever. Many Affordable Care Act (ACA) insurance exchange options have deductibles of $5000 or more. Reminding patients when they schedule their appointments of any balance, and collect-

ing this over the phone or explaining that the patient cannot be seen for a new appointment until the balance is settled, can go a long way toward decreasing receivables.

Practices that do not implement up-front collection processes will see their receivables balloon. Once those patient balances start going beyond 90 days, collecting them successfully will be challenging. Collecting after the provider has seen the patient or performed surgery is time-consuming and difficult, resulting in significant delays and a risk of no-payment.

Be prepared that switching from the "we will bill you later" mindset to one of collecting up front is a *big change* for staff. This change is not easy, and it will not happen overnight. Part of the challenge is that effectively collecting at the point of service is not only about "asking for money." It requires a coordinated *plan* that includes

- Clear financial policies for staff to follow
- Technology tools that help them quickly identify the amounts they can collect. (more on these in the next section)
- Scripts and talking points to help them ask for money
- Training that ensures staff know how to ask and collect effectively
- A commitment from the physicians and manager to review collections data and progress on a regular basis (few things boost collections more than when staff know the physicians are paying attention)

The plan must include all five of these elements in order to be truly successful. Without a clear policy, there are no rules for staff to follow. Without tools, they do not know how much to ask for. Without scripts and training they cannot be certain how or who to ask for money from. Someone on the management team must pay attention to how much is being collected because as the adage goes, "Employees *respect* what management *inspects*."

Finally, resistant managers often complain that collecting from patients at the point of ser-

vice will require them to write more refund checks. Although this may be true in a small number of cases, getting the majority of patient payments in the bank, in exchange for writing a few additional checks each month, is well worth it. It is certainly cheaper and more efficient than sending hundreds of statements each month.

8. Provide presurgical counseling and collect a deposit. The process of presurgical financial counseling is helpful to the patient, who needs to understand what he or she owes, as well as to the billing process, because there are many rules and variables in getting reimbursed for surgical procedures.

As discussed earlier, your staff must know these rules and be prepared to discuss them prospectively with the patient so that his or her financial responsibilities are transparent. If staff or the patient is not crystal clear about what is covered and what the patient will owe, the billing team will spend unnecessary time chasing unpaid claims and patient statements.

Use septoplasty (30520) as an example. Payer rules and claim submission guidelines vary widely for this procedure, which might be part of a cosmetic rhinoplasty if function is a concern. Therefore, septoplasty nearly always requires prior authorization. What must the physician document from his or her physical exam of the septum to justify functional surgery? Does the payer require that the patient fail medical therapy first and what therapy(s)? For how long? For which symptoms? Is a CT required to demonstrate the deviation and obstruction?

It is the practice's responsibility to fully understand these rules for the different payers. If staff does not follow plan guidelines, provide the right documentation along with the claim, and obtain prior authorization, the claim will be rejected. Worse, there will be no recourse with the patient. If the plan guidelines are not followed, the patient cannot be billed.

Nearly all of this can be avoided by establishing a proactive, presurgical counseling process. This process is typically coordinated by a full-time surgery coordinator. This person needs his or her own office or at least a quiet and private space in which to talk with patients. The surgery coordinator uses a scheduling worksheet and checklist to ensure all reimbursement criteria are met. To discuss costs with patients, he or she uses a Surgical Cost Quotation that clearly explains what the patient's insurance plan will pay and what the patient will owe. The staff enters insurance plan allowable data for each procedure and patient-specific coverage details; then the patient's portion becomes clear.

Most modern practices collect at least 50% of the patient's responsibility prior to the date of surgery. Some practices require more. In every practice that implements a quotation process, patients are thrilled. The process allows patients to understand what they owe and make an informed decision about how they can pay.

Strategy 3: Adopt Payment Technologies

Effectively implementing presurgical counseling and point-of-service collections requires access to information, and this requires the use of free or low-cost technology tools. Here are six that your practice can use to improve collections and delight patients:

1. Online cost estimators. It used to be nearly impossible to predict what could be collected from patients until an EOB came with the plan's payment. But today, cost estimators provide real-time data about what a patient owes (Figure 5–2). Staff enter the *Current Procedural Terminology* (CPT®) codes for office visits or surgeries into the cost estimator—which is available through a Web browser and offered for free

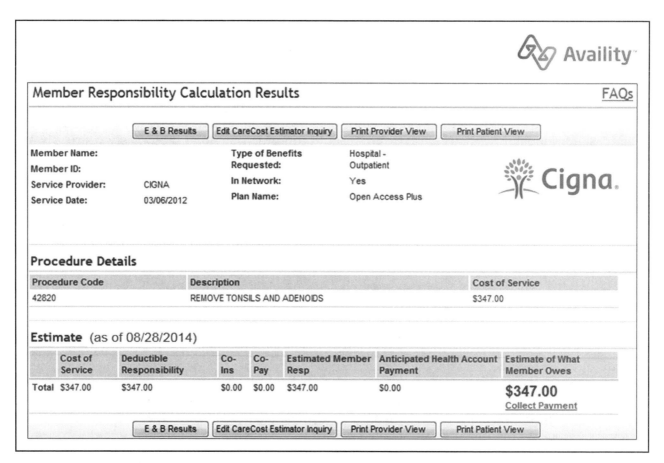

Figure 5–2. Example Payer Cost Estimator. The Cost Estimator from Availity (http://www.availity.com) illustrates what can be collected from a patient who is scheduling tonsillectomy with adenoidectomy. Payers and clearinghouses offer these types of online estimators, at no cost to a practice. Used with permission from Availity.

by various clearinghouses and payers—and the cost estimator calculates exactly what staff can collect from the patient standing at the check-out counter, or speaking with the surgical coordinator.

2. Automated scripting, specific to the patient's coverage rules. An emerging technology is one that enhances the cost estimator and makes it easier for staff to collect. One clearinghouse refers to it as "Patient Access" (Figure 5–3). The

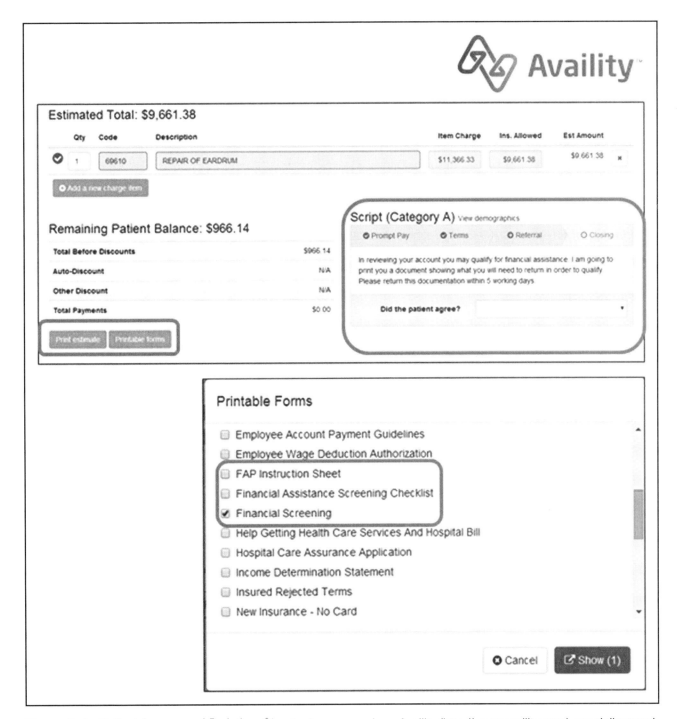

Figure 5–3. Patient Access and Scripting. Clearinghouses such as Availity (http://www.availity.com) can deliver real-time financial data within a script that integrates your practice's financial policies. Such tools boost staff confidence when asking patients for money and can increase point of service collections. Used with permission from Availity.

technology integrates the amount your staff can collect with patient-friendly language that is specific to the patient's plan coverage, and specific to your practice's financial and collection policies. By entering your policies into the system as part of the setup process, the technology is customized to the practice. The result is a highly individualized script that staff read to the patient at the point of service or surgical counseling. The script empowers staff to collect, even if they are unsure how to ask for money.

3. Online payment processing. Improve payment convenience by using online payment processing. This makes payment processing accessible from every staff person's computer, through a Web browser. Companies such as TransFirst (http://www.transfirst.com) offer online credit card payment processing at very low rates.

4. Automated, recurring billing. How do you pay for Internet-based commercial services every month? By automated, recurring payment. Your practice can offer the same option to patients, giving them a convenient way to pay their bill in installments, and requiring only a one-time setup and virtually no ongoing management by staff.

This tool empowers check-out staff or the surgery coordinator to establish a payment plan before the patient leaves the office. This will decrease reliance on complex spreadsheets or clunky billing system collections modules. The patient's credit card is automatically billed for an agreed upon number of months, until the balance is paid off. TransFirst and PayPal (http://www.paypal.com) both offer an automatic, recurring bill-pay feature. Some practice management system vendors do as well.

5. Online bill pay. Americans love the convenience of paying bills online—46% of those with Internet access pay their bills online or through a banking website.[1] Capitalize on this trend by enabling online bill payment. If your practice management system vendor offers a patient portal, use its online payment feature.

Alternatively, solutions from TransFirst or PayPal are easy to implement and easy to use.

6. Patient financing. CareCredit (http://www.carecredit.com) offers a health care "credit card" that allows patients to finance large deductibles and coinsurances. For a small service fee, your money is off the books and in the bank in 2 business days. CareCredit assumes the credit risk and handles the collections with the patient directly. This is great for patients and great for your bottom line. Financing options include 6- or 12-month interest-free payments, or financing for up to 5 years.

After you have launched these patient payment technology options, do not keep them a secret. Put promotional copy on your website. Make flyers or postcards for the front desk, and posters for the exam rooms. Add information to your "on hold" message. Finally, make sure the front desk, billing office, and surgical counselors are fully trained to use the tools to collect payments.

Strategy 4: Optimize the Billing Team

We are often asked, "How can we optimize the efficiency of the billing staff? What should their priorities be?" Although it is true that each practice has a unique set of circumstances that can impact billing operations, there are certain best practices that we find common in successful practices, and these fall into three primary categories: people, tasks, and analysis.

People

1. Hire problem solvers who have experience in your specialty. Unless you are in a large practice that has experienced supervisors and a solid orientation and training program, stick to hiring people with the right experience and skills for the billing team. That means hiring someone with a proven track record of working in an otolaryngology practice and who can demonstrate reimbursement acumen in the areas of coding,

claim submission, denial management, and accounts receivable follow-up and management.

Ask about subspecialty experience, too. Although all neurotologists and otolaryngic allergists are classified as otolaryngologists, their billing nuances could not be more different. Ask candidates relevant questions about your subspecialty billing issues to identify existing knowledge as well as training needs.

We recommend billing quizzes for all candidates, and case study discussions, for example, provide candidates with an accounts receivable report and ask them to analyze it. You would be surprised how many people who apply for billing office jobs do not know the basics of bilateral billing or E/M code selection, and cannot prioritize the action steps for cleaning up old receivables.

2. Divide follow-up tasks by payer type. As we have discussed throughout this chapter, billing rules and reimbursement guidelines vary by payer. Create a team of internal experts by dividing claim follow-up tasks by payer and allocate the number of payers each person manages depending on the claim volume for each. For instance, one staff member might manage only Medicare and Blue Cross Blue Shield, if the two represent a large share of your payer mix. Dividing responsibilities by payer allows you to hold staff accountable, and ensures there is a "point person" and "subject matter expert" for each plan.

3. Collaborate and communicate. The most ineffective billing teams are the ones who sit in cubicles and rarely communicate or share with one another. The most effective billing teams meet weekly or every other week to discuss payer trends, billing processes, policy changes, and other details related to accounts receivable. Foster collaboration among your team, and together they will achieve great things.

Tasks

1. Review and verify codes. In the most successful practices, physicians—not coders, not EHRs—select codes. We have always been proponents of having physicians select codes because they are the ones delivering the service, and therefore know better than anyone what was performed. The billing team, however, must function as a knowledgeable, "second pair of eyes" to ensure the codes selected comply with CPT rules and payer guidelines. The billing team's role is to verify accuracy and speak with physicians directly if changes are needed.

2. Submit claims electronically, every day. This is, as they say, "billing 101." Successful practices submit accurate, "clean" electronic claims on a daily basis to as many payers as possible because they are processed faster than paper claims. Paper claims should be submitted only to payers who require this method of billing. Electronic claims are paid faster and preferred by most payers including Medicare.

3. Review, fix, and resubmit claims on the edit report—every day. We frequently find that this simple task goes undone in many offices. Here is what should happen: After the billing team transmits the day's claims electronically, the claims are reviewed or "scrubbed" by your electronic clearinghouse to ensure the demographic, insurance, and code information is appropriate before the claim is sent to the insurance company. This ensures that a "clean" claim is passed on to the payer. After the clearinghouse scrubs the practice's electronic claim batch, any missing demographic or insurance data are immediately sent back to the practice to correct. These are easy fixes—name, gender, date of birth—and can be completed quickly, which is why the review, fix, and resubmission of these claims must be done *daily*.

4. Speed up payment posting with electronic remittance advice (ERA). ERA is a way to receive electronic payments directly into your practice management system. It decreases or eliminates the mundane staff task of posting payments all day at a computer.

Ask your vendor about its ERA service and features. It is important that the payments come into your system by "line item" (by each CPT code billed), instead of having all services "lumped" together in one payment. If your vendor's ERA service "lumps" payments, require staff to contact the payer for each payment received to determine the allocation of each payment for each CPT code. Without this additional investigative work, there is no way to determine whether payment is correct.

5. Sign up for payer electronic funds transfer (EFT). This is a staff efficiency tool that gets your money in the bank faster. Instead of receiving a paper check in the mail, payments from payers can be securely transferred to your practice's bank account using EFT. Using EFT reduces the number of checks your staff will have to deposit, and fewer checks reduce the risk of employee theft. Most major payers offer this service, and there is no cost to enroll.

6. Print and mail patient statements every day. Daily statement mailing is better for cash flow than waiting until month's end. Staff can generate patient statements immediately after a payment from the insurance company is posted. As point-of-service collections processes are implemented, the number of patient statements will be reduced.

7. Follow up on current balances quickly. Focus on unpaid claims in the "30 day" column of the accounts receivable report first. If staff stays ahead of the curve and gets the current claims paid quickly, in a short period of time, the number of "very old," outstanding balances will be minimized.

8. Create policies and procedures for how the team must follow up on past due balances. In addition to focusing on the use of claim estimators and improving front-end collection processes, make sure there is an organized process for monitoring and following up on unpaid balances.

To improve efficiency, strive for procedures that leverage technology. Some clearinghouses offer claim status tools that enable staff to access online details about whether a claim was received by the payer and why the claim has not been paid. Not only does the use of such tools speed the follow-up process, but it can eliminate the need for payer phone tag, handwritten notes, and the potential for staff to record verbally provided claim status details inaccurately. Staff simply login, use search and sort parameters to look up a patient's claim status, and obtain the details needed to understand status and take action. Trizetto offers the ease of submitting a corrected claim, appealing the claim, verifying eligibility, and more, with the click of a button (Figure 5–4).

Finally, a complete policy for claim follow-up must include specifics about how to establish payment plans, approve patients for charity care, and handle uninsured and underinsured patients who ask about cash discounts. Physicians should be actively involved in reviewing and approving such policies.

Analysis

As noted in the beginning of this chapter, billing is a detailed business, and the billing team must be willing to dive deep into analyzing the details of reports, EOBs, and data. Such deep dives are essential for not only getting claims paid, but for analyzing rejection patterns and denial trends and making a plan to address them through process change and front-end staff training.

Here are 6 analysis tasks the billing team must complete:

1. Verify that payer payments are correct, according to contract. Enter all contracted payment schedules into the practice management system and hold billing staff accountable for verifying that payments match contracted amounts. Some systems do this automatically and alert staff to payments that do not match. Other systems require staff to review the payment amount against the payment loaded into the system. Either way, the billing team must be held accountable for ensuring the practice is accurately paid.

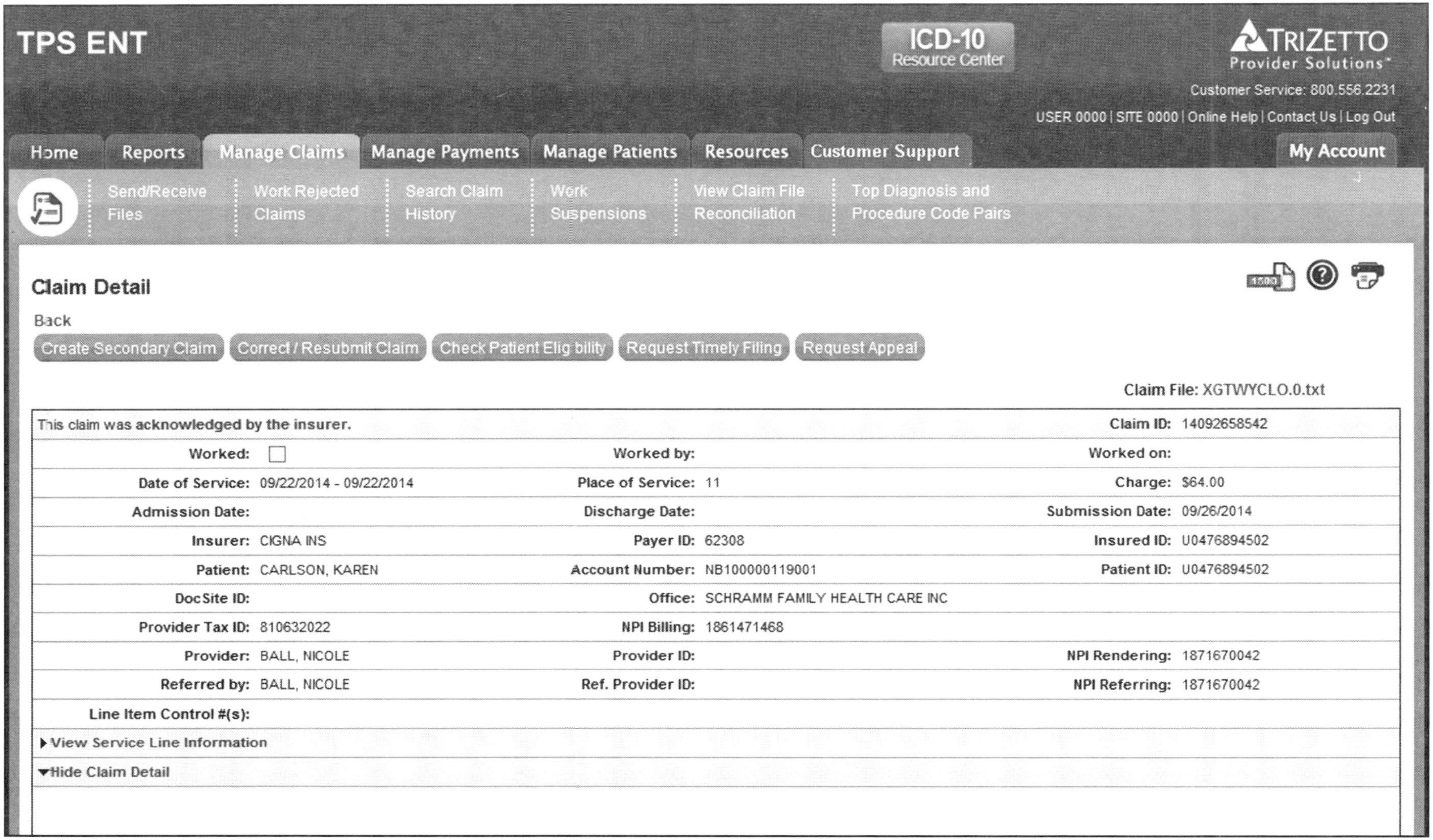

Figure 5–4. Online Claim Inquiry. Clearinghouses such as Trizetto (http://www.trizetto.com) improve billing staff efficiency with tools such as Claim Inquiry. Staff can look up claim status, determine actions needed, click to correct/resubmit a claim, request an appeal, and much more. Used with permission from Trizetto.

41

2. Track and report key metrics monthly. Review the following monthly parameters against the healthy benchmarks noted below:

- Days in Receivable. The number of days, on average, it takes to get an account paid. Divide total receivables by average daily charges (annual charges/365).. In a healthy practice, this is 30 to 45 days.
- Percent of accounts receivable greater than 90 days. In a healthy practice, this is 15% or less.
- Net Collection Percentage. This measures the practice's effectiveness in collecting legitimate reimbursement and helps you understand the percentage of collectible money that has been left on the table for avoidable reasons (such as no preauthorization). Divide Total Receipts (net of refunds) by Charges minus Contractual Adjustments. In a healthy practice, this is 95% or more.

3. Analyze the accounts receivable report monthly. This analysis is akin to peeling an onion. Staff should start with high-level report data and peel away layers to get down to payer-specific patterns and issues. Table 5–2 shows a basic accounts receivable report, available in any PMS. Make sure this report is generated by "date of service," not "date of posting" and that "pre-pays" such as presurgical deposits are isolated from actual insurance and patient receivables.

Billing staff can initiate account follow-up by drilling into the claims in the "30–60 day" column. This column typically has the biggest rewards, because the claims are still fairly "young" and there is opportunity to correct and resubmit them.

4. Review and analyze EOBs. Appropriate analysis of each EOB is critical to ensure the practice was paid according to contract terms, and to drive the next steps in the revenue cycle, such as billing a secondary payer or sending a

Table 5–2. ENT Associates Aged Accounts Receivable Report

ENT Associates Aged Accounts Receivable Report							
	Pre	0–30	30–60	60–90	90–120	120+	Total
Pt. Resp. A/R	$12,456	$16,000	$18,000	$9,000	$9,000	$40,000	$92,000
Pt. Resp. %	N/A	17.4%	19.6%	9.8%	9.8%	43.5%	100%
Insurance A/R	N/A	$346,000	$74,000	$11,000	$13,500	$27,500	$472,000
Insurance %	N/A	64.2%	16.3%	3.5%	4%	12%	100%
Total A/R	$12,456	$362,000	$92,000	$20,000	$22,500	$67,500	$564,000
Total A/R %	N/A	64.2%	16.3%	3.5%	4%	12%	100%
		Healthy: 50% or MORE of receivables are here			Healthy: 15% or LESS of receivables are here		
This Month's Days in Receivable	[Total Receivables ÷ 365] ÷ 365 = _____ Healthy: 30–45 "Days"						

Note. The accounts receivable report is a key diagnostic for identifying billing and collections problems.

statement to the patient for payment of the balance. Another important aspect of EOB analysis is to determine any primary third-party claim follow-up, such as appealing services denied for inappropriate bundling, medical necessity, low pay appeals, incorrect coding, and inappropriate reporting of services during the global period. Involve physicians and other providers in denial appeals for medical necessity and coding denials.

EOBs are also a great diagnostic tool for evaluating whether billing processes are working. On a quarterly basis, ask billing staff to review a random stack of EOBs and analyze them for denial trends that identify front-end, process-related problems such as

- Demographic errors
- Eligibility-related denials
- Wrong primary/secondary insurance company
- No referral authorization
- No coverage at time of service

Hold the team accountable for devising and implementing solutions to prevent these errors in the future.

5. Review the adjustments report quarterly. The adjustments report provides details about the amounts "written off" and to what category. Common adjustment categories include contractual adjustments for each individual payer, no referral, prior authorization not obtained, bad debt, and charity care. The most useful adjustments reports are those that are highly detailed. If yours is not, talk to your vendor about setting up more granular adjustment reporting categories.

Analyzing this report sheds light on rejection patterns and can lead the billing team to address issues that cause claim rejection patterns before they become acute.

6. Analyze the credit balance report monthly. Credit balances are those that your practice owes patients or insurance companies and you are required to refund them to the appro-

priate party. Stay on top of these refunds by having the billing team generate a credit balance report monthly to review, validate, and submit a request for a refund to the practice manager or financial manager. Process refunds monthly—getting behind can become expensive.

Educate and Empower Staff

As Benjamin Franklin wisely said: "An investment in knowledge always pays the best interest." When it comes to billing and collections, this could not be truer.

In our work with hundreds of otolaryngology practices nationwide, we find a common thread among the practices that have cash flow problems, accounts receivable issues, and coding and billing errors; they do not provide the knowledge, essential publications, training, or ongoing education to those performing billing and collections tasks.

The result is a group of well-intentioned folks in the billing office who try to do their best, but aren't very successful. Many of them pretty defeated. In nearly every case their failings are not a result of low intellect or malicious intent; they are the result of not being provided with the right information, tools, and ongoing knowledge necessary to do their job well.

When we begin explaining some of the tips and information provided in this chapter, the faces of these employees visibly change and their eyes widen. They become sponges for the new information. Here's what we recommend for educating and empowering your team:

1. Always have a budget line for staff training and education. Thinking that you "can't afford" to provide ongoing staff education is silly and shortsighted. To put things in perspective: You can "save" a few thousand dollars on the tuition and airfare required to send someone to a regional coding/billing workshop, but you stand to lose at least that much on *one* big surgical claim if it's not submitted correctly. Small

practices should budget $3000 to $4000 per year (including travel expenses) and larger ones $5000 or more.

2. Provide a new CPT coding book, every year. It is astounding how many billing staff are hobbling along with coding books that are several years old because the practice will not pay for the new edition each year. Do not let your practice fall into this trap. Buy the book and arm your team with the latest codes and information annually.

3. Send at least one staff (and a physician) to an annual ENT-specific coding and reimbursement workshop. There are so many reasons this is a good annual investment. Your staff will not only learn otolaryngology-specific coding, but they will meet and learn from other participants experiencing similar issues and will get the latest changes to codes and rules. Once home, the staff person should be expected to summarize the most important things learned and discuss them with the entire team.

4. Encourage webinar attendance. Medicare, ENT-specific programs, clearinghouse companies, and payers offer valuable education for free, online. Encourage team attendance at these events, or divide the responsibility and ask the staff person who attends to send a summary e-mail to the team.

5. Encourage e-newsletter sign-ups and regular online reading. Make it part of your team's job to stay current by reading. There are many resources available for free. We suggest the following for staff: https://www.CMS.gov, http://www.PhysiciansPractice.com, http://www.entnet.org, http://www.MedicalOfficeMgr.com, http://www.MGMA.com and https://www.AAPC.com.

6. Foster sharing in staff meetings. Divide learning opportunities among the staff and ask for reports of what was learned. This enables your team to participate in more webinars and workshops than if everyone had to attend all of them and empowers staff who do attend to distill and teach-back the information to colleagues. When all teach, all learn.

Conclusion

Billing is a detail-laden and critical component of practice management. The 5 strategies discussed provide an interconnected framework that supports a healthy cash flow. Whether you are new to practice or are already thriving, using the tactics described will improve the efficiency of the billing process, the productivity of staff, and the volume of collections. As you make improvements, use the Billing Strategies Self-Assessment at the end of this chapter to identify gaps and stay on track (Table 5–3).

Table 5–3. Billing Strategies Self-Assessment

Our Practice . . .	Yes	No
1. Preregisters at least 90% of all new patients through a patient portal or by phone. (That means all demographic and insurance information is entered into the computer system *prior to* the patient's arrival for their first appointment.)		
2. Re-registers every established patient who is seen in the office, by verifying and/or updating demographic and insurance information in the computer.		
3. Verifies eligibility and benefits for all new and established patients, *every day,* and prior to *every surgery*.		
4. Knows which procedures require precertification or preauthorization, and obtains it 100% of the time it is required.		
5. Posts all office visit services by end of day.		
6. Uses cost estimators to calculate what patients owe, before they leave the office.		
7. Collects copays and unmet deductible amounts from patients before they leave the office.		
8. Collects presurgical deposits from patients, prior to the date of surgery.		
9. Sets up automated, recurring payment plans using the patient's credit card, prior to surgery, or prior to the patient leaving the office.		
10. Offers patient financing options to help patients settle their bill.		
11. Sends claims for all surgeries and hospital services within 48 hours.		
12. Electronically submits claims every day.		
13. Reviews and corrects claims that hit the clearinghouse "front-end edit" report *every day.* Then resubmits the corrected claims *that same day*.		
14. Can easily identify plan underpayments because payor reimbursement schedules are loaded into the computer system.		
15. Has Electronic Remittance Advice (ERA) and Electronic Funds Transfer (EFT) for as many plans that offer it.		
16. Uses online tools for precertification, preauthorization, and unpaid claim status.		
17. Has created detailed adjustment categories ("Patient not eligible," "No prior authorization obtained") so we can monitor denial patterns and fix problems.		
18. Analyzes EOB forms to identify denial patterns, then fixes the reasons at the source.		
19. Generates patient statements *on the same day the insurance payment is posted—not* on a monthly or bimonthly billing cycle.		
20. Maintains an average "days in receivable" (the average number of days it takes to receive payment on an account) of *30 to 45 days*.		
21. Maintains an average of *15% or less* of all receivables over 90 days old.		
22. Maintains a "net collection ratio" (the percentage of collectible money, not adjustments, that is actually collected) of *95% or higher*.		

Note. Assess your practice to determine whether billing process improvements are needed. A modern otolaryngology practice can answer "yes" to all of these statements. If yours cannot, focus on changing each "no" to "yes," and you will see fewer claim denials and overdue receivables.

Reference

1. Western Union Payments Money Mindset Index, March 25, 2013. http://ir.westernunion.com/News/Press-Releases/Press-Release-Details/2013/Western-Union-Survey-Reveals-Increasing-Consumer-Adoption-of-Mobile-Technologies-for-Bill-Payments/default.aspx. Accessed September 9, 2014.

CHAPTER 6

Successful Navigation of the Appeals Process

R. Cheyenne Brinson

Introduction

Effective navigation of the appeals process is a critical aspect of billing and practice management. Failure to have a successful strategy for appeals will result in lost revenue and negatively impact the productivity of the clinician and office staff. Appeals can often seem arbitrary and hopeless, leaving the clinician feeling powerless. However, this chapter explores general concepts and specific strategies for managing the appeals process successfully.

Should I Appeal?

In short, usually if claims are coded correctly, all denials should be appealable. There are 3 general elements of submitting a "clean claim" as reviewed below: (1) satisfaction of medical necessity guidelines to justify a given intervention, (2) appropriate medical documentation and coding of the care provided, and (3) accurate "front-end" office management. Any rejected claim that successfully meets these criteria should be appealed.

The life cycle of the appeals begins before submission of the claim with proper documentation of the medical care and appropriate coding/ claim submission. Many denials can be avoided by

understanding medical necessity guidelines prior to the case. Most payers publish medical policies on their respective websites. It is imperative to document the rationale for surgery in the patient's medical records, most commonly in the office visit where the decision for surgery was made. In addition to a discussion of the medical condition and the risks/benefits/alternatives to the surgery, an important element of this note, from a billing perspective, is documentation of "failure of conservative treatment" (the key buzzwords for most medical policies) and other requirements from the payers.

The second important element of avoiding an appeal event is fully documenting the medical care that was provided to justify the claim being submitted including the office visit and procedures. From a practical standpoint, it is advisable to build the electronic health record (EHR) template based on combined payer guidelines as they are typically similar. Using the most stringent payer guidelines and adding any other payer requirements garners a template that covers all the required elements. The operative report should also include any elements required by the payers. Best practice indicates to use payer language in the "Indications for Surgery" paragraph of the operative note to highlight all of the required medical necessity elements.

Finally, many claims are delayed or rejected because of front-end issues, including obtaining referrals and preauthorizations, verifying a patient has active insurance, updating changes in a patient's insurance plan, accurately recording the patient's demographic information, submitting claims in a timely manner, and promptly transmitting any documentation requested by the insurance carrier. These steps are performed by the administrative team members, not the provider. Optimization requires proper training and supervision, including a system for identifying and correcting errors.

My Claim Is Denied

Most payers have an appeal process and virtually all request a payer-specific form to be completed. These appeal forms are typically located on the payer's website. For best results, follow payer-directed guidelines, including completion of the appeal form. Simply mailing an appeal letter usually will not yield a successful appeal. Instead of a letter, most payer appeals forms ask the reason for the appeal. The use of concise appeal language is advised as there may be a limit on the number of characters that are available to explain the appeal reason.

Many clearinghouses today have the ability to generate appeal forms prepopulated with patient demographic and claim information. This is a significant time saver and a best practice to use these tools provided by the clearinghouse. Oftentimes, these services are premium services and additional fees will apply. The return on investment (ROI) for these premium services more than pays for the nominal monthly fee. Using automation in the appeals process greatly reduces the necessary staff time needed for appeals.

Another time saver is to create templates of standard appeal language. Depending on the practice management system and/or clearinghouse, these templates may be automated in those systems. If not, save the appeal language as a Microsoft Word (Microsoft Corporation, Redmond WA) document and then copy and paste the language onto the payer's appeal form. Be sure to customize any template you use for the specific patient appeal.

Appeal Language

The American Academy of Otolaryngology-Head and Neck Surgery (AAO-HNS) has a number of template appeal letters available for download at http://www.entnet.org/Practice/Appeal-Template-letters.cfm. This language can be cut and pasted onto the payer appeal form. A sample appeal letter for septoplasty denial is as follows:

Dear [Medical Director]:

Please consider this letter a formal request for reconsideration of a denial received for a septoplasty on [Patient's Name] on [Date of Service] by [Name of Physician].

The [claim] [precertification] for the [septoplasty] was billed with CPT® code 30520 - Septoplasty or submucous resection, with or without cartilage scoring, contouring, or replacement with graft.

If the precertification or the claim was denied because the patient's condition was not chronic for more than a certain period of time, then you might include the **bolded text** below in the appeal letter:

I disagree with [insurer name]'s denial of the septoplasty based on your logic that the [Patient Name]'s condition was not chronic for over 2 months. According to current medical practice, it is more clinically appropriate to document nasal obstruction that persists despite reasonable medical therapy (eg, 4–8 weeks). As a result, I believe that [insurer name]'s denial of this procedure is not justifiable.

If the precertification or the claim was denied because you did not include a photograph of the external nose, then you might include the bolded text below in your template letter:

I disagree with [insurer name]'s denial of this septoplasty as medically unnecessary for [Patient Name] because I did not include a photograph of the patient's external nose. Photographs will often not show a clinically significant septal deviation; only caudal deviations will be evident and photos generally demonstrate external nasal deformities. As such, I believe that [insurer name]'s denial of this procedure is not justifiable.

If the precertification or the claim was denied because you noted that the patient has a posterior septal deviation, which causes a physiologic functional impairment, then you might include the bolded text below in your template letter:

Septoplasty corrects deformities of the partition between the two sides of the nose. I am enclosing the previously submitted claim [or precertification request], the Explanation of Benefits and operative notes.

Please reprocess this [claim] [precertification] for the payment of CPT code 30520. If you require additional information, please contact me at [Phone number].

Thank you for your prompt action.

Source: http://www.entnet.org/content/payer-appeal-letters

When writing appeal language, always use language that ties the information together for the insurance company. For example,

The patient meets the medical necessity guidelines as indicated by the Payer Name Medical Policy, Policy Number, and Policy Name.

Using bullet points, repeat the language in the medical policy demonstrating that the criteria has been met. By clearly outlining how the policy was met, the payer does not have to interpret what was intended and sets a higher appeal success rate.

Appealing Denials of an E/M Service Performed on Same Day as Procedure

One of the most common denials for otolaryngologists is evaluation and management (E/M) service performed on the same day as a procedure.

While the E/M code is appended with a modifier 25, many payers will still deny the E/M service. Assuming the E/M was billed correctly, this denial may be appealable. Depending on the reason for denial, sample appeal language includes:

- *Please review the attached claim and documentation. Reimbursement for the E/M service performed on the same day as a (list procedure here) was incorrectly denied. The E/M service was performed for a separate diagnosis. It is, by definition, a separate service.*
- *Although a different diagnosis is not required for reporting of the E/M services on the same date, the separate diagnosis is appropriate in this circumstance.*
- *The documentation of the E/M service and the procedural note clearly indicate a separate E/M service.*
- *Please reprocess the attached claim and reimburse for both services since it is medically necessary and the documentation supports both services.*

Appealing Denials of Modifier 59

Even codes appended with modifier 59 may be denied. Merely stating that the Correct Coding Initiative (CCI) edits allow codes to be billed together does not ensure payment. Modifier 59 (Distinct Procedural Service) is used to communicate to the payer that this is a *special circumstance* and the procedure is distinct or independent, and, while not ordinarily reported together, you meet the "special requirement" qualifying for payment. Successful appeal language will demonstrate to the payer that it is a:

- different session
- different procedure or surgery
- different site or organ system
- separate incision/excision
- separate injury (or area of injuries in extensive injuries)

Refer to Chapter on modifiers for more information on modifier 59.

Appealing Denials of 31237

Another common denial for otolaryngologists is endoscopic sinus debridement services following endoscopic sinus surgery and a septoplasty and/or inferior turbinate submucous resection procedure. The basis of this denial is that the septoplasty (and/or submucous resection of the inferior turbinate) procedure has a 90-day global period. Current Procedural Terminology (CPT) 31237, therefore, is denied because it falls within the septoplasty global period even though it is being performed for postoperative care after sinus surgery which has a 0-day global period. Imperative to submitting a clean initial claim is a well-documented 31237 procedure note (including the indication for the procedure) and appending modifier 79 to 31237 code, if a septoplasty and/or submucous resection of the inferior turbinate was also performed. However, the claim may still get denied, yet it should be appealed. An example appeal includes:

Re: Denial of CPT 31237-79, 50 (modifier 79 is used for an unrelated procedure in the global period, modifier 50 is used for bilateral procedure)

The endoscopic debridement service (CPT 31237) is not included in the global surgical package or global period for the septoplasty (CPT 30520) performed at the same operative session. The endoscopic sinus debridement service provided, 31237-79, 50, was for care of the patient's sinuses—those procedures performed at the same operative session ([List codes performed such as CPT 31255-50, 31267-50]) have a 0-day global period. I did not perform the endoscopic sinus debridements (31237-79, 50) for postoperative care of the septoplasty (30520).

I performed separate procedures at the same operative session that involve different postoperative global periods. The endoscopic sinus surgery codes ([List codes performed such as 31255, 31267]) have a 0-day global period while the septoplasty (30520) has a 90-day global period. If the patient had undergone only a septoplasty (30520, 90-day global period), I would

not have needed to perform the endoscopic sinus debridement (31237-79, 50).

My contracted rates with xxx (name the payer to whom you are writing) are based on Medicare's fee schedule. Medicare clearly assigns a 0-day global period to the codes I billed ([List codes performed such as 31255, 31267]). Therefore, the endoscopic sinus debridements performed postendoscopic sinus surgery (31237) should be paid. I appended modifier 79 (unrelated procedure in the global period) to show that the endoscopic sinus debridements (31237) are unrelated to the septoplasty (30520), the procedure which has a 90-day global period.

The endoscopic sinus surgery codes I billed, [List codes performed such as 31255 and 31267], do not include any follow-up care after the date of service; therefore, the endoscopic sinus debridements (31237) are billable and should be paid.

Please reprocess the claim for immediate payment.

Appealing Denials of Surgical Navigation Codes

Otolaryngologists performing functional endoscopic sinus surgery (FESS), skull base approaches, and other procedures often use stereotactic computer-assisted navigation (SCAN), or image guidance to assist them in clarifying complex anatomy. This service (+61782 - cranial, extradural) is separately reportable when medical necessity has been documented in the operative note. If the medical necessity is appropriately documented in the operative report, then it is acceptable to appeal a denial of a SCAN. The AAO-HNS provides the following sample template appeal letter:

Please consider this letter a formal request for reconsideration of a denial received for a stereotactic computer-assisted navigation (SCAN) procedure (image guidance) performed on [Patient's Name] on [Date of Service] by [Name of Physician].

The claim for the SCAN procedure was billed with CPT code +61782 cranial, extradural

(List separately in addition to code for primary procedure).

Although CPT code +61782 is a new CPT code and became effective on January 1, 2011, it describes an existing procedure that [Insurer Name] previously covered and reimbursed. The former code for the SCAN procedure was CPT code +61795 - Stereotactic computer assisted volumetric (navigational) procedure, intracranial, extracranial, or spinal (List separately in addition to code for primary procedure); it was deleted because the CPT Editorial Panel split it into three separate add-on codes (+61781 Stereotactic computer-assisted (navigational) procedure; cranial, intradural - , +61782 - Stereotactic computer-assisted (navigational) procedure; cranial, extradural and +61783 - Stereotactic computer-assisted (navigational) procedure; spinal) to differentiate distinct anatomic regions. Of course, one can no longer report a service with a deleted code, but CPT code +61782 is the same procedure that was previously covered by +61795. Therefore, your denial of +61782 as experimental and/or investigational or otherwise considered non-reimbursable is totally illogical. The full allowable amount should be paid for CPT code +61782 because it is an add-on procedure code, and its Medicare fee work relative value already accounts for the procedure never being performed alone.

As you may be aware, SCAN provides the surgeon with 3D real-time positioning within the nasal cavity and paranasal sinuses, allowing him/her to appropriately remove diseased tissue and avoid damage to the orbital, other extracranial and/or intracranial areas. This is particularly useful in patients who have experienced a loss of surgical landmarks and barriers due to previous surgery, sinonasal polyposis, neoplasms, or severe infections/inflammatory processes. The purpose of using stereotactic computer-assisted navigation in sinus surgery is to maximize accuracy and safety of the surgical procedure.

I am enclosing the previously submitted claim, the Explanation of Benefits, operative notes, and the American Academy of Otolaryngology-Head and Neck Surgery's policy statement, Intra-Operative

Use of Computer Aided Surgery and Coding for Stereotactic Computer Assisted Navigation.

Please reprocess this claim for the payment of CPT code +61782. If you require additional information, please contact me at [Phone number].

Link to Intra-Operative Use of Computer Aided Surgery Policy statement: *http://www.entnet.org/Practice/policyIntraOperativeSurgery.cfm*

Link to Coding for Stereotactic Computer Assisted Navigation: *http://www.entnet.org/Practice/Coding-for-Stereotactic-Computer-Assisted-Navigatione.cfm*

Source: http://www.entnet.org/content/payer-appeal-letters

Appealing Denials of an Unlisted Code

There are times an otolaryngologist will perform services where there is no CPT code. These procedures must be reported using an "unlisted" code and will likely be denied; of course, an appeal is warranted. The AAO-HNS provides the following sample template appeal letter:

On [date of service] I performed a [name of service or procedure] on the above-mentioned patient. There is no specific CPT code for this procedure/service; therefore, I am submitting the unlisted procedure code [insert CPT code and descriptor].

The procedure performed on [insert patient name] may be reasonably compared to existing CPT code [code number and description] in terms of physician work and practice expense. [Define here what the procedure entailed and how much more/less difficult it was than the base CPT code].

My charge for (the comparator base existing CPT code) is $_____. I estimated the charge for the submitted unlisted procedure to be [list percent that procedure is less or more difficult than base code] for the reasons mentioned above. Therefore, I have submitted a charge of $_____ for this procedure. Attached, please find a detailed copy of *my operative report/office notes and a claim on the above-mentioned patient.*

Source: http://www.entnet.org/content/ payer-appeal-letters

Appeal Denied

There are occasions when an appeal is denied. Each payer has their own process for second-level appeals. The key to being successful is to follow the payer guidelines and most importantly deadlines. If an appeal is denied, examine the documentation and appeal language. Were the medical necessity guidelines followed? Were CPT guidelines followed? Did the documentation support medical necessity guidelines? If the answer to all of the above is yes, then follow the payer-established chain of command for second-level appeals. If the payer does not budge or does not respond, then you might file a complaint with the state insurance commissioner.

Tracking Appeals

Tracking appeals is a vital element to the appeals process. How appeals are tracked is dependent on the practice management system and/or clearinghouse. Many systems allow a claim to be marked as "appealed" and then are shifted to a worklist of appealed claims. This allows the practice to view outstanding appeals and set a "tickler" for follow-up. If the system does not allow for this type of tracking, revert to a Microsoft Excel spreadsheet that lists the claim, date sent, and date for follow-up.

If the practice is utilizing electronic remittance advice (ERA), then either the practice management system and/or clearinghouse should be able to generate reports based on denial reason codes. Reviewing denial reason codes can ascertain if there are payer issues, coding problems, or other trends. This allows the practice to be proactive in identifying trends and finding solutions to potential problems.

Another best practice is to measure appeal success rate. This will require a Microsoft Excel spreadsheet that lists all appeals submitted and appeals won. The purpose of tracking is to determine if there are payer trends and also to ensure staff are properly appealing denials.

Conclusion

Claim denials are, unfortunately, a part of everyday practice. Successful otolaryngology practices have streamlined internal processes to utilize available technology and tracking. Most appeals can be won the first round with documentation that supports payer-defined medical necessity and clearly articulated appeal language.

CHAPTER 7

Legal Issues: Management Strategies and Avoiding Pitfalls

Patricia S. Hofstra and Elinor Hart Murárová

Introduction

The legal issues that plague physician ear, nose, throat (ENT) practices are numerous. The legalities associated with running an ENT practice, providing patient care and coding and billing are time consuming and can be overwhelming. Thousands of laws and regulations at the federal, state, and local levels govern the practice of medicine. Contractual agreements with third-party payers, vendors, partners, and employees, add to the legal minefield that physician practices must navigate in order to practice medicine and provide patient care. The penalties for failing to comply with legal and regulatory requirements can be civil and criminal fines; imprisonment; loss of ability to participate in federally funded third-party payer programs such as Medicare, Medicaid, and TriCare; and loss of licensure or other disciplinary actions by State Boards regulating the practice of medicine.

This chapter focuses on the legal issues associated with coding and billing and discusses corporate compliance programs as a management strategy to reduce the risk of failing to comply with legal and regulatory requirements. This chapter also provides guidance with respect to preparing for and responding to government and third-party payer audits.

Key Points

- Federal making law and regulations have strict rules on referrals, exchanging anything of value, and providing false claims. Violations of these areas can result in significant penalties.
- The Health Insurance Portability and Accountability Act (HIPAA) establishes standards to protect individual's medical records and personal health information.
- All physicians participating in Medicare and Medicaid need to adopt a compliance program.
- The 4 compliance risk areas associated with physician practice are coding and billing; reasonable and necessary services; documentation; and improper inducements, kickbacks, and self-referrals.
- Four different government contractors review coding, billing, and other documentation to determine if government payment to the health care provider was proper and to recover funds when necessary.

53

Overview of Laws and Regulations

The following provides a brief overview of the laws and regulations that govern physician practices.

Federal Law and Regulations

Social Security Act

The Social Security Act establishes the Medicare and Medicaid laws, rules, and regulations, including the regulations relating to payment for physician services rendered. Medicare has established specific rules for payment of covered benefits for physician services based on fee schedules.

Medicare coverage is limited to items and services that are considered "reasonable and necessary" for the diagnosis or treatment of an illness or injury (and within the scope of a Medicare benefit category). A national coverage determination (NCD) is a US nationwide determination of whether Medicare will pay for an item or service. In the absence of an NCD, an item or service is covered at the discretion of the Medicare contractors based on a local coverage determination (LCD). LCDs vary by region and can be inconsistent.

Medicare billing and coding guidance is also provided through transmittals. The Centers for Medicare and Medicaid Services (CMS) use transmittals to communicate new or changed policies or procedures for billing and coverage. The cover or transmittal page summarizes and specifies the changes. Physician practices are obligated to keep up to date on new or changed policies and procedures for billing, coding, and coverage. Transmittals, NCDs, and LCDs all add to the complexity of physician practice billing and coding.

Anti-Kickback Laws

The federal Anti-Kickback Statute is a criminal statute generally prohibiting the exchange of (or offer to exchange) anything of value, in an effort to induce (or reward) the referral of federal health care program business (42 U.S.C. § 1320a-7b). The Anti-Kickback Statute provides for penalties for individuals and entities on both sides of the prohibited transaction. A single violation

under the Anti-Kickback Statute may result in a fine of up to $25,000 and imprisonment for up to 5 years (42 U.S.C. § 1320a-7b[b]). In addition, convictions for violating the Anti-Kickback Statute result in mandatory exclusion from participation in federal health care programs (42 U.S.C. § 1320a-7[a]). Absent a conviction, individuals who violate the Anti-Kickback Statute may still face exclusion from federal health care programs at the discretion of the Secretary of Health and Human Services (42 U.S.C. § 1320a-7[b]). The government may also assess civil money penalties, which could result in treble damages plus $50,000 for each violation of the Anti-Kickback Statute (42 U.S.C § 1320a-7a[a][7]). Although the Anti-Kickback Statute does not afford a private right of action, the False Claims Act, described below, provides a vehicle whereby individuals may bring qui tam actions alleging violations of the Anti-Kickback Statute. (*See* 31 U.S.C. §§ 3729–3733.)

False Claims Act

The False Claims Act (FCA) provides criminal penalties for knowingly or willfully filing a false claim to a government program. Specifically, the FCA provides, in pertinent part, that

1. Any person who (1) knowingly presents, or causes to be presented, to an officer or employee of the United States Government or a member of the Armed Forces of the United States a false or fraudulent claim for payment or approval; (2) knowingly makes, uses, or causes to be made or used, a false record or statement to get a false or fraudulent claim paid or approved by the Government; (3) conspires to defraud the Government by getting a false or fraudulent claim paid or approved by the Government; . . . or (7) knowingly makes, uses, or causes to be made or used, a false record or statement to conceal, avoid, or decrease an obligation to pay or transmit money or property to the Government, . . . is liable to the United States Government for a civil penalty of not less than $5,000 and not more than $10,000, plus 3 times the amount of damages which the Government sustains because of the act of that person . . .

2. For purposes of this section, the terms "knowing" and "knowingly" mean that a person, with respect to information (1) has actual knowledge of the information; (2) acts in deliberate ignorance of the truth or falsity of the information; or (3) acts in reckless disregard of the truth or falsity of the information, and no proof of specific intent to defraud is required. (31 U.S.C. § 3729)

While the FCA imposes liability only when the claimant acts "knowingly," it does not require that the person submitting the claim have actual knowledge that the claim is false. A person who acts in reckless disregard or in deliberate ignorance of the truth or falsity of the information, also can be found liable under the Act (31 U.S.C. § 3729[b]). Thus, the FCA imposes liability on any person who submits a claim to the federal government that he or she knows (or should know) is false. The FCA also imposes liability on an individual who knowingly submits a false record in order to obtain payment from the government. In addition to its substantive provisions, the FCA provides that private parties may bring an action on behalf of the United States (31 U.S.C. § 3730 [b]). These private parties, known as "qui tam relators," may share in a percentage of the proceeds from an FCA action or settlement.

Self-Referral (Stark) Laws and Regulations

The Stark Law is a limitation on certain physician referrals. The Stark Law prohibits physician referrals of designated health services (DHSs) for Medicare and Medicaid patients if the physician (or an immediate family member) has a financial relationship with that entity (42 U.S.C. § 1395nn). A financial relationship includes ownership, investment interest, and compensation arrangements (42 U.S.C. § 1395nn[h][5]). The term *referral* is defined more broadly than merely recommending a vendor of DHS to a patient. Instead, the term *referral* means, for Medicare Part B services, "the request by a physician for the item or service" and, for all other services, "the request or establishment of a plan of care by a physician which includes the provision of the designated health service." DHS includes clinical laboratory services

as well as the following: physical-therapy services; occupational-therapy services; radiology, including magnetic resonance imaging, computerized axial tomography scans, and ultrasound services; radiation-therapy services and supplies; durable medical equipment and supplies; parenteral and enteral nutrients, equipment, and supplies; prosthetics, orthotics, and prosthetic devices; home health services and supplies; outpatient prescription drugs; and inpatient and outpatient hospital services.

The Stark Law contains several exceptions, which include physician services, in-office ancillary services, ownership in publicly traded securities and mutual funds, rental of office space and equipment, and bona fide employment relationship. Strict compliance with each element of an exception is mandatory. As a general rule, compliance with the Stark exceptions requires written agreements between physicians and health care facilities that set compensation in advance at fair market value and prohibit compensation based on the volume or value of referrals for DHS services. The in-office ancillary services exception applies to physicians ordering DHS in the context of their own practices and is particularly relevant to ENT practices offering CT and other DHS services. To qualify for the in-office ancillary services exception, the practice must be a group practice as defined by the Stark regulations and must meet the supervision, location, and billing requirements of the in-office ancillary services exception. The Stark Law and exceptions are complicated, and practices should seek legal advice from an experienced health care attorney for specific guidance regarding compliance with the Stark Law.

Health Insurance Portability and Accountability Act (HIPAA)

The HIPAA establishes national standards to protect individuals' medical records and other personal health information and applies to health plans, health care clearinghouses, and those health care providers that conduct certain health care transactions electronically. The rule requires appropriate safeguards to protect the privacy of personal health information, and sets limits and conditions on the uses and disclosures that may be made of such information without patient authorization. HIPAA also gives patients rights over their health information, including rights to examine and obtain a copy of their health records, and to request corrections. There are significant financial penalties for failing to comply with HIPAA. (*See* 45 C.F.R. Part 160 *et seq.*; 45 C.F.R. § 164[A], 164[E].)

State and Local Laws

In addition to the above-referenced federal laws, each state has numerous laws and regulations governing physician practices. Most states have anti-kickback and false claims acts similar to federal laws. However, state laws can extend beyond the federals laws. For example, some states consider the routine waiver of copayments and deductibles to be insurance fraud, some states prohibit the corporate practice of medicine, and some states prohibit fee splitting. A discussion of individual state laws is beyond the scope of this chapter, but physicians must understand and comply with the laws of their individual states and local governments in addition to applicable federal laws and regulations.

Compliance Programs

The health care reform law of 2010 mandates that all physicians participating in Medicare and Medicaid adopt a compliance program. In addition, physician practices can reduce the risk of legal and regulatory noncompliance, and potentially mitigate penalties, by adopting and adhering to an effective compliance program. The Department of Health and Human Services, Office of the Inspector General (OIG) has provided Compliance Program guidance for Individual and Small Group practices. (*See* OIG Compliance Program for Individual and Small Group Physician Practices, Dep't of Health & Human Servs., Office of Inspector General, 65 *Fed. Reg.* 59434–59452 [Oct. 5, 2000].) The OIG's guidance outlines 7 basic components of a compliance program. These basic components are:

- Conducting internal monitoring and auditing through the performance of periodic audits
- Implementing compliance and practice standards through the development of written standards and procedures
- Designating a compliance officer or contact(s) to monitor compliance efforts and enforce practice standards
- Conducting appropriate training and education on practice standards and procedures
- Responding appropriately to detected violations through the investigation of allegations and the disclosure of incidents to appropriate government entities
- Developing open lines of communication, such as (1) discussions at staff meetings regarding how to avoid erroneous or fraudulent conduct and (2) community bulletin boards, to keep practice employees updated regarding compliance activities
- Enforcing disciplinary standards through well-publicized guidelines

Compliance Program Audits

A physician practice's bills and medical records should be reviewed for compliance with applicable coding, billing, and documentation requirements on an annual basis or as otherwise required by law, as well as whenever a potential problem is identified. Audits can be conducted by the practice or a qualified outside billing and coding consultant. There is no absolute rule regarding what should be audited, how many charts should be audited, or how the audit should be conducted. However, compliance program audits should be meaningful and designed to identify and address billing and coding issues. If concerns are suspected or identified prior to or during the compliance audit, legal counsel should be consulted immediately.

When Medicare billing and coding errors are found, a corrected claim must be submitted and any overpayment refunded to the payer within 60 days of discovery. Other payers may have different requirements and time frames for correcting claims and refunding overpayments. Whenever a billing or coding error is identified, the practice should review the statutory, regulatory, and contractual requirements for correcting the claim and refunding any overpayment.

Audits can be used to determine whether:

- Bills are correctly coded and accurately reflect the services provided (as documented in the medical records)
- Documentation is being completed correctly
- Services or items provided are reasonable and necessary
- Any incentives for unnecessary services exist

Risk Areas

The OIG has identified and focused on 4 compliance risk areas associated with physician practices. These risks areas include (1) coding and billing; (2) reasonable and necessary services; (3) documentation; and (4) improper inducements, kickbacks, and self-referrals. (*See also supra*, summarizing federal laws relating to improper inducements, kickbacks, and self-referrals.)

Coding and Billing

Coding and billing is the number one risk area identified by the OIG. Specific risk areas associated with coding and billing that have been among the most frequent subjects of investigations and audits by the OIG include:

- Billing for items or services not rendered or not provided as claimed
- Submitting claims for equipment, medical supplies, and services that are not reasonable and necessary
- Double billing resulting in duplicate payment

- Billing for noncovered services as if covered
- Knowing misuse of provider identification numbers, which results in improper billing
- Unbundling (billing for each component of the service instead of billing or using an all-inclusive code)
- Failure to properly use modifiers
- Clustering
- Upcoding the level of service provided

A more detailed discussion of coding and billing risk areas can be found in the audit section of this chapter.

Medical Necessity

Documentation of the medical necessity of services, supplies, and equipment is essential for payment. Billing for services, supplies, and equipment that are not reasonable and necessary involves seeking reimbursement for a service that is not warranted by a patient's documented medical condition (42 U.S.C. § 1395i[a][1][A]: "[N]o payment may be made under part A or part B [of Medicare] for any expenses incurred for items or services which are not reasonable and necessary for the diagnosis or treatment of illness or injury to improve the functioning of the malformed body member"). Thus, a provider may only bill for services that meet the standard of being reasonable and necessary for the diagnosis and treatment of a patient. According to the Medicare reimbursement or insurance plan rules, Medicare and other third-party payers may deny payment for a service that is not properly documented and reasonable and necessary.

Under Medicare, a physician practice may bill in order to receive a denial for services, but only if the denial is needed for reimbursement from the secondary payer and identified as such.

Documentation

The OIG also identifies documentation as a significant risk area. Timely, accurate, and complete documentation is essential for payment. The old adage, "if it is not documented, it wasn't done," is strictly adhered to for payment purposes by governmental and other third-party payers. The medical record is therefore used by payers to validate (1) the site of the service, (2) the appropriateness of the services provided, (3) the accuracy of the billing, and (4) the identity of the caregiver (ie, the service provider).

Medical record documentation is also used by plaintiffs and defendants in medical malpractice cases. Medical malpractice litigation is built around the medical record. The medical record provides the primary objective record of the patient's condition and the care provided.

Practices must ensure accurate medical record documentation including the following for malpractice risk management and payment purposes:

- Complete and legible medical records
- The reason for the encounter; any relevant history; physical examination findings; prior diagnostic test results; assessment, clinical impression, or diagnosis; plan of care; and date and legible identity of the provider in each patient encounter
- The rationale for ordering diagnostic and other ancillary services
- CPT® and ICD codes used for claims submission supported by documentation contained in the medical record
- Identified appropriate health risk factors (The patient's progress, his or her response to, and any changes in, treatment, and any revision in diagnosis must be documented.)

Government Audits

Four different government contractors review coding, billing, and other documentation to determine whether the government's payment to a health care provider was proper. These contractors are:

- Medicare Administrative Contractors (MACs), who process and pay claims
- Recovery Audit Contractors (RACs), who identify on a postpayment basis improper payments
- Zone Program Integrity Contractors (ZPICs), who investigate potential fraud
- Comprehensive Error Rate Testing (CERT) Contractors, who review claims used to annually estimate Medicare's improper payment rate

MACs

MACs conduct postpayment claims reviews on a small percentage of paid claims to determine if the payments were proper based on the underlying documentation. MACs use the findings from postpayment claims reviews to help prevent future payment errors, for example, by reviewing claims received from specific providers or for specific services with a history of improper payments to determine whether additional action is needed to prevent similar improper payments in the future.

RACs

RACs conduct postpayment claim reviews to identify improper payments not previously identified through other reviews. RACs tend to focus auditing efforts on physician practices whose billings for Medicare services trend higher than the majority of providers and suppliers in their community. RAC may use automated reviews (where NO medical record is involved in the review) in situations where the RAC's algorithm determines that the claim contains an overpayment. RACs are paid from funds recovered from health care providers. RACs tend to focus on claims with the highest risk of improper payments. When a RAC audit determines that a provider has been overpaid, a demand letter is sent to the provider by the RAC, requesting a refund of the overpayment. There is a limited appeal process for the provider. If a timely refund is not made, the alleged overpayment can be automatically deducted from future Medicare payments to the provider. RACs may refer providers with suspicious billing practices to ZPICs if the RAC suspects fraud.

ZPICs

ZPICs look for fraud and abuse through data analysis and data mining, conduct medical reviews in support of benefit integrity, support law enforcement, investigate complaints, recommend recovery of Medicare funds through administrative action, and refer appropriate cases to law enforcement.

Cases are brought to the attention of ZPICs in 2 ways: reactive and proactive. Reactive cases originate from complaints, and proactive cases originate from trending and targeted review data analysis. (*See, eg,* Ctrs. for Medicare & Medicaid Servs., Medicare Program Integrity Manual, Chpt. 4–Benefit Integrity, § 4.2.2 [Rev. 495, 12-13-13], *available at* http://www.cms.gov/Regulations-and-Guidance/Guidance/Manuals/downloads/pim83c04.pdf [hereinafter "Medicare Program Integrity Manual"]; *see also* Hofstra, P., *Medicare's ZPIC Audits: The Auditor's New Stomping Ground*, Med. Practice Mgmt., 139–42 [Nov./Dec. 2010] [hereinafter "Hofstra 2010"].)

Data analysis is the ZPIC's first step in determining whether patterns of claims submission and payment indicate potential problems. ZPIC's use sophisticated audit tools that lead to referrals to the ZPIC's Benefit Integrity Unity (BIU) for fraud and abuse investigations. Data analysis includes identification of aberrancies in billing patterns within homogeneous groups of claims that might suggest improper billing or payment. Although ZPIC audits are most frequently done off site, the ZPIC has the right and ability to conduct the audit at the provider's service site.

ZPIC's medical reviews focus on making coverage and/or coding determinations and reducing the billing error rate through medical review and provider notification, education, and feedback. The ZPIC evaluates the medical record to determine if there is evidence in the medical record that the service submitted was actually provided and if the service was medically reasonable and necessary. (*See* Medicare Program Integrity Manual § 4.18.3; Hofstra 2010.) The ZPIC documents the errors found and communicates these to the provider in a written format, when the review does not find evidence of potential fraud. A referral may be made for additional provider education

and follow-up, if appropriate. (*See* Medicare Program Integrity Manual § 4.19; Hofstra 2010.)

If the medical records do not support services billed by the provider, the ZPIC will downcode or deny payment, in part or in whole, for the service. (*See* Medicare Program Integrity Manual § 4.19.) The ZPIC is required to thoroughly document the rationale utilized to make the medical review decision.

Based on the medical review, if a provider appears to have knowingly and intentionally furnished services that are not covered or filed claims for services not furnished as billed or made any false statement on the claim or supporting documentation to receive payment, the provider is referred to the BIU for possible fraud investigation. (*See id.* § 4.19.1.) The BIU is a team of investigators and auditors with experience and existing relationships with law enforcement. The BIU's goals are to identify, prioritize, investigate, and resolve fraud and abuse claims; protect the Medicare Trust Fund by finding overpayments; perform high-quality investigations; educate beneficiaries, law enforcement, and payer employees to prevent fraud and abuse; and keep CMS updated on fraud schemes.

Examples of patterns and trends which result in referral to the BIU include medical records having obvious or nearly identical documentation, sequences of codes that evidence a trend to use the high-end codes more frequently than would normally be expected, and patterns of billing more hours of care than would normally be expected on a given workday. (*Id.* § 4.3.)

The focus of the BIU is to address situations of potential fraud, waste, and abuse. (*Id.*) The BIU may determine that the resolution of an investigation does not warrant referral for criminal, civil monetary penalties or sanctions and that an educational meeting with the provider is more appropriate. In that case, the BIU informs the provider of questionable or improper practices, the correct procedure to be followed, and the fact that continuation of the improper practice may result in administrative sanctions. (*Id.*) If the alleged improper practices continue, the BIU is required to consult with the OIG regarding a potential action for sanctions.

When cases are referred to the OIG, the OIG will usually exercise one or more of the following options with respect to a case: conduct a criminal or civil investigation, refer the case back to the BIU for administrative action/recovery of overpayment with no further investigation, refer the case back to the BIU for administrative action/recoupment of overpayment after conducting an investigation, consult with the Assistant US Attorney's Office regarding prosecution, or refer the case to another law enforcement agency for investigation. (*Id.* § 4.18.1.)

In addition to the referral of cases to the OIG, BIU units are obligated to minimize potential loss to the Medicare Trust Fund and prevent future improper payment. Options to prevent future improper payment include placing the provider's claims on prepayment review and suspending payment pending further development of the case. (*Id.*)

ZPICs may extrapolate findings based on an extrapolation formula when making a determination of overpayments. (*See id.* § 4.33; *see also* Hofstra 2010.) The ZPIC will notify the provider of any determination of overpayment and will forward the letter to the fiscal intermediary (FI) for review and confirmation. A formal demand letter will be issued by the FI, and the demand letter will notify the provider of the any appeal rights. In cases of suspected fraud, the provider's first notification may be from law enforcement rather than the ZPIC or the FI.

There is no limit to the number of cases that a ZPIC can review, no restriction on how far the ZPIC can look back to identify overpayments, and no time frames for conducting the review, unlike the restrictions placed on RACs. Also unlike RACs, ZPICS are not paid on a contingency fee basis. (Fotheringill LM, ZPICs: Bite Worse Than RAC Bark, Sept. 2, 2009, http://racmonitor.com.)

CERT Contractors

Finally, Comprehensive Error Rate Testing (CERT) contractors conduct postpayment claim reviews on a nationwide random sample of claims, which are used to annually estimate the national Medicare fee-for-service improper payment rates. These reviews are used to estimate the national Medicare improper payment rate, and to estimate the improper payment rate for each MAC and by type of service and provider.

Private Payer Audits

In addition to federal and state government audits, other third-party payers conduct payment audits to assure proper payments. Although any billed service can be audited, government and private payers most frequently audit ENT providers to ensure that the services provided were medically necessary, that the provider's documentation supports the level of service billed, that multiple procedures performed on the same day on the same patient are billed correctly, that evaluation and management services are properly billed, that modifiers are used appropriately, and that services are billed under the correct provider's NPI. Providers, who are statistical outliers for their specialty based on the payer's computer algorithms, are most likely to be audited. For example, a provider who bills every patient for a level 4 visit, bills using a modifier 25 or 57 for every case, or bills every patient for cerumen removal using a microscope has an increased chance of being audited.

Under certain circumstances, applicable to both government payers and private payers, improper billing whether negligent or intentional, is considered insurance fraud and a criminal act (Table 7–1).

Overpayments

A health care provider must refund any overpayments made by governmental payers on behalf of state and federal health plan beneficiaries, regardless of the cause of the overpayment, even in the absence of a request for a refund. Failure to refund an overpayment made by a governmental payer in a timely manner could lead to civil and criminal penalties, as well as exclusion from participation as a provider in government health plans. Refunds of overpayments must be made within

Table 7–1. Contractor Type

	Medicare Administrative Contractor (MAC)	Zone Program Integrity Contractor (ZPIC)	Comprehensive Error Rate Testing (CERT) Contractor	Recovery Audit Contractor (RAC)
Primary purpose of contractor claims reviews	To better ensure payment accuracy and better ensure that providers with a history of a sustained or high level of billing errors comply with Medicare billing requirements	To identify and investigate patterns of billing that indicate potentially fraudulent claims and providers	To annually estimate the national Medicare fee-for-service (FFS) improper payment rate	To identify Medicare FFS claim underpayments and overpayments not previously identified through MAC claims processing or other contractor reviews
Basis for selecting claims for postpayment review	Claims from providers with a history of improper billing Data analyses of paid claims to identify patterns of payments that may be improper	Claims submitted by providers flagged as high risk by CMS's Fraud Prevention System Referrals from other contractors Fraud hotline Data analyses of paid claims to identify patterns of billing by a provider or group of providers that suggests potential fraud	Random sample selected from claims processed	Data analyses of all paid claims to identify services with payments most likely to be made improperly CMS approves the RAs' selection of services and the coverage and payment criteria to be applied to them in advance of review

Source: Gov't Accountability Office, *Medicare Program Integrity: Increased Oversight and Guidance Could Improve Effectiveness and Efficiency of Postpayment Claims Reviews*, GAO-14-474, Table 1 (July 2014), *available at* http://www.gao.gov/assets/670/664879.pdf.

60 days after the practice becomes aware of the overpayment. The calculation of overpayments is complicated by the Medicare rules, which state that all other payers come before Medicare in determining who is the primary, secondary, or tertiary payer.

With respect to a nongovernmental third-party payer, when an overpayment has been made the provider must establish whether a contract exists between the payer and the provider that addresses the issue of insurance overpayment. If

such a contract exists, the terms of that contract govern the legal rights and obligations of the parties. If no contract exists, or the contract does not address the issue of overpayments, then the law relating to restitution applies to the situation.

The law relating to restitution also applies to patients who make overpayments. Restitution is an equitable concept applied by courts based on what is generally accepted as fair or valid, rather than a precise legal principle. The rule of restitution is that when a payer pays money it does not owe, the payer is entitled to have the money returned. The rule of restitution is based on an assumption that the payee is receiving a windfall at the same time that the payer is sustaining a loss, which is unfair. Although there are certain exceptions to the principle of restitution, such as the voluntary payment doctrine, when a provider receives more than full payment for services rendered to a patient (usually because of multiple payers on a single claim), the provider is unjustly enriched and, therefore, would not meet any of the exceptions to the general rule. A health care provider is entitled to payment of the bill and anything over and above that amount constitutes a windfall and must be returned.

Any overpayment made to a health care provider that is not refunded to the payer or a patient may be considered unclaimed property and must be reported as such to the state. Holders of unclaimed property are prohibited by law from taking unclaimed property and recognizing it as business income. State law may require businesses, including physician practices, even those holding no unclaimed property, to report and deliver unclaimed property to the state on an annual basis. A business that fails to report and deliver unclaimed property to the state may be required to pay interest to the state on the unclaimed property and may be subject to civil and criminal penalties. Providers in possession of unclaimed property have a responsibility to perform due diligence tasks as the holder of unclaimed property.

Conclusion

It is virtually impossible in one chapter to address all of the legal issues facing ENT practices. Best practice management strategies for reducing risks related to coding and billing include being aware of the requirements for accurate coding and billing for care, adopting and adhering to an effective compliance program, conducting meaningful audits and following up to assure that any concerns identified in the audit process are addressed, refunding overpayments in a timely manner as may be legally required, educating and training staff, and appropriately documenting the care provided. Seeking advice and guidance from qualified and experienced health care legal counsel and coding consultants early and often, while seemingly expensive, can result in substantial savings in the long run. Legal counsel and coding consultants can also help minimize the agony of governmental and third-party payer audits.

CHAPTER 8

Billing Guidelines for Nonphysician Practitioners and Teaching Physicians

Sarah Wiskerchen

Introduction

Increasing patient care demands have made it essential for otolaryngologists to look beyond traditional care models and incorporate nonphysician practitioners into their practice teams. In academic settings, physicians may be supported by both residents and nonphysician practitioners. With these changes it is critical that physicians, practitioners, and billing staff understand and effectively apply the unique billing rules that exist for office and hospital settings, both for private and academic practices.

Key Points

Within this chapter we will outline

- The types of nonpractitioners typically used in an otolaryngology practice
- The importance of Scope of Practice rules in nonpractitioner billing
- Medicare billing guidelines for direct, incident-to, and split/shared services

- How groups can research other payer (non-Medicare) guidelines for nonphysician practitioners
- Medicare teaching physician guidelines

Types of Nonphysician Practitioners in an Otolaryngology Practice

The term *nonphysician practitioner* can have varied meanings in an otolaryngology practice. Oftentimes it is used to describe audiologists and speech therapists, for which billing rules are described elsewhere in this book. Within this chapter, the term *nonpractitioner* is used to describe 3 provider categories: physician assistants, nurse practitioners, and clinical nurse specialists. The title physician assistant is commonly abbreviated as PA, nurse practitioner as NP, and clinical nurse specialist as CNS. Collectively we use the abbreviation NPP for nonphysician practitioner.

Both nurse practitioners and clinical nurse specialists are classified as advanced practice registered nurses (APRNs) and both require Master of Science in Nursing degrees. Nurse practitioners are certified through the American Academy of

63

Nurse Practitioners, and clinical nurse specialists are certified through the American Nurses Credentialing Center. Nurse practitioners are more commonly used in the private otolaryngology practice setting than clinical nurse specialists.

Understanding Scope of Practice for Nonphysician Practitioners

When considering the hire of a physician assistant, nurse practitioner, or clinical nurse specialist, state Scope of Practice guidelines provide the foundation for what services the NPP can perform. Scope of practice guidelines are set at the state level by legislative and regulatory process. Physician assistant rules are typically enforced through a state's medical board, and nurse practitioner and clinical nurse specialist scope of practice rules are enforced through the state's board of nursing. In addition to determining what services the nonphysician practitioners can perform, the laws and regulations describe requirements for physician supervision and prescribing practices. Although there has been some progress in recent years toward greater regulatory consistency across states, hiring entities should not assume that all state rules are the same. The regulations for PAs do not always match those for NPs, even within the same state. Scope of practice regulations for clinical nurse specialists are not as consistent across states as they are for nurse practitioners.

Medicare Billing Guidelines for Nonphysician Practitioners

When billing for NPPs, Medicare's guidelines are often used as a reference point because the rules are provided in writing. Chapter 15 of the *Medicare Benefit Policy Manual* and Chapter 12 of the *Medicare Claims Processing Manual* are essential documents to review and use. URL links to these manuals are referenced later in this chapter. As guidelines evolve, the manuals may be updated periodically, it is essential to subscribe

to Medicare's Transmittal document program, which alerts both Medicare Administrative Carriers (MACs) and providers to policy changes that affect the manual text.

Direct Billing

The first billing method is termed "Direct." When a provider completes Medicare credentialing and obtains his or her own national provider identifier (NPI) number and provider transaction access number (PTAN), services that the provider performs can be billed in his or her name, and payments for those services are assigned (paid) to the employer organization. When a PA, NP, or CNS performs and reports a service using the Direct method, the claim is allowed at 85% of the MPFS (Medicare Physician Fee Schedule) allowable.

Many practices prefer the Direct billing method because it offers a high degree of flexibility. As long as the practitioner complies with state scope of practice and physician supervisory requirements, the NPP is not restricted from seeing new patients or new problems, and direct supervision by a physician is not always required.

Direct billing can be used in both the office and hospital settings. In the office, an NPP could see patients independently, following state scope of practice and supervision guidelines, and report the service to Medicare under his or her own credentials. No modifier is required to designate that an NPP performed the service, because their name and provider numbers are specified on the claim.

In the hospital setting, assistance at surgery is always performed using the Direct billing method when it is provided by an NPP that is employed by the practice. In some cases the NPP may be formally employed by the facility; however, the cost of the NPP must be borne by the practice or department to support professional billing by the NPP. Medicare instructs providers to designate the NPP's surgical assistance using modifier AS with the surgical *Current Procedural Terminology* (CPT®) code(s). Note that all surgical assistance services are billable, but payers may have specific guidelines about reimbursement on specific CPT codes (not all codes may be paid).

Incident-To Billing

Incident-to is a billing concept that applies to various types of medical staff, but in this chapter we address how it applies to NPPs in a physician practice setting. Under incident-to billing rules, the patient encounter must meet specific criteria, including

- The services are an integral, although incidental, part of the provider's professional service.
- The services are of a type commonly furnished in providers' offices or clinics (*incident-to does not apply in an ASC or hospital setting*).
- "The provider must initiate the course of treatment of which the service being performed by the NPP is an incidental part, and there must be subsequent services by the physician of a frequency that reflect continuing active participation in and management of the course of treatment." This requirement is often described as setting the *plan of care*.
- The supervising physician must be physically present within the office where the incident-to service is provided (direct supervision).

All of the incident-to requirements must be met simultaneously. For example, if an NPP saw a new Medicare patient independently, that service could not be reported incident-to even if a physician was present in the office, because the plan of care had not been previously set. Alternately, if the NPP saw an established patient with an established problem, but no physician was in the office at that time, the service could not be reported incident-to because the physician presence rule was not met.

According to section 60.1 in Chapter 15 of the *Medicare Benefit Policy Manual*, "Direct supervision in the office setting does not mean that the physician must be present in the same room with his or her aide. However, the physician must be present in the office suite and immediately available to provide assistance and direction throughout the time the aide is performing services."

With incident-to reporting, services are reported in the name of an onsite-supervising physician, and the claim is allowed at 100% of the Medicare Physician Fee Schedule. In a group practice setting, the onsite supervising physician may be different than the physician who set the plan of care, but the name of the onsite supervising physician must be reported on the claim.

Split/Shared Billing

Another policy that impacts NPP billing for Medicare patients is that of Split/Shared Evaluation and Management (E/M) services. A Split/Shared E/M service is one where the NPP and the physician both see the patient, and may see the patient together, but neither performs the entire service. Although this approach may aide the physician, practices must understand Medicare's billing and documentation rules for these scenarios.

In the office setting, when the physician and NPP perform an encounter together but neither performs the entire visit, Medicare's incident-to guidelines take precedence over split/shared reporting. If incident-to criteria are met, including the patient or problem's established status (eg, established patient with an established problem where the NPP is carrying out the physician's predetermined plan of care and not changing the plan of care), the encounter may be billed in the name of the physician. If incident-to criteria are not met (ie, new patient or established patient with a new problem), the visit does not meet incident-to guidelines and must be reported in the name of the NPP, and is subject to the decreased reimbursement associated with direct billing. If the physician wishes to report such a visit in his or her own name, he or she must perform and document all components of the E/M service independently, which results in repeat work.

When a hospital E/M service is shared between a physician and an NPP from the same group practice, and the physician provides any face-to-face portion of the E/M encounter with the patient, the service may be billed under either the physician's or the NPP's NPI number. For example, if an NPP sees the hospital patient alone, and the physician also sees the patient the same day, when each provider documents the services they performed their work can be combined and reported by the physician. If only the NPP sees the

hospital patient, then it is billed as a direct service in his or her own name.

Table 8–1 and Table 8–2 display potential ENT scenarios for direct, incident-to, and split/shared billing that involve a nonphysician practitioner.

Table 8–1. NPP Billing Scenarios: Clinic Setting

Clinic Setting	Billing Options
1. The NPP sees a new Medicare patient independently. He or she performs and documents the history, exam, and medical decision making. The physician is physically present in the office but is not involved in any assessment of the patient.	Report the service using the NPP's NPI because the service does not meet the incident to plan-of-care requirement. Expect allowable at 85% of the MPFS. (Direct)
2. The NPP sees an established Medicare patient who was seen last month by a physician within the group practice. The patient's condition has not changed, and no modification is made to the plan of care. A physician is present in the office, but is not asked to see the patient.	Two options: (1) Report service using the NPP's NPI and expect allowable at 85% of the MPFS. (Direct) (2) Report service using the onsite physician's NPI and expect allowable at 100% of the MPFS. (Incident-to)
3. The NPP sees an established Medicare patient who was seen last month by a physician within the group practice. The patient's condition has not changed, and no modification is made to the plan of care. The physician is not present in the office.	Report service using the NPP's NPI because the physician direct supervision requirement is not met. Expect allowable at 85% of the MPFS. (Direct)
4. The NPP does the history and exam of a new patient and discusses the case with the physician. The physician then goes into the exam room (with or without the NPP), performs a brief history and brief exam and determines the final diagnosis and plan. The NPP dictates or inputs the note in the EHR.	Two options: (1) Report service using the NPP's NPI because this service does not meet incident-to or split/shared guidelines. Expect allowable at 85% of MPFS. (Direct) (2) Report service using physician's NPI but only at the E/M level performed by the physician.
5. In scenario 4, what if the NPP enters his/her information in the EMR and the physician does his/her own EMR documentation. Can we combine the notes and bill under the physician?	No, not for an office encounter.
6. The NPP does a full history, full exam and determines the diagnosis and plan on a new patient. The physician then sees the patient, retakes the entire history, performs the entire exam, and confirms the diagnosis and plan with the patient. NPP dictates or inputs his own documentation, and physician dictates or inputs his own documentation.	Report service using physician's NPI at the level of his/her documentation because the physician performed the entire service. Expect allowable at 100% of the MPFS. This scenario requires duplication of the history, exam, and decision making by the physician and is not efficient. The NPP may not be considered a "scribe" in this scenario because scribes do not ask questions or perform an exam.

Table 8–2. NPP Billing Scenarios: Hospital Setting

Hospital Setting	Billing Options
1. The NPP sees a new Medicare patient independently. He or she performs and documents the history, exam, and medical decision making. The physician is not involved in any assessment of the patient.	Report the service using the NPP's NPI. Expect allowable at 85% of the MPFS. (Direct)
2. The NPP sees an established Medicare patient who was seen last month by a physician within the group practice. The patient's condition has not changed, and no modification is made to the plan of care. The physician is not involved in any assessment of the patient.	Report service using the NPP's NPI. Expect allowable at 85% of the MPFS. (Direct) Incident-to does not apply in the hospital setting.
3. The NPP independently performs the history and exam of a new patient. Later the same day the physician sees the patient alone or with the NPP. Both the NPP and the physician dictate or input their notes in the EHR.	Report service using physician's NPI. Expect allowable at 100% of the MPFS. (Split/Shared)
4. The NPP assists the physician at surgery in a nonacademic facility.	Report services using the NPP's NPI. Expect allowable at 85% of the MPFS for services that Medicare has approved for assistant coverage. Apply modifier AS to signify assistance by an NPP. Keep in mind that the MPFS for surgical assistance is 16% of the standard allowable; collectively this will result in allowance of 13.6% for surgical assistance by an NPP.
5. The NPP assists the physician at surgery in a teaching facility when no qualified resident is available (and the ENT department has a resident teaching program).	Report services using the NPP's NPI. Expect allowable at 85% of the MPFS for services that Medicare has approved for assistant coverage. Apply modifier AS to signify assistance by an NPP when no qualified resident was available. Verify with your Medicare MAC whether modifier 82 should also be appended.

Researching Other Payer Billing Rules for Nonphysician Practitioners

Because Medicare's billing policies are clearly defined and available in writing, they are often adopted by physician practices as a standard for all payers. For the most accurate reporting, physician groups should research both state-specific Medicaid guidelines and payer-specific rules to confirm how they compare to Medicare's policies. Key questions include

- Does the payer independently credential NPPs, and in which categories (PA, NP, CNS)?
- Do they adhere to Medicare's incident-to guidelines for all NPP types?
- Do they adhere to Medicare's guidelines for split/shared services for all NPP types?

- If no to any of the 3 questions, what billing rules do they require for NPPs, by type?
- Should the physician or group use any special modifiers to designate NPP services? If yes, what are they?
- How will the group be paid for each approved billing method?

Medicare's Teaching Physician Rules

Medicare's teaching physician rules apply when a physician supervises residents in an approved graduate medical education (GME) setting, and seeks to bill for their participation in the care that includes the residents. Section 100 within Chapter 12 of the *Medicare Claims Processing Manual* provides detailed definitions and rules pertaining to teaching physicians that should be reviewed by all academic practices and physicians. Key elements of the requirements include these concepts:

- **Critical or Key Portion:** Medicare sets standards for the degree of physician involvement in resident care, measured as the "critical or key portion." These standards must be met in order for physicians to bill for their participation and supervision.
- **Teaching Setting:** In section 100 of Chapter 12 of the *Medicare Claims Processing Manual*, Medicare defines this is as "Any provider, hospital-based provider, or non-provider setting in which Medicare payment for the services of residents is made by the fiscal intermediary under the direct graduate medical education payment methodology." Attending physician services in a teaching setting are paid by the Part B Medicare Administrative Carrier (MAC), while facility fees are paid by the Part A Medicare Administrative Contractor (MAC).
- **Documentation Requirements:** Medicare standards require that documentation for

teaching physician services must detail the service furnished, the participation of the teaching physician in providing the service, and whether the teaching physician was physically present. The manual states that "Documentation may be dictated and typed or hand-written, or computer-generated and typed or handwritten." Section 100 describes details for use of macros in an electronic health record, including, "The note in the electronic medical record must sufficiently describe the specific services furnished to the specific patient on the specific date. It is insufficient documentation if both the resident and the teaching physician use macros only."

- **Physically Present:** Medicare describes that to meet the requirement of "physically present" the teaching physician must be located in the same room (or partitioned or curtained area, if the room is subdivided to accommodate multiple patients) as the patient and/or performs a face-to-face service.

Medicare's teaching physician rules describe that physician services are paid under the MPFS if they are

- Personally furnished by a physician who is not a resident
- Furnished by a resident where a teaching physician was physically present during the critical or key portions of the service
- Certain E/M services furnished by a resident under "Exceptions for E/M Services Furnished in Certain Primary Care Centers" (section 100.1.1.C)

Evaluation and Management Services in the Teaching Setting

Medicare adheres to American Medical Association (AMA) Current Procedural Terminology (CPT) code definitions of E/M services, and their applicable guidelines. When reporting E/M services that involve a resident, the attending/teaching physician must document the following:

- That they performed the service or were physically present during the key or critical portions of the service when performed by the resident
- Their participation in the management of the patient

When these criteria are met, the practice is allowed to combine the documentation of the resident and the teaching physician when assigning CPT codes to be billed by the teaching physician. In addition, this note must include any changes in the patient's condition and clinical course. Refer to your institutional guidelines regarding date of service reporting requirements. Medicare's teaching guidelines do not specifically state which date must be used when a patient is admitted late at night by the resident and seen by the attending on the following calendar day.

Section 100.1.1A of Chapter 12 of the *Medicare Claims Processing Manual* outlines 4 documentation and billing scenarios for E/M services performed by a teaching physician alone or with a resident, as well as scenarios for how the patient care scenarios can be documented to acknowledge that the physical presence and key or critical participation requirements were met.

Surgical Procedures in the Teaching Setting

Section 100.1.2 of Chapter 12 states: "In order to bill for surgical, high-risk, or other complex procedures, the teaching physician must be present during all critical and key portions of the procedure and be immediately available to furnish services during the entire procedure."

The guidelines explain that the teaching physician is responsible for the "preoperative, operative and postoperative care of the beneficiary," but also allow the teaching physician to determine which postoperative visits require his or her

physical presence. Essential language of the surgical rule states the following:

> *During non-critical or non-key portions of the surgery, if the teaching surgeon is not physically present, he/she must be immediately available to return to the procedure, i.e., he/she cannot be performing another procedure. If circumstances prevent a teaching physician from being immediately available, then he/she must arrange for another qualified surgeon to be immediately available to assist with the procedure, if needed.*

If the physician participates in two overlapping surgeries, the critical or key components of each cannot be performed simultaneously. During the non-key or noncritical portion of the procedures, if the physician is not immediately available, he or she must assign a qualified physician to immediately assist the resident should help be needed.

In the case of an endoscopy (eg, direct laryngoscopy), the teaching physician must be present during the entire viewing. This begins when the endoscope is inserted, and ends with its removal. "Viewing the entire procedure through a monitor in another room does not meet the teaching physician presence requirement."

For minor procedures (requiring fewer than five minutes), the teaching physician must be present for the entire procedure if he or she seeks to bill.

Billing for Surgical Assistance in a Teaching Setting

Under Medicare's rules, the surgical assistance performed by a resident is reimbursed to the teaching facility through graduate medical education (GME) funding or other cost reporting. When a qualified resident is not available to provide surgical assistance in a teaching setting, the assistance of a second physician is reported using CPT modifier 82, defined as: Assistant Surgeon (when qualified resident surgeon not available). For example, if a qualified resident is not available to assist with a cervical lymphadenectomy (modified radical neck dissection), the claim would be reported as displayed in Table 8–3.

Restrictions of resident work hours have limited resident availability to provide surgical assistance, and at times this support is provided instead by NPPs. Table 8–4 displays how the cervical lymphadenectomy claim would be formatted if it was instead assisted by an NPP.

Academic practices are urged to also seek guidance from their compliance department regarding their institution's interpretation and requirements for teaching physician billing and documentation requirements.

Conclusion

Understanding billing for nonphysician practitioners is critical when these individuals are employed and providing services for a physician. The key aspect is to determine when the provider needs to bill under their own NPI number and accept the reduced fee and those instances when it can be billed as the physician at the full, allowable amount. Understanding state policy is critical as well, in regard to the individual practitioners.

When working with resident physicians, grasping Medicare guidelines to determine when visits and procedures can be reimbursed and how to properly document is critical. When necessary, work with your individual or hospital coding team to verify the proper language in documentation.

Resources

Medicare Benefit Policy Manual: **Chapter 15— Covered Medical and Other Health Services**
https://www.cms.gov/Regulations-and-guidance/Guidance/Manuals/downloads/bp102c15.pdf

Section 60   Services and Supplies, describes Incident-to guidelines

Section 30.2 Teaching Physician Services

Section 30.3 Interns and Residents

Medicare Claims Processing Manual: **Chapter 12 —Physicians/Nonphysician Practitioners**
http://www.cms.gov/Regulations-and-Guidance/Guidance/Manuals/downloads/clm104c12.pdf

Table 8–3. Surgical Assistance in a Teaching Facility When No Qualified Resident Is Available—Physician

Primary Surgeon	Assistant Surgeon—Teaching Setting, Qualified Resident Not Available
38724	38724-82

Table 8–4. Surgical Assistance in a Teaching Facility When No Qualified Resident Is Available—NPP

Primary Surgeon	Assisting NPP—Teaching Setting, Qualified Resident Not Available
38724	38724-AS (some Medicare MACs may also require modifier 82 in this scenario)

CHAPTER 9

The Office Visit

Betsy Nicoletti and Kimberley J. Pollock

Introduction

Evaluation and management (E/M) services include office visits, consultations, hospital services, nursing home services, critical care services, home services, and emergency department services and are described in the first section of the *Current Procedural Terminology* (CPT®) book. Most of these services are defined with a description of the nature of the presenting problem, and a level of history, exam, and medical decision making. Some also have the typical time associated for the service. CPT does not fully describe the elements associated with E/M codes; therefore, the Centers for Medicare and Medicaid Services (CMS) published guidelines in 1995 and 1997 to provide more specific information about using E/M codes. Physicians and qualified nonphysician practitioners (NPPs) may use either the CMS 1995 or the 1997 Documentation Guidelines to select a level of service for these E/M services.

The E/M service codes are in the 99201–99499 code range. Although they include services provided in many settings, this chapter will discuss codes used to report office services. There are three types of visits commonly reported by otolaryngologists in the office setting, described by CPT as category of codes. The category of an E/M code is the fourth digit in the code. The office code categories primarily used are new patient (9920x), established patient (9921x), and consultation (9924x).

Specialty Versus Subspecialty Designation

The provider specialty designation is critical in defining a new patient (9920x) in E/M coding because a new patient is one who has not been seen by a physician of the same specialty and subspecialty in the same practice in the prior 3 years. CMS has only one specialty designation for otolaryngology and does not recognize otolaryngology subspecialties such as otology or head and neck surgery. The "same group practice" is typically the same tax identification number.

Because CMS and other payers recognize only the single specialty designation of otolaryngology when processing claims, a patient seen by a partner otolaryngologist within the 3-year time period must be reported as an established patient (9921x). Although a practice may have physicians who specialize in otology-neurotology, rhinology, laryngology, pediatric otolaryngology, facial plastics and reconstructive surgery, and head and neck oncologic surgery, the payers usually recognize all of these subspecialties with one specialty designation of otolaryngology. This is important when deciding if a patient is new or established to the physician. That said, your practice may be able to contractually arrange with payers the recognition of otolaryngology subspecialties for coding purposes.

73

New (9920x) Versus Established (9921x) Patients

New patient visits are reported with 99201–99205 series of codes. CPT defines these codes as the correct code to use for a physician office and outpatient department settings. CPT and CMS have slightly different definitions of a new patient. Most payers, however, follow CMS's definition when processing claims. CMS describes a new patient this way:

> Interpret the phrase "new patient" to mean a patient who has not received any professional services, i.e., E/M service or other face-to-face service (e.g., surgical procedure) from the physician or physician group practice (same physician specialty) within the previous 3 years. For example, if a professional component of a previous procedure is billed in a 3 year time period, e.g., a lab interpretation is billed and no E/M service or other face-to-face service with the patient is performed, then this patient remains a new patient for the initial visit. An interpretation of a diagnostic test, reading an x-ray or EKG etc., in the absence of an E/M service or other face-to-face service with the patient does not affect the designation of a new patient.[1]

For example, if the provider performs an E/M service on a new patient (9920x) and sees the patient back in follow-up then the follow-up visit is coded as an established patient (9921x). If the provider performs a procedure without an E/M service (eg, impacted cerumen removal so the audiologist can do the hearing test) then the patient is an established patient (9921x) when he or she returns to see that provider or any of the otolaryngology partners the following week for evaluation of hearing loss. The impacted cerumen removal counts as a face-to-face visit.

CPT adds the concept of "exact same subspecialty" to the definition of a new patient. The CPT description recognizes subspecialties, although most payers do not process claims with this definition. "Solely for the purposes of distinguishing between new and established patients, profes-

sional services are those face-to-face services rendered by a physician and reported by a specific CPT code(s). A new patient is one who has not received any professional services from the physician or another physician of the exactly same specialty and subspecialty who belongs to the same group practice within the past three years."[2]

CMS also states that its policy is to pay for physicians in a group of the same specialty as if they were one physician. Practically speaking, this means patients who are seen by more than one subspecialist in the same otolaryngology practice will be an established patient visit code (9921x) to the second physician, if seen within 3 years.

Location, or site of service where the patient was seen, is not a descriptor in the new patient designation. A new patient is one who has not been seen by the physician in any location for a face-to-face service. If the physician sees the patient in the emergency department and the patient follows up in the office, then that patient is an established patient in the office. If the follow-up appointment in the office is with the same specialty partner of the physician who saw the patient in the emergency department visit, it is still an established patient visit. The reason is that physicians in a group of the same specialty are considered one physician. If an otolaryngologist leaves one practice and moves to another otolaryngology practice and a patient sees that physician in the new practice, the patient is established (9921x) if seen in either practice in the past 3 years. Changing tax ID or practice group practice affiliation does not constitute use of a new patient code (9920x).

Additionally, a new problem does not equate to a new patient code. Often an established patient will return for an unrelated new problem. If that patient has been seen by that physician or by another same specialty partner in that group within 3 years since the prior visit, then the visit is reported with established patient visit codes, even though it is a new problem.

Understanding the definition of a new patient (9920x) makes clear the definition of an established patient. An established patient (9921x) is one seen by the physician or a same specialty partner for any problem, in any location, having any face-to-face service in the past 3 years.

Use these codes for office services provided out of global period. Established patient services are reported with codes 99211–99215.

Consultations (9924x)

CMS stopped recognizing consultation codes in 2010. The Medicare Advantage plans quickly followed suit. However, some state Medicaid programs and many commercial insurance carriers still recognize the consultation codes.

A consultation is a type of evaluation and management service provided at the request of another physician or appropriate source to either recommend care for a specific condition or to determine whether to accept responsibility for ongoing management of the patient's entire care or for the care of a specific condition or problem.[3] CPT provides the following as examples of an "other appropriate source" for consultations: physician assistant, nurse practitioner, doctor of chiropractic, physical therapist, occupational therapist, speech-language pathologist, psychologist, social worker, lawyer, or insurance company.

Consultation codes should not be reported by a physician who has agreed to accept the patient in a transfer of care before an initial evaluation. A consultation requires a 3-step process, all of which require documentation.

First, in order to report a consultation there must be a request for the service documented in the medical record. The consulting physician would be prudent to also document the request in their own medical record as part of their evaluation. This may be done as part of the "chief complaint" or at the beginning of the "history of present illness" sections. Second, the written or oral request for consultation is documented in the patient's medical record by the referring individual and in the consultant's report. The physician must then perform and document the evaluation. Finally, a separate report must be returned to the requesting clinician.

In summary, the familiar R's of a consultation include a *request* from a health care professional who has a national provider identification number, an opinion *rendered* by the consulting

physician, and a separate *report* returned to the requesting clinician.

Outpatient consultation codes are reported with the series 99241–99245 to payers that recognize the consultation codes. These codes are not defined as new or established, and may be reported on a new or an established patient as long as the criteria for a consultation are met. For Medicare, and payers who also do not recognize the consultation codes, use the appropriate new patient (9920x) or established patient (9921x) code.

Practically, the overwhelming majority of consultations occur with new patients. However, CPT states: "If an additional request for an opinion or advice regarding the same or a new problem is received from another physician or other appropriate source and documented in the medical record, the office consultation codes may be used again." Although CPT says a second consultation code may be reported regardless of the time period between visits, many payers will not recognize subsequent consultation codes billed in a 3-year period.

Otolaryngology practices should research which of their private payers still recognize the consult codes, and use these consultation codes when appropriate as these codes best describe the service provided and generally reimburse at a higher rate. This is particularly useful for otolaryngologists because there are so many subspecialties in the field, and all are considered general otolaryngologists by Medicare and most private payers when processing claims.

E/M Levels of Service Based on History, Exam, and Medical Decision Making

Physicians and other health care providers who report E/M services base the level of the service on the 3 key components: history, exam, and medical decision making. Time can also be used instead. Physicians should also consider the nature of the presenting problem when selecting a code using the 3 key components. The CPT book provides charts that show the nature of the presenting problem and the level of history, exam, and medical decision making that are required for each level of service. The description of the code also includes a description of the components and whether 2 of the 3 or all 3 key components are required. For example, 99203 (level 3 new patient office visit) requires all 3 of the key components be at or exceed the documentation requirements. CPT 99203 requires a detailed history, a detailed exam, and low-complexity medical decision making. The definition of a detailed history, detailed exam, and low-complexity medical decision making are found in the CPT book and in the Documentation Guidelines jointly developed by Medicare and the American Medical Association (AMA).

There are 2 sets of guidelines in use: the 1995 and the 1997 guidelines. Payers should use whichever set is most beneficial to the provider on a note-by-note basis when auditing a record. The guidelines are similar except for the exam component. The 1997 exam guidelines include organ system–specific exams, including an exam for the ears, nose, and throat system. This exam will work best for most outpatient and office E/M services. However, otolaryngologists may use either the 1995 or 1997 exam, and for some inpatient services the 1995 multispecialty exam might work best.

History Component

The history component includes 4 parts. These are the chief complaint (CC), history of the present illness (HPI), the review of systems (ROS) and past medical, family, and social history (PFSH). (See Table 9–1.)

A chief complaint is a short statement describing the symptom, problem, condition, diagnosis, or other factor that is the reason for the encounter, and is oftentimes stated in the patient's own words.

The history of present illness is a chronological description of the development of the patient's present illness from the first sign and/or symptom to the present. CPT states the HPI includes the following 7 elements:

- location
- quality
- severity

Table 9–1. Types of History and CPT (Medicare) Documentation Requirements

Types of History	CPT Requirements (Medicare)
Problem focused	Chief complaint Brief HPI (1–3 HPI elements)
Expanded problem focused	Chief complaint Brief history (1–3 HPI elements) Problem pertinent ROS (1 system in the ROS)
Detailed	Chief complaint Extended HPI (at least 4 HPI elements) Extended ROS (2–9 systems in the ROS) Pertinent past, family, or social history (1 of past, family or social history)
Comprehensive	Chief complaint Extended HPI (at least 4 HPI elements) Complete ROS (at least 10 systems in the ROS) Complete PFSH (all 3 PFSH for new patient and consultation codes; any 2 of 3 for the established patient visit code)

- timing
- context
- modifying factors
- associated sign/symptoms

Medicare adds an 8th element: duration.

The review of systems (ROS) is an inventory of body systems obtained through a series of questions seeking to identify signs and/or symptoms that the patient may be experiencing or has experienced. CPT says there are 14 systems:

1) Constitutional symptoms, 2) Eyes, 3) Ears, nose, mouth, throat, 4) Cardiovascular, 5) Respiratory, 6) Gastrointestinal, 7) Genitourinary, 8) Musculoskeletal, 9) Integumentary (skin and/or breast), 10) Neurological, 11) Psychiatric, 12) Endocrine, 13) Hematologic/lymphatic, 14) Allergic/immunologic.

The past history includes such conditions as prior major illnesses and injuries, operations, hospitalizations, current medications, allergies (eg, drug, food), age-appropriate immunization status, and age-appropriate feeding/dietary status.

Family history includes health status or cause of death of parents, siblings, and children; specific diseases related to problems identified in the CC or HPI and/or ROS; and diseases of family members that may be hereditary or place the patient at risk.

Finally, the social history includes marital status and/or living arrangements; current employment; occupational history; military; use of drugs, alcohol, and tobacco; level of education; sexual history; and other relevant social factors.

Examination

The physical exam is defined differently in each set of guidelines. Both the 1995 and 1997 guidelines are presented in Table 9–2 and Table 9–3. The 1997 guidelines provide a platform for an otolaryngology specific ears, nose, and throat system exam. The CMS 1997 ears, nose, and throat system exam is described in Table 9–3.

Medical Decision Making

Medical decision making (MDM) is composed of 3 components: (1) the number of management options or diagnoses addressed at the visit, (2) the amount and/or complexity of data to be reviewed, and (3) the risk of complications and/or morbidity or mortality. (CMS bases this on the table of risk.) Each of these elements requires

Table 9–2. Types of Examination and CPT (Medicare 1995) Documentation Guidelines

Categories for the Levels of Exam	CPT Requirements (Medicare 1995 Guidelines)
Problem focused	A limited examination of the affected body area or organ system (one body area or organ system)
Expanded problem focused	A limited examination of the affected body area or organ system and other symptomatic or related organ system(s) (limited exam of 2–7 body areas or organ systems)
Detailed	An extended examination of the affected body area(s) and other symptomatic or related organ system(s) (extended exam of 2–7 body areas are organ systems)
Comprehensive	A general multisystem examination or a complete examination of a single-organ system (8 organ systems)

Table 9–3. Medicare's 1997 Ear, Nose and Throat Examination

System/Body Area	Elements of Examination
Constitutional	• Measurement of any three of the following seven vital signs 1) sitting or standing blood pressure, 2) supine blood pressure, 3) pulse rate and regularity, 4) respiration, 5) temperature, 6) height, 7) weight (May be measured and recorded by ancillary staff) • General appearance of patient (e.g., development, nutrition, body habitus, deformities, attention to grooming) • Assessment of ability to communicate (e.g., Use of sign language or other communication aids) and quality of voice.
Head and Face	• Inspection of head and face (e.g., overall appearance, scars, lesions and masses) • Palpation and/or percussion of face with notation of presence or absence of sinus tenderness • Examination of salivary glands • Assessment of facial strength
Eyes	• Test ocular motility including primary gaze alignment
Ears, Nose, Mouth and Throat	• Otoscopic examination of external auditory canals and tympanic membranes including pneumo-otoscopy with and notation of mobility of membranes • Assessment of hearing with tuning forks and clinical speech reception thresholds (e.g., whispered voice, finger rub) • External inspection of ears and nose (e.g., overall appearance, scars, lesions and masses) • Inspection of nasal mucosa, septum and turbinates • Inspection of lips, teeth and gums • Examination of oropharynx: oral mucosa, hard and soft palates, tongue, tonsils and posterior pharynx (e.g.; asymmetry, lesions, hydration of mucosal surfaces) • Inspection of pharyngeal walls and pyriform sinuses (e.g., pooling of saliva, asymmetry, lesions) • Examination by mirror of larynx including the condition of the epiglottis, false vocal cords, true vocal cords and mobility of larynx (use of mirror not required in children) • Examination by mirror of nasopharynx including appearance of the mucosa, adenoids, posterior choanae and eustachian tubes (use of mirror not required in children)
Neck	• Examination of neck (e.g., masses, overall appearance, symmetry, tracheal position crepitus) • Examination of thyroid (e.g., enlargement, tenderness, mass)
Respiratory	• Inspection of chest including symmetry, expansion and/or assessment of respiratory effort (e.g., intercostal retractions, use of accessory muscles, diaphragmatic movement) • Auscultation of lungs (e.g., breath sounds, adventitious sounds, rubs)
Cardiovascular	• Auscultation of heart with notation of abnormal sounds and murmurs • Examination of peripheral vascular system by observation (e.g., swelling, varicosities) and palpation (e.g., pulses, temperature, edema, tenderness)
Lymphatic	• Palpation of lymph nodes in neck, axillae, groin and/or other location

Table 9–3. *continued*

System/Body Area	Elements of Examination
Neurological/Psychiatric	• Test cranial nerves with notation of any deficits Brief assessment of mental status, including • Orientation to time, place and person • Mood and affect (e.g., depression, anxiety, agitation)

Content and Documentation Requirements	

Level of Exam	Perform and Document
Problem Focused	• One to five elements identified by a bullet.
Expanded Problem Focused	• At least six elements identified by a bullet.
Detailed	• At least twelve elements identified by a bullet.
Comprehensive	• Perform all elements identified by a bullet; document every element in each box with a shaded border and at least one element in each box with an unshaded border.

documentation, typically as a narrative discussion in the "Assessment/Plan" section of the note. The 4 types of medical decision making are categorized as straightforward, low, moderate and high. The types of medical decision making and the inherent 3 elements are shown in Table 9–4. One must meet or exceed 2 of the 3 elements to choose the type of decision making.

CMS's general guidelines for choosing the number of diagnoses or management options include the following:

• Diagnosed problems are considered less complex than undiagnosed problems.
• New versus established problems relate to the perspective of the examiner, not the patient.
• The more problems addressed at the visit, the more complex the MDM.
• Established worsening problems are considered more complex than known, stable, improving, or minor problems.

CMS's general guidelines for the amount of data reviewed include the following:

• Note that ordering or reviewing labs, x-rays, or medical tests increases the level of MDM.
• Note that personally reviewing a tracing or independently providing an interpretation of a radiographic study increases the level of MDM.
• Note that if you obtain medical information from old records or a patient's caregiver (not with the patient at the time of the visit), document what was obtained as well as your summary of the records reviewed.
• Document discussions regarding diagnostic tests with the physician who performed or interpreted the test.
• Document consults and referrals to other health care professionals.

CMS's general guidelines for the risk of complications, morbidity, and/or mortality are described in the lengthy Table of Risk and include consideration of the patient's presenting problem, diagnostic procedure(s) ordered, or management option(s) selected. The single highest risk element

Table 9–4. Medical Decision-Making Table

	Straightforward	Low Complexity	Moderate Complexity	High Complexity
1. Amount and/ or complexity of data to be reviewed	Minimal or none	Limited	Moderate	Extensive
2. Number of diagnoses or management options	Minimal	Limited	Multiple	Extensive
3. Risk of complications and/or morbidity or mortality	Minimal	Low	Moderate	High

that describes the patient's condition sets the level of risk (minimal, low, moderate, high).

Category and Level of Codes

Elements of the history, examination, and medical decision making are required to achieve a certain CPT level for an office visit. Note the requirements differ for new versus established patients. (See Tables 9–5, 9–6, and 9–7.)

Choosing an E/M Code Based on Time

A physician may use time to select an E/M code in the office when more than 50% of the billing provider's face-to-face time with the patient was spent in counseling. CPT defines this as "for coding purposes, face-to-face time for these services is defined as only that time face-to-face with the patient and/or family."[4] Counseling is described by CPT as a discussion with the patient and/or family concerning one or more of the following areas:

- Diagnosis results, impressions, and/or recommended diagnostic studies

- Prognosis
- Risks and benefits of management (treatment) options
- Instructions for management (treatment) and/or follow-up
- Importance of compliance with chosen management (treatment) options
- Risk factor production
- Patient and family education[5]

Time spent reviewing records, obtaining the patient's history, coordinating care, making phone calls, or arranging for diagnostic tests out of the examination room may not be included in the time for selecting an office visit code. Both CPT and CMS prohibit this out of the exam room time from being included in the total time, when time is used to select a code. Use time to select an E/M code in the office when more than 50% of the billing provider's total face-to-face time was spent in the discussion described above and this is documented in the medical record. For example, state: "I spent 25 minutes face-to-face with the patient and over half of the time was spent in discussion of the risks and benefits of conservative treatment versus surgery." Or, "I spent 15 minutes face-to-face with patient, all of it discussing the allergic triggers for her asthma and how to remove them

Table 9-5. Documentation Requirements for Office/Outpatient Consultation Codes (9924x)

Office Consultation	99241	99242	99243	99244	99245
History*	Problem focused	Expanded problem focused	Detailed	Comprehensive	Comprehensive
Exam*	Problem focused	Expanded problem focused	Detailed	Comprehensive	Comprehensive
Medical decision making*	Straightforward	Straightforward	Low	Moderate	High

Note. *Documentation must meet or exceed all 3 of the 3 key components.

Table 9-6. Documentation Requirements for New Patient Codes (9920x)

New Patient	99201	99202	99203	99204	99205
History*	Problem focused	Expanded problem focused	Detailed	Comprehensive	Comprehensive
Exam*	Problem focused	Expanded problem focused	Detailed	Comprehensive	Comprehensive
Medical decision making*	Straightforward	Straightforward	Low	Moderate	High

Note. *Documentation must meet or exceed all 3 of the 3 key components.

Table 9-7. Documentation Requirements for Established Patient Visit Codes (9921x)

Established Patient	99211	99212	99213	99214	99215
History*	Does not require presence of physician or other qualified health care professional	Problem focused	Expanded problem focused	Detailed	Comprehensive
Exam*		Problem focused	Expanded problem focused	Detailed	Comprehensive
Medical decision making*		Straightforward	Low	Moderate	High

Note. *Documentation must meet or exceed 2 of the 3 key components (typically MDM is 1 of the 2 components).

from her environment." In these cases, time is the trump card, and physician does not need to consider the 3 key component documentation such as number of systems reviewed, elements, and bullets documented. The code is chosen based on the provider's total face-to-face time with the patient when greater than 50% of that time is spent counseling.

Typical total face-to-face times associated with the office visit codes are shown in Table 9–8.

Billing a Procedure With an E/M Code

In certain circumstances, an E/M service may be reported on the same day as a procedure. If both an E/M service and a procedure are reported on the same calendar date, and the procedure has 0 or 10 global days append modifier 25 to the E/M service. A minor procedure is considered a procedure that has 0 or 10 global days, including nasal endoscopy (31231) and flexible fiberoptic laryngoscopy (31575). If the purpose of the visit is to evaluate the patient's condition, and in the course of that evaluation the procedure is required, then both the E/M and procedure services may be reported.

However, if the purpose of the visit is to perform the procedure then report only the procedure code and not also the E/M code. For example,

report only the procedure code when the patient is scheduled for an in-office balloon sinus ostium dilation and there is not a separate condition (eg, ear infection) that would warrant an E/M service on the same day.

When reporting both the E/M and procedure codes, append modifier 25 to the E/M service and provide separately identifiable documentation for both the E/M and the procedure. The definition of modifier 25 is "significant separately identifiable evaluation and management service by the same physician or other qualified healthcare professional on the same day of the procedure or other service."[6]

CMS, however, says that the payment for the procedure includes the decision for the minor surgical procedure, and an E/M service should only be reported when it is separate and distinct. The chapter guidelines in the National Correct Coding Initiative (NCCI) manual states, (Chapter 11, Letter R.): "The decision to perform a minor surgical procedure is included in the payment for the minor surgical procedure and should not be reported separately as an E&M service. However, a significant and separately identifiable E&M service unrelated to the decision to perform the minor surgical procedure is separately reportable with modifier 25."[7]

The *Medicare Claims Processing Manual* (100-04) Section 40.1 (B) states this about E/M services before a procedure: "These services may be paid

Table 9–8. Face-to-Face Time Requirements for Office/Outpatient Codes

Level of Code	Face-to-Face Time Requirement for the Level of Code		
	Consultation (9924x)	New (9920x)	Established (9921x)
992x1	15	10	5
992x2	30	20	10
992x3	40	30	15
992x4	60	45	25
992x5	80	60	40

for separately: The initial consultation or evaluation of the problem by the surgeon to determine the need for surgery. Please note that this policy only applies to major surgical procedures. The initial evaluation is always included in the allowance for a minor surgical procedure . . . "[8]

For a scheduled procedure, report only the procedure and no E/M code unless the patient requires evaluation and management of a distinct separate problem. For example, when the medical records states "patient presents today for a biopsy," report only the biopsy CPT code. If the record indicates that the patient presented with the condition that needed evaluation, and as a result of that evaluation the procedure was performed, then CPT allows reporting of both the E/M service (with modifier 25) and the procedure code. However, many Medicare contractors and private payers have policies that may not always follow CPT roles.

Postoperative Global Periods

The global surgical package is a concept developed by Medicare in 1992 which bundles into the physician payment for a CPT code certain services including preoperative, intraoperative, and postoperative care. The Medicare Physician Fee Schedule Data Base assigns each surgical CPT code a 0, 10-, or 90-day global period. That means payment for follow-up and related care for the procedure is included in the payment. A separate E/M service may be billed in addition to the surgical service when performed on the day of the procedure, if the E/M service meets the criteria for use of modifier 25 or 57, and the day before the surgical procedure if the E/M service meets the criteria for use of modifier 57. Refer to Chapter 11, "Demystifying Modifiers," for more information.

The global surgical package rules are based on both CPT and Medicare guidelines. CPT does allow a surgeon to bill for some postop E/M services provided they are not typical follow-up care, while CMS's policy is that no related services during the postop period are reportable unless a return trip to the operating room is required. Use

modifier 57 on an E/M service when it was the visit at which the decision for surgery was made, and the surgeon is performing a major surgical procedure (90-day global period) that day or the next day. Typically modifier 57 is appended to the E/M code when an urgent 90-day global period procedure will be performed the same day or the next calendar day. For example, a new patient is seen in the office for a neck abscess and is taken to the operating room the next day for an incision and drainage. Modifier 57 is necessary on the office E/M service to show this was when the decision to perform a major procedure took place; modifier 57 will prevent the E/M service from being bundled into the procedure code.

Modifier 24 is used to indicate that an unrelated E/M service took place during the global period. It requires a different diagnosis. For example, modifier 24 would be appended to an E/M code for patient who presents with an unrelated ear infection within a 90-day period following tonsillectomy performed by the same provider. Using a different diagnosis and modifier 24 allows payment for an unrelated E/M service during the global period.

What about the preoperative history and physical exam? Is that a separately reportable service? Once the decision for surgery is made and the patient is scheduled for surgery, a return visit for the purpose of performing a history and physical exam, completing paperwork, and providing informed consent is not separately reportable. Both CPT and CMS consider that part of the global package. This visit for the intent of completing a history and physical and obtaining informed consent is not separately reported.

Conclusion

Otolaryngologists provide a high percentage of patient services in their offices. Although E/M guidelines are complex and potentially confusing, a mastery of this information is imperative to proper coding. Reviewing the rules related to these services will serve the practice in both generating revenue and optimizing compliance.

References

1. Centers for Medicare and Medicaid Services. CMS Internet Manual, 100-04, *Medicare Claims Processing Manual*, Chapter 12, Section 30.6.7 A. https://www.cms.gov/Regulations-and-Guidance/Guidance/Manuals/Downloads/clm104c12.pdf. Accessed February 17, 2015.
2. *Current Procedural Terminology*. Professional Edition. Chicago, IL: American Medical Association; 2014:4.
3. *Current Procedural Terminology*. Professional Edition. Chicago, IL: American Medical Association; 2014:19.
4. *Current Procedural Terminology*. Professional Edition. Chicago, IL: American Medical Association; 2014:8.
5. *Current Procedural Terminology*. Professional Edition. Chicago, IL: American Medical Association; 2014:4.
6. *Current Procedural Terminology*. Professional Edition. Chicago, IL: American Medical Association; 2014:645.
7. National Correct Coding Initiative, Centers for Medicare and Medicaid Services (CMS), Chapter 11, Letter R. https://www.cms.gov/Regulations-and-Guidance/Guidance/Manuals/Downloads/clm104c12.pdf. Accessed February 17, 2015.
8. CMS Internet Manual, 100-04, *Medicare Claims Processing Manual*, Chapter 12, Section 40.1 B. Centers for Medicare and Medicaid Services.

CHAPTER 10

Coding for Hospital Care

Betsy Nicoletti and Kimberley J. Pollock

Introduction

Otolaryngologists admitting patients to the hospital often wonder whether the service is part of the global surgical package or whether it can be separately reported, and paid, in addition to the payment for the surgical procedure. If the service can be billed separately from the global package, or if it is a nonsurgical patient, the question then becomes what type of evaluation and management (E/M) code should be billed. E/M services provided in the hospital are reported with many different categories of codes. This chapter will describe when to use the most common inpatient E/M codes billed by otolaryngologists: initial hospital care codes (often called admission codes), consultations, observation services, and emergency department codes.

Key Points

- Typically one E/M code per day, per specialty (otolaryngology), is reported. For example, if a patient is seen in the office and admitted to the hospital then only one E/M code is reported. Typically, the initial hospital care code, 9922x, is reported in this scenario. All of the hospital care codes are defined by *Current Procedural Terminology* (CPT®) as "per day" codes and multiple visits per day may not be reported by an individual provider.

- The lowest level of initial hospital care codes, 99221, requires documentation of at least a Detailed history and Detailed exam. This can present a problem for some providers who are not familiar with E/M coding because essential information such as a review of systems or extensive exam is oftentimes not documented. It is important for otolaryngologists to be familiar with E/M coding guidelines.

- Medicare's global surgical package for 90-day postoperative global period procedures, such as a thyroidectomy or glossectomy, includes the admission (9922x), daily visits (9923x), and discharge (99238, 99239). If the procedure performed has a 0-day postoperative global period, such as a tracheostomy (31500) or direct laryngoscopy (31525), then subsequent hospital care (9923x) may be reported for daily visits subsequent to the procedure.

- A "routine" admission history and physical (H&P) is included in the global surgical package for all codes and should not be separately reported with an inpatient or outpatient code.

- Modifiers 25 (Significant, Separately Identifiable Evaluation and Management Service by the Same Physician or Other Qualified Health Care Professional on the Same Day of the Procedure or Other

85

Service) and 57 (Decision for Surgery) will oftentimes be used in the inpatient setting when an urgent procedure is performed after a consultation or admission. Refer to Chapter 11, "Demystifying Modifiers," for more information.

- The category of code, the fourth digit, defines the specific E/M code as inpatient (9922x, 9923x, 9925x) or emergency department (9928x). The level of code, the fifth digit (numbers 1 through 5), is achieved based on the provider's documentation of the 3 key components: history, examination, and medical decision making.

General Concepts

Before deciding what category of E/M code to select, the otolaryngologist must first know if the E/M service is part of the global surgical package or if it can be billed separately. Centers for Medicare and Medicaid Services (CMS) assigns a minor procedure with a 0 or 10-day postoperative global period while major procedures have a 90-day postoperative global period. An E/M service provided on the same day as a minor surgical procedure (a procedure with a 0- or 10-day postoperative global period) that is separate and distinct from the procedure may be reported with modifier 25 (see Chapter 11 on modifiers). If a surgeon sees a patient and at that visit determines that the patient will need major surgery (a procedure with a 90-day postoperative global period), and schedules the surgery for that day or the next calendar day, that E/M service is separately reportable with modifier 57. However, if the patient is admitted for the purpose of a previously scheduled procedure, then only the surgical procedure code should be reported.

E/M services related to the surgical procedure that are performed in the hospital, or office, during the postoperative period of a procedure with a 10- or 90-day postoperative global period are not separately reportable as this is considered "typical follow-up care." These services are included in the global surgical package payment for the CPT code billed. This includes subsequent hospital visits and the discharge service performed by the surgeon after the surgery in the hospital for any services within the surgical CPT code's postoperative global period.

No matter what category of code is reported, typically only one E/M service may be reported per day by a provider of the same specialty in the same practice. All of the hospital care codes are defined by CPT as "per day" codes, and multiple visits per day may not be reported by an individual provider.

The category of code, fourth digit of E/M code, the physician reports should match the status selected by the facility. That is, if the patient is assigned inpatient status by the facility, then the physician reports an inpatient code. If the patient is placed in observation status by the facility, then the physician reports either observation codes or office/outpatient codes, depending on the patient's insurance and whether the physician is the admitting or the consulting physician. The status of the patient can change even after the patient is discharged from the hospital. Although only a physician (not a case manager or utilization reviewer) can admit a patient to either inpatient or outpatient status, the facility must select the status based on the level of care the patient requires. This is why case managers will often approach physicians and ask them to change the status of the patient during the admission. It is important for the physician's office staff to check the status of the patient before submitting a claim.

In 2013 CMS developed a 2-midnight rule in an attempt to clarify whether services to patients are inpatient or observation status. If a physician expects that a patient will be in the hospital for at least 2 midnights, then inpatient status is generally appropriate. A stay of less than 2 midnights, unless the patient dies or is transferred to another facility, is generally considered to be an outpatient service. CMS has only 2 classifications of admission status, outpatient and inpatient; CMS does not have an "observation" status and considers observation to be "outpatient." Other payers do recognize the observation status which makes it confusing for providers. CMS requires an admitting order be generated by a physician with admitting privileges, who is knowledgeable about the patient's condition, for the admission.

Initial Hospital Care (99221–99223)

The category of code selected varies based on the status of the patient and whether the otolaryngologist is the admitting or consulting physician. Looking at Table 10–1, the category of code to select is fairly straightforward when the otolaryngologist is the admitting physician. The initial hospital care visit, which is billed for the day that the physician has a billable face-to-face service with the patient, is reported with the initial hospital care codes (99221–99223). For Medicare, modifier AI is appended to the code to tell Medicare that the claim is for the admitting physician. The

3 key components required for documentation of each initial hospital care code level are shown in Table 10–2.

Please refer to Chapter 9, "The Office Visit," for specific information on the level of code documentation required for the History, Examination, and Medical Decision Making components.

Subsequent Hospital Care (99231–99233)

On subsequent days, for patients who are not in a postoperative global period for the provider, the subsequent hospital care codes (99231–99233) are reported. CPT says that all levels of subsequent hospital care include reviewing the medical record and reviewing the results of diagnostic studies and changes in the patient's status (ie, changes in history, physical condition, and response to manage-

Table 10–1 Coding for Inpatients

In This Place of Service—Status of Patient	For This Payer	Use This Category of Code
In the hospital, inpatient status, consultation—first visit this admission	If Medicare	Initial hospital service, 99221–99223 with no modifier
	If Commercial	Inpatient consultation codes 99251–99255
In the hospital, inpatient status—initial service by admitting physician	If Medicare	Initial hospital service, 99221–99223 with AI modifier
	If Commercial	Initial hospital service, 99221–99223 with no modifier
In the hospital, inpatient status—follow-up visit	For all payers	Subsequent hospital visits 99231–99233
In the hospital, inpatient status—part of global surgery	For all payers	No separate charge
In the hospital, inpatient status—discharge day by admitting physician	For all payers	Discharge code 99238, 99239
In the hospital, inpatient status—discharge day by consulting physician	For all payers	Subsequent hospital care 99231–99233

ment) since the last assessment by the physician. The 3 key components required for documentation of each subsequent hospital care code level are shown in Table 10–3.

While CPT does not define "interval," Medicare says that interval means that the past, family and social history does not need to be reviewed.

Remember, one E/M code per day per specialty (otolaryngology) is reported. Only one subsequent hospital care code (9923x) is reported when two different otolaryngologists see the same patient on the same day even for different problems (eg, dizziness and tongue cancer). One otolaryngologist will bill for the combined documentation of both physicians.

If an outside otolaryngologist is covering for the attending otolaryngologist, then the outside physician may separately report the subsequent hospital care code when he or she sees the patient

on rounds assuming the visit is billable (eg, the patient is not in a global period). If, however, the patient is in a global period and the attending otolaryngologist would not have billed for the visit, then the outside rounding otolaryngologist should not bill for the visit. The attending otolaryngologist has been paid for all postoperative care related to the procedure whether he or she personally provides it or not.

Discharge Day Management (99238–99239)

For discharge from the hospital, either 99238 (hospital discharge day management that takes 30 minutes or less) or 99239 (hospital discharge day management that takes more than 30 min-

Table 10–2. Documentation Requirements for Initial Hospital Care Codes (9922x)

	99221	99222	99223
History*	Detailed or comprehensive	Comprehensive	Comprehensive
Exam*	Detailed or comprehensive	Comprehensive	Comprehensive
Medical decision making*	Straightforward or low	Moderate	High

Note. *Must meet all 3 of the 3 key criteria to choose code.

Table 10–3. Documentation Requirements for Subsequent Hospital Care Codes (9924x)

	99231	99232	99233
History*	Problem focused (interval)	Expanded problem focused (interval)	Detailed (interval)
Exam*	Problem focused	Expanded problem focused	Detailed
Medical decision making*	Straightforward or low	Moderate	High

Note. *Must meet 2 of the 3 key criteria to choose code.

utes) are reported. The hospital discharge day management codes are used to report the total duration of time spent by a physician for the final hospital discharge of a patient when not included in the global surgical package. The codes include the final examination of the patient and discussion of the hospital stay, instructions for continuing care to all relevant caregivers, and preparation of discharge records, prescriptions, and referral forms. The total time spent by the physician on that date of service, even if not continuous, may be summed to report the appropriate code.

Report 99238 when the discharge service requires 30 minutes or less time or 99239 when the time is greater than 30 minutes. Remember, to document the time in the note if reporting 99239. Only one physician, the discharging physician of record who may or may not be the attending/admitting physician, may report a discharge day management code. All other physicians will report a subsequent hospital care code (9923x).

Inpatient Consultations (99251–99255)

If the otolaryngologist is the consulting physician, then the category of code billed for the service on a patient with inpatient status varies by the insurance company. Medicare stopped recognizing consultation codes in 2010 and most Medicare Advantage plans quickly followed suit. Many private insurers, however, and some state Med-

icaid programs still do recognize the consultation codes. So the consulting otolaryngologist and coding staff need to know if the patient's insurance does or does not recognize the consultation codes. The initial hospital care codes without modifier AI (99221–99223) are used for Medicare, or any insurance company that does not recognize consultation codes. The inpatient consultation codes (99251–99255) may still be reported for patients whose insurance company still recognizes consultation codes. These inpatient consultation services may be reported on new or established patients, but only once per admission by the consulting physician.

The 3 key components required for documentation of each inpatient consultation code level are shown in Table 10–4.

On subsequent days of the admission, after the initial consultation, the otolaryngologist reports subsequent hospital visit codes (99231–99233), including on the day of discharge.

Observation Status, Admitting Physician (99217, 99218–99220, 99224–99226)

The category of code reported by a physician for a patient who is in observation status also varies depending on the patient's insurance and whether or not the otolaryngologist is the admitting or consulting physician. The admitting physician reports initial observation care codes, 99218–99220, when the service is not included in the global surgical

Table 10–4. Documentation Requirements for Inpatient Consultation Codes (9925x)

	99251	99252	99253	99254	99255
History*	Problem focused	Expanded problem focused	Detailed	Comprehensive	Comprehensive
Exam*	Problem focused	Expanded problem focused	Detailed	Comprehensive	Comprehensive
Medical decision making*	Straightforward	Straightforward	Low	Moderate	High

Note. *Must meet all 3 of the 3 key criteria to choose code.

package and the patient is discharged on a different date of service. While the patient remains in observation, the admitting otolaryngologist reports subsequent observation codes, 99224–99226. On the final day of admission the admitting physician reports observation care discharge, 99217.

Observation Status, Consulting Physician

If the otolaryngologist is the consulting physician to a patient in observation status (Table 10–5) and the patient has Medicare or another insurance that does not recognize consultations, then the

consulting physician reports a new or established patient visit for the initial encounter (new 99201–99205, established 99211–99215). This is confusing to some physicians who wonder why they are using office visits for a patient who is physically located in the hospital. The reason is these codes are defined by CPT as "office or other outpatient services." Since observation is considered an outpatient service, it is correct to use the office and other outpatient services codes for a patient under observation. On subsequent days, the consulting physician continues to report office or other outpatient services, and in this case the patient is an established patient (9921x) since the physician saw the patient the day before. Keep in mind the defi-

Table 10–5. Coding for Patients in Observation Status

In This Place of Service—Status of Patient	For This Payer	Use This Category of Code
Patient in observation status, admitting physician—initial service	For all payers	Observation codes 99218–99220, 99234–99236—admit and discharge or same calendar date
Patient in observation status, admitting physician—subsequent visit	For all payers	Subsequent observation codes 99224–99226
Patient in observation status, admitting physician—discharge visit	For all payers	Observation discharge 99217
Patient in observation status, consulting physician—initial service	If Medicare	New or established patient 99201–99205, 99211–99215
	If Commercial	Office/outpatient consultation 99241–99245
Patient in observation status, consulting physician—subsequent day	If Medicare	Established patient 99211–99215
	If Commercial	Subsequent observation codes 99224–99226
Patient in observation status, consulting physician—discharge day	If Medicare	Established patient 99211–99215
	If Commercial	Subsequent observation codes 99224–99226

nition of a new patient. A new patient (9920x) is a patient who has not been seen by that physician or by another physician in same group who is the same specialty, and exact same subspecialty, in the past 3 years. Remember, most payers consider an otolaryngologist's specialty to be "surgery" and the subspecialty to be "otolaryngology"; they do not recognize the subspecialties of otology, head/neck surgery, etc, to be separate specialties.

If the patient was seen in the office, or in any location in the past 3 years, then the first day of observation status by the consulting physician is an established patient visit (9921x) for a patient whose insurance does not accept consults. On the day of discharge, an established patient visit is also reported by the consulting physician if the patient is seen.

For patients in observation who do have an insurance that still recognizes consultations, then the outpatient consultations codes (99241–99245) are reported for the initial consultation service provided by the otolaryngologist. On subsequent days and for discharge, the subsequent observation care codes are reported (99224–99226), according to CPT. That said, Medicare will allow only the admitting physician to bill the subsequent observation codes so the consulting physician would report an established patient visit code (9921x).

Admission and Discharge on the Same Calendar Date (99234–99236)

There is a third series of codes called "observation or inpatient care services (including admission and discharge services)" (99234–99236). These services may be reported for a patient who has inpatient or observation status, but are more typically reported for a patient in observation status. These codes may not be used by the otolaryngologist for a patient who is in the global period, because the observation and discharge services are part of the global surgical package.

These codes are reported for services provided to a patient who is admitted on one calendar day and is discharged later that same calendar day. In order to report 99234–99236, the physician must see the patient at admission and discharge from observation, and there should be 2 distinct notes documenting the 2 separate services. For Medicare patients the patient must be in observation status longer than 8 hours in order to report these codes. Notice that these codes are not for a 24-hour period but are for a single calendar date.

Emergency Department Visits (9928x)

If an otolaryngologist is called to the emergency department (ED) to see a patient who is subsequently discharged from the ED, the category of code also depends on the patient's insurance. If the patient has an insurance that still recognizes the consultation codes, the office or other outpatient consultation codes are reported (99241–99245). If the patient's insurance does not recognize consultations, the emergency department visit codes are reported (99281–99285) (Table 10–6). The 3 key components required for documentation of each emergency department code level are shown in Table 10–7.

Table 10–6. Coding for Patients Seen in the Emergency Department

In This Place of Service—Status of Patient	For This Payer	Use This Category of Code
Emergency department—in consultation	If Medicare	Emergency department visits 99281–99285
	If Commercial	Office/outpatient consultation 99241–99245

Table 10–7. Documentation Requirements for Emergency Department Codes (9928x)

	99281	99282	99283	99284	99285
History*	Problem focused	Expanded problem focused	Expanded problem focused	Detailed	Comprehensive
Exam*	Problem focused	Expanded problem focused	Expanded problem focused	Detailed	Comprehensive
Medical decision making*	Straightforward	Low	Moderate	Moderate	High

Note. *Must meet all 3 of the 3 key criteria to choose code.

If a patient is seen by the otolaryngologist in the ED and admitted by another service (eg, general surgery trauma), and the otolaryngologist does not see the patient in the inpatient setting that same calendar day, then the otolaryngologist reports the outpatient consultation code (9924x) if non-Medicare or the emergency department code (9928x) if Medicare. If the patient is admitted to observation by another physician and the otolaryngologist does not see the patient again on the same calendar day, then the otolaryngologist codes for the service provided in the ED (9924x if non-Medicare, 9928x if Medicare). If the otolaryngologist does see the patient in the ED and in observation as a consultant, on the same calendar day, then report the outpatient consultation code (9924x) if non-Medicare or outpatient new patient (9920x) or established patient visit (9921x) if Medicare.

If the patient is seen by the otolaryngologist in the ED and the otolaryngologist admits the patient to the inpatient setting, then an initial hospital care is reported (9922x) and modifier AI is appended if Medicare.

Conclusion

After determining that the E/M service is not part of the global surgical package, the next step is selecting the correct category of code. Use the charts in this chapter to guide this selection. The physician's billing and coding staff must check the facility status of the patient prior to submitting the claim in order to match the physician's code selection with the facility status.

CHAPTER 11

Demystifying Modifiers

Kimberley J. Pollock

Introduction

Modifiers are 2-digit codes that are appended to *Current Procedural Terminology* (CPT®) codes. Modifiers are used to indicate to a payer that the service provided has been altered or enhanced by some specific circumstance but not changed in its basic definition. They are used to explain certain specific circumstances to a payer, streamline payments through the claims processing system, and also may affect the amount of payment.

The American Medical Association (AMA) developed, and continues to maintain, the Health care Common Procedure Coding System (HCPCS) Level I code set that includes numeric modifiers. CPT codes are also known as HCPCS Level I codes. The complete listing of CPT modifiers can be found in the *CPT Manual* in Appendix A. CPT eliminated the dash (-) prior to the modifier several years ago. As a result, modifiers are listed using only the 2-digit code without a dash (example: 24, not -24).

The Centers for Medicare and Medicaid Services (CMS) developed and maintains the HCPCS Level II code set which includes alphabetic modifiers (eg, AS, RT). Medicare's payment guidelines for many modifiers such as bilateral procedures (modifier 50), multiple procedures (modifier 51), 2 surgeons (modifier 62), and assistant surgeon (modifiers 80, 82, AS) are published in the Physician Fee Schedule files that are available to the public. Alternatively, this information is pub-lished in an annual AMA publication called *Medicare RBRVS: The Physicians' Guide*.

Oftentimes, otolaryngologists use modifiers incorrectly and the misuse is manifested in claim denials, payer inquiries, refund requests, and unpaid claims. Assigning correct modifiers is important to an efficient revenue cycle in an otolaryngology (ENT) practice.

This chapter will discuss the common modifiers used by ENT practices, how to apply them for everyday use, and pertinent payer reimbursement implications.

Key Points

- Common CPT (HCPCS Level I) modifiers used in otolaryngology can be divided into 3 types. These are modifiers that are appended to (1) evaluation and management (E/M) codes, (2) surgical CPT codes, and (3) diagnostic testing codes. Some modifiers, including 52, 76, and 77, may be appended to different types of codes. Table 11–1 summarizes the types of CPT modifiers used commonly in otolaryngology practices. These will be discussed in greater detail later in this chapter.
- Some modifiers result in a payment reduction or even additional payment; therefore, it is imperative that they be

93

Table 11–1. Common CPT (HCPCS Level I) Modifiers Used in Otolaryngology

| E/M Code Modifiers | Surgical Code Modifiers | | | | Diagnostic Testing Code Modifiers |
	Same-Day Service	Surgeon Role	Complexity	Global Period	
24	50	62	22	58	26
25	51	66	52	76	52
57	53	80		77	
	59	81		78	
	63	82		79	
	76				
	77				

used appropriately so an overpayment does not occur. Utilization of these modifiers is monitored by payers including Medicare. The Office of the Inspector General (OIG) has published reports on overuse of modifiers 25 and 59. Modifiers oftentimes have appeared on the OIG's annual work plan and some are considered "red flags" in terms of utilization and might trigger manual review of the claim and documentation.

- Occasionally the CPT guidelines for using a specific modifier differ from a payer's guidelines. These will be addressed in the discussion below when pertinent.
- HCPCS Level II modifiers common to otolaryngology practices include AI, AS, GC, RT, LT, TC, and the modifier 59 subset modifiers -X{EPSU}. These will also be discussed in more detail in this chapter.

Evaluation and Management Code Modifiers

Three E/M code modifiers are commonly used in otolaryngology: 24, 25, and 57.

Modifier 24: Unrelated Evaluation and Management Service by the Same Physician or Other Qualified Health Care Professional During a Postoperative Period

CPT says: The physician or other qualified health care professional may need to indicate that an evaluation and management service was performed during a postoperative period for a reason(s) unrelated to the original procedure. This circumstance may be reported by adding modifier 24 to the appropriate level of E/M service.

There may be circumstances when a patient is seen in the postoperative global period for a problem that is unrelated to the procedure performed. Typically, these problems have a different diagnosis than the diagnosis code billed for the surgical procedure(s) performed. E/M services unrelated to the procedure may be reported with modifier 24 appended to the appropriate E/M code. Modifier 24 allows payment for an unrelated E/M service.

Do not report an E/M code in the global period if the service is related to the procedure originally performed. For example, if a patient is seen in the office 7 days after a tonsillectomy for oozing from the surgical site, then this service is included in the global surgical package for the tonsillectomy and not separately billed. However, if the patient was seen for ear drainage and acute otitis media is diagnosed, then the E/M service may be reported with modifier 24. The new diagnosis, acute otitis media, is linked on the claim to the E/M code that is appended with modifier 24 to show the patient was seen for a completely different diagnosis.

Coding tips and payer interpretation of modifier 24 are shown in Table 11–2.

Examples of modifier 24 include the following:

1. Patient returns for postop appointment after a tonsillectomy. Mom says patient is still having allergic rhinitis symptoms so this is investigated further and a nasal steroid is prescribed (9921x-24, diagnosis is allergic rhinitis). Also, record 99024 (postop visit, no charge) in the practice's information system and it will have a $0 charge because it is included in the global surgical package.
2. A patient is admitted 3 days after a tonsillectomy for dehydration. Append modifier 24 to the appropriate E/M code and use a diagnosis of dehydration.
3. A patient is seen in the office 6 weeks after a thyroidectomy for dizziness that just started last week (9921x-24, diagnosis is dizziness).

Modifier 25: Significant, Separately Identifiable Evaluation and Management Service by the Same Physician or Other Qualified Health Care Professional on the Same Day of the Procedure or Other Service

CPT Definition of Modifier 25

CPT says: It may be necessary to indicate that on the day a procedure or service identified by a CPT code was performed, the patient's condition required a significant, separately identifiable E/M service above and beyond the other service provided or beyond the usual preoperative and postoperative care associated with the procedure that was performed. A significant, separately identifiable E/M service is defined or substantiated by documentation that satisfies the relevant criteria for the respective E/M service to be reported (see Evaluation and Management Services Guidelines for instructions on determining level of E/M service). The E/M service may be prompted by the symptom or condition for which the procedure and/or service was provided. As such, different diagnoses are not required for reporting of the E/M services on the same date. This circumstance may be reported by adding modifier 25 to the appropriate level of E/M service. Note: This modifier is not used to report an E/M service

Table 11–2. Coding Tips and Reimbursement Implications for Modifier 24

Coding Tips	Reimbursement Implications
• Append modifier 24 to the **unrelated E/M service** that was performed in the postoperative global period of a procedure performed for a different condition or diagnosis.	• Protects the E/M service from being bundled into the global surgical package of the unrelated procedure previously performed.
• If there is more than one diagnosis code on the claim, be sure to properly link (or correlate) the unrelated diagnosis code with the E/M code reported.	• Payment is allowed.

that resulted in a decision to perform surgery (see modifier 57). For significant, separately identifiable non-E/M services, see modifier 59.

Medicare's Definition of Modifier 25

The above CPT definition and instruction differ from Medicare's interpretation of modifier 25. Medicare says that the global surgical package for minor procedures, meaning those codes with a 0- or 10-day postoperative period, also includes E/M services on the day of the procedure that are related to the surgery. Append modifier 25 to an E/M code to tell the payer that a significant, separately identifiable E/M service was performed on the same day as a minor procedure.

Controversy About Modifier 25

All surgical procedure codes have an inherent E/M component for preservice physician work. The controversy is when does the E/M service performed go "above and beyond" the E/M service included in the procedure code? And, does the documentation support that additional work and effort? These are not easy questions to answer. Medicare says a visit by the same physician on the same day as a minor surgery or endoscopy is included in the procedure's global surgical package, unless a significant, separately identifiable service is also performed (then modifier 25 is appended to the E/M code).

While both CPT and Medicare say that different diagnoses are not required for reporting the E/M service on the same date as the procedure, the documentation must support the necessity for both codes. Additionally, the significant, separately identifiable E/M service documentation must be independent from the procedure performed and documented. For example, the procedure should not be documented in the body of the E/M note as this does not show separate services. Separate E/M and procedure notes are recommended to show that the E/M service was significant and separately identifiable.

When to Use Modifier 25

If the purpose of the visit was to perform the procedure, then report only the procedure. If only the

procedure is documented, then only the procedure is reported. Advent of the electronic health record (EHR) has essentially forced providers to document an E/M service for every encounter even if the purpose of the visit was to perform the procedure (eg, remove impacted cerumen, excise a skin lesion). This is a risk area that practices face and providers should be encouraged to override the EHR recommendation that every patient is billed an E/M service on the same day as a procedure.

The American Academy of Otolaryngology-Head and Neck Surgery's (AAO-HNS) Clinical Indicators are a useful tool to determine the indications including history and exam appropriate for performing a procedure.

Payers monitor the use of modifier 25 and some regularly send providers a profile report comparing use of modifier 25 to same specialty peers. These reports should be read carefully and acted upon as they are typically precursors to a payer audit.

Coding Tips and Reimbursement Implications for Use of Modifier 25

Table 11–3 includes some coding tips and reimbursement implications for modifier 25.

Examples of modifier 25 include the following:

1. New patient, 67-year-old female smoker, is seen for a 6-month history of persistent hoarseness. The documentation reflects the patient's breathing to be normal but her voice is raspy. The mirror exam is inconclusive. A flexible fiberoptic laryngoscopy (FFL) is performed for further evaluation. An E/M and separate procedure notes are documented.

   Codes:

   9920x-25   New patient visit

   31575   Flexible fiberoptic laryngoscopy (0-day global)

   The decision to perform the minor procedure was made as a result of the provider's evaluation of the patient; therefore, both codes are supported and modifier 25 is appended to the E/M code.

Table 11–3. Coding Tips and Reimbursement Implications for Modifier 25

Coding Tips	Reimbursement Implications
• Append modifier 25 to the E/M code, not the surgical procedure code • A different diagnosis for the E/M and procedure codes is not required	• Protects the E/M service from being bundled into the global surgical package for the minor procedure also billed

2. New patient is asked to see the otolaryngologist by the pediatrician in consultation for severe throat pain, change in voice, and trismus. Upon examination the patient is diagnosed with a peritonsillar abscess and is taken to the operating room later the same day for incision and drainage.

   Codes:

   9924x-25   Outpatient consultation (office as place of service)

   42700   I&D (10-day global, operating room as place of service)

   The decision to perform the minor procedure was made as a result of the otolaryngologist's evaluation of the patient; therefore, both codes are supported and modifier 25 is appended to the E/M code. Modifier 57 is not appended to the E/M code because the surgical procedure (42700) is a minor procedure (10-day global period). Modifier 57, to be discussed in the next section, is appended when the decision is made to perform a major surgical procedure (90-day global) the same day or day after the E/M service is provided.

3. An established patient seen 2 weeks ago returns for scheduled excision of suspicious looking skin lesion. Both E/M and procedure notes are documented.

   Codes:

   Excision of skin lesion code (and repair code if appropriate) only

   The decision to excise the skin lesion was made at the previous visit. The purpose of today's visit is to excision the skin lesion;

therefore, a separate E/M code appended with modifier 25 is not justified.

4. A patient returns for removal of bilateral impacted cerumen. He wears hearing aids and regularly comes to the office for ear cleaning. The medical assistant did a full review of systems, re-reviewed the past, family, and social history. The otolaryngologist performed a usual complete head and neck exam.

   Codes:

   69210-50 only

   The purpose of the visit was to remove impacted cerumen; therefore, only the procedure is billed. A different condition was not evaluated to warrant a separate E/M code with modifier 25. Refer to Chapter 16, "Office Otology," for more information on use of CPT 69210.

5. Established patient returns for follow-up of persistent hoarseness after 2 weeks of voice rest. Her mirror exam is now within normal limits. However, she now complains of green nasal drainage so endoscopy is performed; acute maxillary sinusitis is diagnosed and an antibiotic is prescribed. Separate E/M and procedure notes are documented in the EHR.

   Codes:

   9921x-25   Established patient visit (diagnosis code: hoarseness)

   31231   Nasal endoscopy (diagnosis code: acute maxillary sinusitis)

   Two separate, unrelated diagnoses were evaluated. The E/M code is appended with modifier 25 and the diagnosis code billed is hoarseness.

The nasal endoscopy code is reported with a diagnosis of acute maxillary sinusitis. It is essential, for proper coding and reimbursement, that the appropriate diagnosis code be linked to the respective CPT code. The otolaryngologist, rather than a check-out clerk, should perform the linking activity to ensure accuracy.

6. Established patient returns for follow-up of persistent hoarseness after 2 weeks of voice rest. After an appropriate history was taken, a flexible fiberoptic laryngoscopy was performed, and the exam is within normal limits. The patient is instructed to return as needed.

    Codes:

    31575   FFL only

    A significant, separately identifiable E/M service is not described warranting use of modifier 25. There is no documentation of the patient's breathing or voice quality or a mirror exam; the FFL was used for the exam. There is also no change in the plan of care that could justify reporting an E/M code.

7. Established patient returns for follow-up of persistent hoarseness after 2 weeks of voice rest. After an appropriate history is taken, the patient's breathing is normal but her voice is assessed to be worse. The mirror exam of the larynx is inconclusive. A flexible fiberoptic laryngoscopy is performed, and the anatomical findings are worse than the previous exam.

Speech therapy is now prescribed and the patient is asked to return in 4 weeks. Separate E/M and procedure notes are documented.

Codes:

9921x-25   Established patient visit
            (diagnosis code: hoarseness)

31575   FFL (diagnosis code:
            hoarseness)

Even though only one diagnosis is documented and billed, both the E/M code appended with modifier 25 and the procedure code are justified. The plan of care has changed due to the condition that supports the separate E/M code.

Modifier 57: Decision for Surgery

CPT says: An E/M service that resulted in the initial decision to perform the surgery may be identified by adding modifier 57 to the appropriate level of E/M service.

Medicare says: The global surgical package for major procedures, those with a 90-day postoperative period, also includes any E/M services the day before and the day of the procedure that are related to the surgery. Append modifier 57 to an E/M code to tell the payer that the decision-making service was performed in the preoperative global period.

Table 11–4 lists key coding tips and reimbursement implications for modifier 57.

Table 11–4. Coding Tips and Reimbursement Implications for Modifier 57

Coding Tips	Reimbursement Implications
• Append modifier 57 to the E/M code (not the surgical procedure code) to reflect a surgery decision-making E/M service was performed on the day before or the day of a major procedure (Medicare defines this as a procedure with a global period of 90 days). Typically, the procedure is unplanned or urgent.	• Protects the E/M service from being bundled into the global surgical package of the unrelated procedure previously performed.
• Do not use modifier 57 on an E/M code to report a routine preop visit or history/physical. This service is included the global surgical package for the code(s) performed and billed.	• Allows payment for the E/M as well as the procedure.

Examples of modifier 57 include the following:

1. A non-Medicare patient is seen in the emergency room at the request of Dr. ER to evaluate a deep neck abscess. The consultation service (9924x-57) is performed and the patient is taken to the operating room for incision and drainage (I&D) (21501).
2. A non-Medicare patient is admitted from the otolaryngologist's office to the hospital to treat a deep neck abscess with IV antibiotics and subsequently seen in the hospital on the same day to perform the admission history and physical (H&P) (9922x-57). The abscess requires incision and drainage (I&D) the next day (21501).

Surgery CPT Code Modifiers

There are several CPT modifiers that may be appended to surgery codes. Discussion follows about the modifiers most commonly used in otolaryngology. Surgery code modifiers may be divided into 4 types: same day, complexity, global period, and surgeon role modifiers.

Same-Day Service Modifiers

Same-day service modifiers are those that are appended to a CPT code(s) when the service(s) are performed on the same calendar day.

Modifier 50: Bilateral Procedure

CPT says: Unless otherwise identified in the listings, bilateral procedures that are performed at the same session should be identified by adding modifier 50 to the appropriate 5-digit code.

Codes that allow modifier 50 are those procedures performed on anatomical structures that have laterality, or bilateral body parts, such as the sinuses and ears.

However, some CPT codes already describe bilateral procedures so modifier 50 should not be appended to these codes. For example, the code for nasal endoscopy (31231) states *Nasal endoscopy,*

diagnostic, unilateral or bilateral (separate procedure). It is not appropriate to report 31231 with modifier 50 because the code specifically says "unilateral or bilateral."

Although some CPT codes do not explicitly say the procedure is bilateral, it is implied because of other CPT instructions or the anatomical location on which the procedure performed is not considered a bilateral body part. For example, the tonsillectomy and adenoidectomy codes (42820–42836) represent inherently bilateral procedures so it is not appropriate to append modifier 50 to any of these codes. In fact, a CPT Assistant (February 1998) says that if the procedure is performed unilaterally, then the appropriate code is reported with modifier 52 (reduced services).

Another example is a septoplasty (30520). The septum is an anatomical structure without laterality unlike the ears or sinuses. Therefore, it would not be appropriate to append modifier 50 to 30520 even though both sides of the septum are straightened in the procedure. Other structures that are considered "central," or without laterality, include the larynx and tongue. Typically modifier 50 is not appended to these codes.

The Medicare Physician Fee Schedule (MPFS) details which CPT codes are payable with modifier 50. The bilateral surgery indicators used in the MPFS, the definitions, and ENT examples are listed in Table 11–5. Refer to the MPFS for information on all CPT codes.

Be careful because occasionally there is a discrepancy between what CPT says about a code being unilateral or bilateral compared to the MPFS payment allowance. For example, CPT 30930 (Fracture nasal inferior turbinate(s), therapeutic) should not be billed with modifier 50 according to CPT guidelines. The word "turbinate(s)" means singular or plural turbinate. However, the MPFS lists 30930 as payable when billed with modifier 50. Physicians are expected to follow CPT coding guidelines and code correctly (meaning bill 30930 without modifier 50) even though the payer guidelines mistakenly allow modifier 50 payment on the code.

Tips for using modifier 50 are shown in Table 11–6.

The 2 usual ways of reporting bilateral procedures are shown in Table 11–7 and Table 11–8.

Table 11–5. Medicare's Bilateral Surgery Indicators and ENT Examples

Indicator Number	Medicare's Definition	ENT Examples
0	"The 150% payment adjustment does not apply. When a procedure is reported with a modifier 50 or modifiers LT and RT base the payment for both sides on the lesser of the total charge or the fee schedule for a single code. For example, code XXXXX 50 is billed at $200. The allowed amount on a single code XXXXX is $125.00. Medicare will allow $125 for both services. Payment in full for both services is inappropriate because of physiology or anatomy, or the code description is for a unilateral code and a bilateral code exists."	30520, 31541 and most larynx procedure codes, 41220 and most tongue procedure codes
1	"The 150% payment adjustment does apply. When the service is submitted with modifier 50, the LT and RT or with 2 units of service, then Medicare will allow the lower of the billed amount for both services or will allow 150% of the allowed amount for a single service. Medicare will allow the bilateral adjustment before the multiple procedure payment adjustment when the provider submits other services subject to the multiple surgery rules."	69436 and most ear procedure codes, 31237–31297 and most sinus procedure codes, 38720–38724 (neck dissection codes)
2	"The allowed amount is for a service performed bilaterally. Medicare could allow the lower of the actual charge or the fee schedule for a single service. The procedure code descriptor is bilateral, or unilateral or bilateral or the service is usually performed bilaterally. When billing for a procedure with a 2 indicator use one number of service and one line of service. Medicare will reject the services as unprocessable."	69210
3	"The Medicare allowed amount is for 2 units of service. If the service is submitted using a modifier 50 or the RT/LT or two units of service, then Medicare will allow the fee schedule for both services. Apply the multiple surgery rules prior to applying the multiple payment reduction rules. Services in this category are generally radiology or other diagnostic tests and are not subject to the special payment rules for bilateral surgeries."	Generally radiology codes

Table 11–6. Tips for Using Modifier 50

Do	Don't
• Use modifier 50 to identify that a code was performed bilaterally. • Survey payers to determine how to format bilateral procedures on the claim: (1) Medicare requires the "bundled" format with 69436-50 on one line, or (2) other payers may require the "line-item" format with 69436 on one line followed by 69436-50 on the second line. • Watch reimbursement closely to ensure bilateral procedures are paid appropriately. • Expect 100% reimbursement of the payer allowable on first stand-alone procedure code and 50% reimbursement on second stand-alone procedure code.	• Allow the payers to "forget" to reimburse appropriately for bilateral procedures. Watch payments carefully to ensure the bilateral procedure was paid appropriately. • Use when the CPT procedure code states "unilateral or bilateral" (eg, 30801, 30802, 31231).

Table 11–7. Bundled Format for Modifier 50

CPT Code/ Modifier(s)	Description	Units	Fee Reported	Fee Expected
Bundled Format (use for Medicare and other payers who prefer this format)					
69436-50	Bilateral tympanostomy (requiring insertion of ventilating tube), general anesthesia	1	200%	150%

Table 11–8. Line-Item Format for Modifier 50

CPT Code/ Modifier(s)	Description	Units	Fee Reported	Fee Expected
Line-Item Format (use if format required by payer or payer format preference is unknown)					
69436	Right tympanostomy (requiring insertion of ventilating tube), general anesthesia	1	100%	100%
69436-50	Left tympanostomy (requiring insertion of ventilating tube), general anesthesia	1	100%	50%

Because modifier 50 is a payment modifier, not an informational modifier, it is important to know the payer's preference for bilateral procedure billing to ensure appropriate reimbursement. Medicare requires the "bundled" format as shown in Table 11–7. If the payer's preference is unknown, use the line-item format as shown in Table 11–8.

Modifier 51: Multiple Procedures

CPT says: When multiple procedures, other than E/M services, Physical Medicine and Rehabilitation services or provision of supplies (eg, vaccines), are performed at the same session by the same individual, the primary procedure or service may be reported as listed. The additional procedure(s) or service(s) may be identified by appending modifier 51 to the additional procedure or service code(s). Note: This modifier should not be appended to designated "add-on" codes (see Appendix D in the *CPT Manual*).

Modifier 51 is appended to secondary stand-alone procedure codes. It is never appended to add-on codes as designated by the "+" symbol or codes exempt from modifier as identified by the Ø symbol. Remember to list codes in descending value order with the highest code(s) listed first.

For example, if a septoplasty and right tympanostomy tube placement is performed the appropriate codes and modifiers are 30520 and 69436-51. The septoplasty has a higher value than the tube placement; therefore, 30520 is listed first and 69436 is appended with modifier 51 because it is a secondary (lower valued) stand-alone procedure.

Medicare says: It is not necessary to report modifier 51 on the claim; the processing system has hard-coded logic to append the modifier to the correct procedure code. Medicare pays for multiple surgeries by ranking from the highest physician fee schedule amount to the lowest physician fee schedule amount. For example, 100% for the highest valued procedure, then 50%

of the physician fee schedule amount for each of the lower-valued codes. This multiple surgery pricing logic also applies to assistant surgeon services. The multiple procedure payment reduction also applies to bilateral services (modifier 50) performed on the same day with other procedures. MPFS lists for each CPT code whether the code is subject to Medicare's multiple procedure payment formula (MPPF).

Payers apply a multiple procedure payment reduction to secondary stand-alone procedures to account for overlapping pre-, intra-, and postoperative care. As noted above, Medicare's MPPF reimburses 100% of the allowable for the first procedure and 50% of the allowable for all secondary stand-alone procedures. Other payers may have a different MPPF such as 100%, 50%, 25%, 25%. It is important to know the payer's MPPF, preferably before the managed care contract is signed.

It is not necessary to also append modifier 51 when modifier 50 (bilateral procedures) or 59 (distinct procedural service) is used as it would be redundant information to the payer. For example, Table 11–9 shows the appropriate format for bilateral endoscopic maxillary antrostomies (31256-50) and bilateral endoscopic anterior ethmoidectomies (31254-50) when the payer requires bilateral procedures to be bundled on one line.

Table 11–10 shows the appropriate format for bilateral endoscopic maxillary antrostomies (31256-50) and bilateral endoscopic anterior ethmoidectomies (31254-50) when the payer requires bilateral procedures to be listed in line-item format.

Table 11–9. Bundled Format for Bilateral and Multiple Procedures Applied

Bundled Format	Comments (assume Medicare MPPF)
31254-50	Reimbursement should be 150% of the payer allowable (100% for the first side, 50% for the second side).
31256-50	Modifier 51 is not necessary on the lower valued, secondary stand-alone bilateral procedure codes. Reimbursement should be 100% of the payer allowable (50% for the first side, 50% for the second side). However, Medicare says if a code is reported as a bilateral procedure and is reported with other primary (or stand-alone) procedure codes on the same day, the bilateral adjustment is applied first before applying any applicable multiple procedure reductions. Therefore, Medicare would reimburse 50% of the 150% allowable (or 75% of a single code allowable). Payer explanation of benefits (EOB) forms should be carefully analyzed to ensure accurate reimbursement.

Table 11–10. Line-Item Format for Bilateral and Multiple Procedures

Line-Item Format	Comments
31254	Reimbursement should be 100% of the payer allowable.
31254-50	Modifier 50 is appended to the second of the same CPT codes. Reimbursement should be 50% of the payer allowable.
31256-51	Modifier 51 is appended to the secondary stand-alone procedure code. Reimbursement should be 50% of the payer allowable.
31256-50	Modifier 50 is appended to the second of the same CPT codes. Reimbursement should be 50% of the payer allowable.

Modifier 59: Distinct Procedural Service

CPT says: Under certain circumstances, it may be necessary to indicate that a procedure or service was distinct or independent from other non-E/M services performed on the same day. Modifier 59 is used to identify procedures/services, other than E/M services, that are not normally reported together, but are appropriate under the circumstances. Documentation must support a different session, different procedure or surgery, different site or organ system, separate incision/excision, separate lesion, or separate injury (or area of injury in extensive injuries) not ordinarily encountered or performed on the same day by the same individual. However, when another already established modifier is appropriate, it should be used rather than modifier 59. Only if no more descriptive modifier is available, and the use of modifier 59 best explains the circumstances, should modifier 59 be used. Note: Modifier 59 should not be appended to an E/M service. To report a separate and distinct E/M service with a non-E/M service performed on the same date, see modifier 25.

Modifier 59 identifies lower-valued procedures/services that are not normally reported together with a higher-valued procedure/service but are appropriately billed under the circumstances. This modifier is oftentimes used to bypass Medicare's Correct Coding Initiative

(CCI) procedure-to-procedure claim processing edits that are designed to prevent improper payment when incorrect code combinations are reported.

For example, CPT 31255 describes and endoscopic total ethmoidectomy while 31254 is for an endoscopic anterior ethmoidectomy. Both codes should not be reported for procedures on the same sinus and there is a CCI edit preventing payment for both codes when billed together. A payer would deny 31254-51 if 31255 and 31254-51 were reported together when different procedures were performed on different sides. However, Medicare's CCI edits allow a modifier to bypass the edit so it would be appropriate in this scenario to append the lower-valued code, 31254, with modifier 59 to show distinct procedures were performed on different sides. Some payers may allow use of modifiers RT (right) and LT (left) to be used.

Coding tips and reimbursement implications for use of modifier 59 are listed in Table 11–11.

At the time this chapter was written, Medicare said that modifier 59 was associated with considerable abuse and high levels of manual audit activity; leading to reviews, appeals, and even civil fraud and abuse cases. Therefore, Medicare introduced 4 modifiers as subsets of modifier 59. These known collectively as modifiers X{EPSU}. The individual modifiers and their official descriptions are shown in Table 11–12.

Table 11–11. Coding Tips and Reimbursement Implications for Modifier 59

Coding Tips	Reimbursement Implications

• Used to report:
  ○ a different session
  ○ different procedure or surgery
  ○ different site or organ system
  ○ separate incision or excision
  ○ separate lesion
  ○ or separate injury (or area of injury in extensive injuries), not ordinarily encountered or performed on the same day by the same individual
 	
• Modifier 59 replaces modifier 51 on the lower-valued code to indicate it should be considered a distinctly separate procedure from the higher valued code reported on the same claim.
	• Allows payment
	• Multiple procedure payment reduction(s) will still apply.

Table 11–12. Medicare's Modifier 59 Subset Modifiers

Subset Modifier	Description
XE	Separate encounter, a service that is distinct because it occurred during a separate encounter
XP	Separate practitioner, a service that is distinct because it was performed by a different practitioner
XS	Separate structure, a service that is distinct because it was performed on a separate organ/structure
XU	Unusual non-overlapping service, the use of a service that is distinct because it does not overlap usual components of the main service

At this time, Medicare has not published more definition information about when to use the subset modifiers and is still accepting modifier 59 when appropriate.

Modifier 53: Discontinued Procedure

CPT says: Under certain circumstances, the physician or other qualified health care professional may elect to terminate a surgical or diagnostic procedure. Due to extenuating circumstances or those that threaten the well-being of the patient, it may be necessary to indicate that a surgical or diagnostic procedure was started but discontinued. This circumstance may be reported by adding modifier 53 to the code reported by the individual for the discontinued procedure. Note: This modifier is not used to report the elective cancellation of a procedure prior to the patient's anesthesia induction and/or surgical preparation in the operating suite.

For example, if the patient develops an intraoperative cardiac issue and the anesthesiologist requests the procedure be stopped, the otolaryngologist will append modifier 53 to the CPT code being performed. If the procedure is aborted prior to the start of surgery (eg, making the incision), then bill an appropriate E/M code instead of the surgical CPT code appended with modifier 53.

Reimbursement will vary and the payer will typically require review of the operative report. It is important to document, in the operative report, how much or what percentage of the CPT code/procedure was actually performed prior to ter-

minating the procedure. This will give the payer an idea of what percentage of the allowable to reimburse.

This modifier is not to be used if the procedure was terminated at the otolaryngologist's discretion. For example, if an endoscopic procedure was planned but the surgeon had to convert it to an open procedure, then only the code for the open procedure should be reported. The endoscopic procedure with modifier 53 should not also be reported with the open code.

Modifier 63: Procedure Performed on Infants less than 4 kg

CPT says: Procedures performed on neonates and infants up to a present body weight of 4 kg may involve significantly increased complexity and physician or other qualified health care professional work commonly associated with these patients. This circumstance may be reported by adding modifier 63 to the procedure number. Note: Unless otherwise designated, this modifier may only be appended to procedures/services listed in the 20005–69990 code series. Modifier 63 should not be appended to any CPT codes listed in the Evaluation and Management Services, Anesthesia, Radiology, Pathology/Laboratory, or Medicine sections.

This modifier is appended to a CPT code when the procedure is performed on a neonate or infant that weighs less than 4 kg (8.8 pounds) to account for the significant increase in work intensity specific to this patient population. The patient's actual weight, in kilograms, should be documented in the operative report to support use of modifier 63. Generally, modifier 63 is not reported with codes that are for correction of congenital abnormalities because the additional work that the modifier represents is already inherent in these procedures.

Refer to Appendix F, Summary of CPT Codes Exempt from Modifier 63, in the *CPT Manual* for a complete listing of codes that should not be appended with modifier 63. Two codes specific for otolaryngology that should not be reported with modifier 63 are 30540, *Repair choanal atresia; intranasal*, and 30545, *Repair choanal atresia; transpalatine*.

Payer reimbursement guidelines vary, and the operative report will likely be reviewed prior to payment.

Modifier 76: Repeat Procedure or Service by Same Physician or Other Qualified Health Care Professional

CPT says: It may be necessary to indicate that a procedure or service was repeated by the same physician or other qualified health care professional subsequent to the original procedure or service. This circumstance may be reported by adding modifier 76 to the repeated procedure or service. Note: This modifier should not be appended to an E/M service.

The definition of modifier 76 is rather vague. Some payers say this modifier is never appended to a surgical CPT code; rather it is used to report multiple diagnostic tests (eg, chest x-ray, EKG) on the same calendar day. The *CPT Assistant*, May 2001, says modifier 76 is intended to describe a "re-operation." Would this "re-operation" occur on the same calendar day or occur only during the postoperative global period (meaning starting the day after surgery)? The answer is not clear and payers have different interpretations.

This modifier can be used to indicate the claim/charge is not a duplicate but is for the same procedure that was performed earlier, typically on a different calendar day but may be on the same day. The provider's usual fee is billed for the procedure and payer reimbursement will likely be reduced to account for any overlapping

global period between the original procedure and the current procedure.

An example might be a re-do septoplasty (30520-76, 90 day global) 6 weeks after the original septoplasty because the patient was hit in the face with a basketball.

Modifier 77: Repeat Procedure by Another Physician or Other Qualified Health Care Professional

CPT says: It may be necessary to indicate that a basic procedure or service was repeated by another physician or other qualified health care professional subsequent to the original procedure or service. This circumstance may be reported by adding modifier 77 to the repeated procedure or service. Note: This modifier should not be appended to an E/M service.

See above discussion for modifier 76. Modifier 77 typically applies when the same service is provided by a same specialty partner since the practice has been paid for global care.

Complexity Modifiers

CPT says a code describes the "operation per se" which is extremely vague with regard to variances for procedure difficulty. In reality, for any given procedure, there could typically be a range of work effort required to provide the service. CPT provides 2 modifiers, 22 and 52, to reflect a way to inform a payer about the physician work variance.

Medicare says the payment allowable for codes/services represents the average or usual work effort required to provide a service. Thus, Medicare instructs the individual carriers to increase or decrease the payment for a service only under very unusual circumstances based upon review of medical records and other documentation.

Modifier 22: Increased Procedural Services

CPT says: When the work required to provide a service is substantially greater than typically required, it may be identified by adding modifier 22 to the usual procedure code. Documentation must support the substantial additional work and the reason for the additional work (ie, increased intensity, time, technical difficulty of procedure, severity of patient's condition, physical and mental effort required).

This modifier is not to be used with E/M codes. It is typically appended to surgical CPT codes when additional work involves significant additional work and complexity than the usual procedure. Sometimes a procedure is a little more difficult and sometimes it is a little less difficult; the physician's average procedure should be taken into account prior to using modifier 22. Consider using modifier 22 on the code, or codes, when the service is significantly more difficult.

The documentation must support the significant additional work and the reason for the work such as time, increased technical difficulty, or patient condition. The documentation should also quantify the percentage additional difficulty and/or the amount of additional time. A separate "complexity paragraph," at the beginning of the operative note, is the best place for this additional documentation. The body of the operative report should also reflect and support the additional work. There must be a compelling reason for how the service differs from the usual procedure for a payer to approve additional reimbursement.

Increase the billed fee by an appropriate amount reflective of the additional work. Also, send the claim electronically but indicate "additional information available upon request" in field 19 of the CMS 1500 form. The payer will typically send a request asking for additional information, meaning the operative report. Sending a paper claim with the operative report before the payer wants it is usually ineffective; a payer typically wants the information when *they* want it, not when you want to send it.

Medicare says that the procedure is valued for the average service and there could typically be a range of work effort to provide the service. Most payers, including Medicare, will manually review the claim before considering paying an additional amount for the added complexity. Medicare typically reimburses an addition 20% of the allowable with good documentation and rationale.

It is difficult to justify reporting modifier 22 on a high volume of cases. If the surgeon does a great deal of very difficult cases, then these difficult cases become the "usual" or "typical" case for that surgeon. Overuse of modifier 22 can be a red flag and trigger an audit.

Use of modifier 22 may delay any payment due to the claim being manually reviewed or while undergoing an appeal effort for additional payment. Monitor payments closely to determine whether the modifier successfully increased payment.

Examples in otolaryngology where modifier 22 may be appropriate include, but are not limited to

1. An endoscopic modified Lothrop procedure was performed involving drilling out a stenotic frontal sinus ostium and partial septectomy (31276-22).
2. A modified radical neck dissection was performed on a patient who has had previous radiation therapy to the area and there is extensive scar tissue and adhesions complicating the operative field (38724-22).

Modifier 52: Reduced Services

CPT says: Under certain circumstances a service or procedure is partially reduced or eliminated at the discretion of the physician or other qualified health care professional. Under these circumstances the service provided can be identified by its usual procedure number and the addition of modifier 52, signifying that the service is reduced. This provides a means of reporting reduced services without disturbing the identification of the basic service.

Sometimes a service is partially reduced due to the provider's discretion. Modifier 52 allows for the service to be reported, in a reduced fashion, without disturbing the meaning of the basic service. Do not append modifier 52 to an E/M service if the relative key components were not documented; rather use an unlisted E/M code instead (99499).

CPT says that all audiologic function tests (92550–92597) include testing of both ears. Append modifier 52 to the code when a test is performed only on one ear instead of 2 ears. Another example of using modifier 52 is to report a unilateral tonsillectomy. The *CPT Assistant* from February 1998 states the codes for tonsillectomy and adenoidectomy (42820–42836) are intended to represent bilateral procedures. It is not appropriate to append modifier 50 when performed bilaterally. Therefore, if the procedure is performed unilaterally, then the appropriate code would be reported with modifier 52.

Payer guidelines vary on whether a reduction in payment is applied. Again, send the claim electronically but indicate the reason for modifier 52, such as "hearing test on one ear," in field 19 of the CMS 1500 form.

Global Period Modifiers

Modifier 58: Staged or Related Procedure or Service by the Same Physician or Other Qualified Health Care Professional During the Postoperative Period

CPT says: It may be necessary to indicate that the performance of a procedure or service during the postoperative period was (a) planned or anticipated (staged); (b) more extensive than the original procedure; or (c) for therapy following a surgical procedure. This circumstance may be reported by adding modifier 58 to the staged or related procedure. Note: For treatment of a problem that requires a return to the operating/procedure room (eg, unanticipated clinical condition), see modifier 78.

Each operative report should reflect in the Indications for Surgery paragraph the planned nature

of the procedures, and the date of the previous surgery to support use of modifier 58. Do not use modifier 58 for treatment of surgical complications such as a posttonsillectomy bleed or cerebrospinal fluid leak after a skull base procedure. Instead, use modifier 78 when a return to the operating room is required to treat a surgical complication.

Modifier 58 is not used for an endoscopic sinus debridement (31237) after endoscopic sinus surgery (31254–31288, 0-day global period) when in a global period of a septoplasty (30520, 90-day global period) and/or inferior turbinate submucous resection (30140, 90-day global period) at the same operative session. Instead, use modifier 79 for the endoscopic debridement because the debridement is unrelated to the procedure for which the 90-day global period applies.

Table 11–13 lists coding tips and reimbursement implications for using modifier 58.

Examples of modifier 58 include, but are not limited to, the following:

1. Division and inset of a forehead flap (CPT 15731 performed 6 weeks earlier) in planned multiple stages of reconstruction after Mohs surgery was performed to remove a nasal skin cancer (15630-58). The division and inset was a prospectively planned second stage of surgery to reconstruct the nasal defect.
2. Re-excision, on a different day in the 10-day postop global period, of a malignant skin

Table 11–13. Coding Tips and Reimbursement Implications for Modifier 58

Coding Tips	Reimbursement Implications
• Used when a subsequent procedure is performed that was (1) planned or anticipated (staged) (2) more extensive than the original procedure (3) for therapy following a surgical procedure • The modifier is necessary only if the subsequent surgery is within the global period. • Append modifier 58 to the procedure code(s) performed in the global period of the first procedure. Do not append the modifier to the code(s) for the first procedure billed.	• Use of the modifier protects reimbursement for subsequent procedure during global period. • Global period resets with the date of the subsequent case. • Reimbursement should be at 100% of the payer allowable.

lesion where margins were found to be positive on final pathology report (116xx-58). Although the re-excision was not prospectively planned, it was anticipated that re-excision would be performed if the pathology report showed positive margins.

3. Removal of remaining thyroid tissue for malignancy, with limited (central) neck dissection, in the global period after a partial thyroidectomy (60252-58). This is an example of a more extensive procedure performed after the original procedure to treat the same problem.

Modifier 78: Unplanned Return to the Operating/Procedure Room by the Same Physician or Other Qualified Health Care Professional Following Initial Procedure for a Related Procedure During the Postoperative Period

CPT says: It may be necessary to indicate that another procedure was performed during the postoperative period of the initial procedure (unplanned procedure following initial procedure). When this procedure is related to the first, and requires the use of an operating/procedure room, it may be reported by adding modifier 78 to the related procedure. (For repeat procedures, see modifier 76.)

Modifier 78 is used to indicate that another related but unplanned procedure was performed in the operating room during the postoperative period of the original procedure. Recall that Medicare's global surgical package includes any services performed in the global period that are related to the initial procedure unless it requires a return to the operating room. An operating or procedure room is an ambulatory surgery center (ASC), catheterization lab, or endoscopy suite but not a treatment room in the physician's office or the emergency room.

The "same physician or other qualified health care professional" is defined as one who is the same specialty (otolaryngology) in the same group practice. The group has been paid for postoperative care; therefore, if the patient is returned to the operating room for a related procedure by a same specialty partner, then modifier 78 is appended.

Although the postoperative period does not start until the next calendar day, some payers may require use of modifier 78 when the unplanned procedure occurs on the same day as the original procedure.

Table 11–14 lists coding tips and reimbursement implications for using modifier 78.

An example of modifier 78 is taking a patient back to the operating room for control of a post-tonsillectomy bleed in the 90-day global period. If the patient is treated in the office setting, then this service is included in the global surgical package according to Medicare. Other payer policies might vary; it is best to have written confirmation from a payer that related procedures performed in the office are billable.

If the control requires a return to the operating room, then the appropriate surgical code (eg, 42962) is reported with modifier 78. If the partner otolaryngologist is on call and takes the patient to

Table 11–14. Coding Tips and Reimbursement Implications for Modifier 78

Coding Tips	Reimbursement Implications
• Append modifier 78 to the subsequent surgical procedure performed in the operating room in the global period of a previous related procedure.	• The modifier protects reimbursement for the subsequent procedure performed during global period. • Payment is usually for the intraoperative service only (eg, typically the usual allowable is reduced by 20% to 30%). • A new postoperative period does not begin when using modifier 78.

the operating room, then the partner will report the appropriate code with modifier 78 just as if the original surgeon would.

Modifier 79: Unrelated Procedure or Service by the Same Physician or Other Qualified Health Care Professional During the Postoperative Period

CPT says: The individual may need to indicate that the performance of a procedure or service during the postoperative period was unrelated to the original procedure. This circumstance may be reported by using modifier 79. (For repeat procedures on the same day, see modifier 76.)

If the service is considered related to the previous procedure, it is considered part of the global surgical package.

A common application in otolaryngology is performing an endoscopic sinus debridement (31237) after endoscopic sinus surgery (eg, 31254-31288, 0-day global) and a septoplasty (30520, 90-day global) and/or inferior turbinate submucous resection (30140, 90-day global). The sinus debridement is not related to the septoplasty or inferior turbinate procedure; therefore, it may be separately reported but requires modifier 79 to trigger payment by the payer. Modifier 58 (staged procedure) is not accurate because the sinus debridement is not related to the procedures for which the 90-day global applies (the septoplasty or inferior turbinate submucous resection in this example). Be sure the diagnosis code reported for 31237 is related to the sinuses (eg, chronic sinusitis)

rather than related to the septoplasty or turbinate pathology.

Another example is a patient is seen at the first postop visit after a tympanoplasty (eg, 69631) and now complains of hoarseness likely due to the endotracheal tube used for anesthesia. A flexible fiberoptic laryngoscopy (31575-79) is performed.

If the postoperative procedure is related to the original surgery, such as performing a flexible fiberoptic laryngoscopy after thyroid surgery to check the status of the laryngeal nerve, then it is not separately reported.

Table 11–15 lists coding tips and reimbursement implications for using modifier 79.

Modifiers 76 and 77

Refer to the previous discussion in the Same-Day Service Modifier section.

Surgeon Role Modifiers

There are occasions when more than one surgeon participates in a procedure code and this necessitates use of a surgeon role modifier. This section will discuss utilization of the co-surgeon modifier, 62, as well as the 3 assistant surgeon modifiers, 80, 81, and 82.

Modifier 62: Two Surgeons

CPT says: When 2 surgeons work together as primary surgeons performing distinct part(s) of a

Table 11–15. Coding Tips and Reimbursement Implications for Modifier 79

Coding Tips	Reimbursement Implications
• Append modifier 79 to the unrelated surgical procedure code performed in the global period of a prior procedure. • The modifier may be appended to a procedure code performed in the office or hospital setting.	• The modifier protects reimbursement for the subsequent unrelated procedure performed during the postoperative global period of the previous procedure. • Payment should be at 100% of the allowable for the unrelated procedure. • A new postoperative global period begins for the service reported with modifier 79.

procedure, each surgeon should report his or her distinct operative work by adding modifier 62 to the procedure code and any associated add-on code(s) for that procedure as long as both surgeons continue to work together as primary surgeons. Each surgeon should report the co-surgery once using the same procedure code. If additional procedure(s) (including add-on procedure(s) are performed during the same surgical session, separate code(s) may also be reported with modifier 62 added. Note: If a co-surgeon acts as an assistant in the performance of additional procedure(s), other than those reported with the modifier 62, during the same surgical session, those services may be reported using separate procedure code(s) with modifier 80 or modifier 82 added, as appropriate.

To summarize, this modifier is used when 2 surgeons perform different parts of the same CPT code and neither surgeon performs the entire code/procedure. Recall that the global package for all surgical CPT codes includes the intraoperative services of making the incision or the approach to get to the level of pathology, performing the resection or correcting the problem, as well as the usual closure to repair the operative tract. The exception to this guideline is the skull base surgery codes (61580–61616) which include separate approach and definitive (resection) services.

A common example, in otolaryngology, of 2 surgeons sharing the same CPT code is the endoscopic endonasal resection of a pituitary tumor, 62165. The code includes the approach, the tumor resection, and the closure. It is considered cosurgery, or use of modifier 62 on the same CPT code (62165), when the otolaryngologist performs the approach while the neurosurgeon resects the tumor and the otolaryngologist closes. When the procedure is performed through the nose in an open manner using a microscope, then 61548-62 is reported by both the otolaryngologist and neurosurgeon. If a separate abdominal fat graft is harvested for the closure, then the surgeon may report the code (20926) without modifier 62 because 2 surgeons did not perform the graft harvest. CPT 20926 is appended with modifier 51 (multiple procedures).

In some cases, 2 surgeons perform the primary procedure code together (code is appended with modifier 62) then one of the surgeons stays to assist for the rest of the codes/procedure (then the other codes are appended with an appropriate assistant surgeon modifier). It is imperative that each surgeon's operative report clearly reflect the individual work performed.

If 2 surgeons perform different procedures reported by different CPT codes, then the cosurgery modifier does not apply. For example, the pediatric otolaryngologist places bilateral tympanostomy tubes in a child (69436-50) at the same operative session as the urologist performs a circumcision. Each surgeon bills his or her own CPT code(s); this is not considered cosurgery with use modifier 62 because the surgeons are not sharing a CPT code.

There may be instances where the otolaryngologist and neurosurgeon perform a case together but each surgeon will report his or her own CPT code even if the procedures are performed through the same incision. For example, the otolaryngologist does the craniofacial approach to the anterior skull base (61580) while the neurosurgeon resects the intradural tumor (61601). Each surgeon will report his or her own CPT code and modifier 62 does not apply since the surgeons are not sharing a code.

When modifier 62 is used, both surgeons must dictate separate operative reports. Each surgeon lists him-/herself as the primary surgeon then lists the other surgeon as a "cosurgeon." Each surgeon should document only what he or she did and say that the other surgeon will document his or her portion of the procedure in a separate operative note.

The Medicare Physician Fee Schedule shows which CPT codes are payable with modifier 62. Medicare reimburses 62.5% of the allowable to each surgeon. Each surgeon has pre- and postoperative responsibilities for the patient.

Medicare says the 2 surgeons must be of different specialties (eg, otolaryngology and neurosurgery), but CPT does not make that distinction. Remember, Medicare and most payers do not recognize the subspecialties of otolaryngology such as neurotology, facial plastics, rhinology, laryngology, pediatric otolaryngology, or head and neck oncology. It is usually difficult to justify 2 surgeons of the same specialty doing different parts of the same CPT code. Therefore, it is oftentimes difficult to get paid when 2 otolaryngologists bill the same CPT code with modifier 62.

However, an exception might be when 2 otolaryngologists perform a free flap together. One surgeon is harvesting the flap while the other is preparing the recipient site. If 2 surgeons of different specialties did the procedure, then each reports the free flap code with modifier 62. One could argue that 2 surgeons of the same specialty are providing the exact same level of service and both should be paid (both dictate their own operative report describing their own separate service). These exceptions must be justified and will be approved on a case-by-case basis with the payer; extensive appeals of denials may be required as well.

Table 11–16 shows several common cosurgery scenarios in ENT.

Modifier 66: Surgical Team

CPT says: Under some circumstances, highly complex procedures (requiring the concomitant services of several physicians or other qualified health care professionals, often of different specialties, plus other highly skilled, specially trained personnel, various types of complex equipment) are carried out under the "surgical team" concept. Such circumstances may be identified by each participating individual with the addition of modifier 66 to the basic procedure number used for reporting services.

Table 11–16. Common Cosurgery (Modifier 62) Scenarios in ENT

Examples	Billed Fee	Expected Payment
Otolaryngologist does the transnasal/trans-sphenoidal approach for neurosurgery to remove a pituitary tumor. Both surgeons report 61548-62. Otolaryngologist does not separately report codes for septoplasty and/or endoscopic sinus surgery because the approach is included in 62165.	100% of usual fee	62.5% each physician
Same scenario as above but the procedure is performed endoscopically. Both surgeons report 62165-62. Otolaryngologist does not separately report codes for septoplasty and/or endoscopic sinus surgery because the approach is included in 62165.	100% of usual fee	62.5% each physician
Otolaryngologist does the cervical approach for the spine surgeon's anterior cervical discectomy/decompression and fusion. Both surgeons report 22551-62. The spine surgeon will report additional codes for the instrumentation and bone graft procedures. Otolaryngologist may report these same codes with an appropriate assistant surgeon modifier (80, 82) if performed.	100% of usual fee	62.5% each physician
Otolaryngologist and neurosurgeon perform a translabyrinthine/transmastoid excision of an acoustic neuroma (cerebellopontine angle tumor, vestibular schwannoma). Both surgeons report 61526-62. Other codes such as those for microdissection (69990) and/or abdominal fat graft (20926) may be reported as appropriate.	100% of usual fee	62.5% each physician
Otolaryngologist and neurosurgeon perform a retrosigmoid/suboccipital approach for excision of an acoustic neuroma (cerebellopontine angle tumor, vestibular schwannoma). Both surgeons report 61520-62. Other codes such as those for microdissection (69990) and/or abdominal fat graft (20926) may be reported as appropriate.	100% of usual fee	62.5% each physician

This modifier is used if a team of surgeons (more than 2 surgeons of different specialties) is required to perform a specific procedure code. Each surgeon reports the same code with modifier 66.

This modifier is rarely used because is it not common in otolaryngology where 3 surgeons would perform different parts of the same CPT code.

Reimbursement for modifier 66 is usually determined on a case-by-case basis by the payer. The Medicare Physician Fee Schedule shows which CPT codes are payable with modifier 66.

Modifier 80: Assistant Surgeon

CPT says: Surgical assistant services may be identified by adding modifier 80 to the usual procedure number(s).

The assistant may be of any specialty such as otolaryngology or family practice. The otolaryngologist dictates the operative note and identifies the role/work performed by the assistant. For example, the primary surgeon might document "due to the complexity of the case, an assistant was required for suction, retraction and irrigation throughout the case."

The assistant surgeon submits the same CPT codes as the primary surgeon appended with modifier 80. The assistant surgeon's fee is typically reduced by about 50% of the fee if billed as a primary surgeon. For example, if the physician's usual fee for the CPT code as a primary surgeon is $1,000 then he or she would bill $500 as an assistant surgeon (modifier 80). The billed fee is a symbol of the physician's "value" or "worth." Clearly the value or worth of an assistant surgeon is not the same as the value for the primary surgeon; this is why the assistant's fee is reduced.

All CPT codes may be billed with modifier 80; however, payment is dependent on payer guidelines. Medicare reimburses 16% of the code allowable; bilateral (modifier 50) and multiple procedure discounts also apply. Medicare requires use of modifier AS for PAs, NPs, and CNSs; other payer guidelines may vary (more information about modifier AS is in the HCPCS Level II modifier section of this chapter).

Medicare will not pay an assistant-at-surgery for surgical procedures in which a physician is used as an assistant-at-surgery in fewer than 5% of the cases for that procedure nationally (this is determined through manual reviews). The MPFS lists for each CPT code whether payment for assistant services is allowed. Each code is assigned a payment status of 0, 1, or 2:

0 = Payment restrictions for assistants at surgery applies to this procedure unless supporting documentation is submitted to establish medical necessity.

1 = Statutory payment restriction for assistants at surgery applies to this procedure. Assistant at Surgery may not be paid.

2 = Payment restrictions for assistants at surgery does not apply to this procedure. Assistant at Surgery may be paid.

For example, a septoplasty (30520) has an assistant surgery payment status of 1 meaning payment is excluded for this code. However, a unilateral thyroid lobectomy (60220) has a payment status of 2 meaning payment for an assistant is allowed.

Modifier 81: Minimum Assistant Surgeon

CPT says: Minimum surgical assistant services are identified by adding modifier 81 to the usual procedure number.

Although a primary operating physician may plan to perform a surgical procedure alone, during an operation circumstances may arise that require the services of an assistant surgeon for a relatively short time. In this instance, the second surgeon provides minimal assistance, for which he/she reports the surgical procedure code appended with the modifier 81. Modifier 81 is used only with surgical CPT codes.

This modifier is not frequently used in otolaryngology. An example might be if the otolaryngologist is doing a complicated mastoidectomy for cholesteatoma removal and requires assistance from his or her partner for a short time to identify the facial nerve. The assistant was involved in the procedure for only a short time.

Modifier 82: Assistant Surgeon (when qualified resident surgeon not available)

CPT says: The unavailability of a qualified resident surgeon is a prerequisite for use of modifier 82 appended to the usual procedure code number(s).

This modifier is appended to the surgical CPT codes billed by an academic otolaryngologist who assists his or her partner because there is not a qualified resident available to assist on the case. The primary surgeon must document in the operative note that due to the unavailability of a qualified resident in this situation the complexity of the case required an assistant. Refer to Medicare's Teaching Physician guidelines for more specific information on use of modifier 82 and for documentation requirements for the primary surgeon. The documentation, billing, and reimbursement information provided above in the modifier 80 discussion also applies for modifier 82.

Diagnostic Testing Code Modifiers

Modifier 26: Professional Component

CPT says: Certain procedures are a combination of a physician or other qualified health care professional component and a technical component. When the physician or other qualified health care professional component is reported separately, the service may be identified by adding modifier 26 to the usual procedure number.

Professional component refers to certain procedures, usually diagnostic testing, that are a combination of a physician component and a technical component. Using modifier 26 identifies the physician's component. The professional component includes reading films, interpreting diagnostic tests, and providing a separate written report.

Surgical procedure codes do not have separate professional and technical components. For example, 31579 (Laryngoscopy, flexible or rigid fiberoptic, with stroboscopy) is a surgical CPT code, and although it may be performed by a speech pathologist and an otolaryngologist, modifier 26 does not apply to this surgical code.

A complete service, one that is reported without modifier 26, is one in which the physician provides the entire service including equipment, supplies, technical personnel, and the physician's professional services. The complete service can be divided into a technical component (HCPCS Level II modifier TC) and a professional component (modifier 26).

In some cases, such as functional endoscopic speech and swallowing testing (92612–92617), a separate CPT code exists to describe the professional component so modifier 26 does not apply.

The physician reports only the professional component of a service when that service is provided in a setting where the physician does not own the equipment, such as a hospital outpatient department. For example, if an otolaryngologist is reading a sleep study on a patient who had an attended sleep study performed at the hospital (and sleep medicine is not doing the interpretation), then the otolaryngologist reports the appropriate sleep study code with modifier 26. The date of service is the day the separate interpretation report was documented.

Use of modifier 26 will be discussed again in Chapter 17, "Audiology," Chapter 21, "Office Sleep Medicine," and Chapter 22, "In-Office Imaging."

Modifier 52: Reduced Services

The CPT definition of this modifier was previously discussed as it pertains to a complexity surgery CPT code. However, this modifier also has the applicability for audiologic diagnostic testing. All audiometric tests include testing of both ears. Append modifier 52 to the code if a test is performed on one ear instead of 2 ears.

For example, the patient is known to have no hearing in one ear so only the contralateral ear is tested; append the appropriate audiologic testing code with modifier 52.

HCPCS Level II Modifiers

HCPCS Level II modifiers are part of the national code set which is maintained by CMS. These are not official CPT modifiers and may not be recognized by all payers. In addition to the X{EPSU} modifiers previously discussed, other HCPCS Level II modifiers common to otolaryngology are discussed below.

Modifier AI: Principal Physician of Record

Medicare requires the admitting physician of record to append modifier AI to the initial hospital care E/M code (99221–99223). This is an informational modifier and does not affect payment.

Modifier AS: Assistant at Surgery

Medicare says to use the modifier AS for assistant at surgery services provided by a Physician Assistant (PA), Nurse Practitioner (NP), or Clinical Nurse Specialist (CNS). These services are always direct-billed by the PA or NP and are never billed "incident to" the physician. (Refer to Chapter 8, "Billing Guidelines for Nonphysician Practitioners and Teaching Physicians," for more information.) A MD/DO should not report a code with modifier AS; rather, a physician uses modifier 80 or 82 as appropriate.

Medicare allows 85% of the 16% assistant surgeon allowable to be paid for modifier AS; therefore, approximately 13.6% is allowed for the assistant at surgery services provided by a PA or NP (applicable multiple procedure reductions will also apply). All CPT codes may be billed with modifier AS; however, payment is dependent on payer guidelines. Refer to the previous modifier 80 discussion on which CPT codes are payable with modifier AS.

Modifier RT: Right Side (Used to Identify Procedures Performed on the Right Side of the Body) and Modifier LT: Left Side (Used to Identify Procedures Performed on the Left Side of the Body)

Medicare says to use modifier RT when the body contains a right and left anatomical part of the body and a service is performed on the right side of the body; use modifier LT when the service is performed on the left side. Use of modifier RT

may help to provide more information to a payer particularly if different procedure codes were performed on either side.

This modifier is not necessary when a procedure is performed only on one side of an anatomic structure with laterality. For example, it is not necessary to report 69433-RT when a right tympanostomy tube is placed under local anesthesia.

When bilateral procedures are performed, Medicare will recognize the code billed with modifier 50 (eg, 31256-50) or the codes listed separately with the RT and LT modifiers (eg, 31256-RT and 31256-LT). Reimbursement for both sides will be the same, at 150% of the allowable, regardless of format.

Use of modifiers RT and LT may be effective when performing different procedures on different sides so the payer will not bundle the lower-valued code into the higher-valued code. For example, when a right endoscopic total ethmoidectomy is performed (31255-RT) but only an endoscopic anterior ethmoidectomy was performed on the left side (31254-LT). Alternatively, a CPT modifier could be used such as 31255 and 31254-59. It is also acceptable to use both the CPT modifier and the HCPCS Level II modifiers such as 31255-RT and 31254-59, LT.

Modifier TC: Technical Component

Medicare says: Under certain circumstances, a charge may be made for the technical component alone. Under those circumstances the technical component charge is identified by adding modifier TC to the usual procedure number.

Modifier TC is used when the otolaryngologist provides only the technical component of a diagnostic test that has both professional (modifier 26) and technical components. The technical component includes the necessary equipment, supplies, and auxiliary personnel (eg, technician, nurse) to perform the test.

For example, a patient is referred by a neurologist for a basic vestibular evaluation (92540), and this will be performed by the otolaryngologist's audiology technician. (The otolaryngologist is in the office supervising the audiology technician.) The neurologist will interpret the electronystagmogram (ENG). The performing otolaryngologist will bill 92540-TC, for the technical component involved in performing the diagnostic test, and the neurologist will bill 92540-26, for the professional component of reading the ENG.

If the provider performs both the professional and technical components of the diagnostic test, such as the audiologist doing 92540, then the code is billed without a modifier. This is called "global billing." Payment for the professional (modifier 26) and technical (modifier TC) components equals the payment for the "global" service; there is no financial incentive to billing either way.

Modifier GC: This Service Has Been Performed in Part by a Resident Under the Direction of a Teaching Physician

Medicare's teaching physician guidelines are well defined in various CMS resources at https://

www.cms.gov. Medicare requires modifier GC be appended to any CPT code when the resident performs a service in a teaching facility under the supervision of a teaching physician. The service provided may be an E/M code or a surgical procedure code. Modifier GC is informational only and does not affect payment.

Summary

A summary of the CPT modifiers discussed in this chapter, with the associated Medicare reimbursement implication, is shown in Table 11–17.

The medical record should support use of the modifier billed. Accurate utilization of modifiers is essential to ensure optimal payments.

Table 11–17. Summary of CPT Modifiers and Medicare Payment Implication

CPT Modifier	CPT Description	Medicare Payment Implication
22	Increased Procedural Services	By report; often paid at an additional 20% if justified and sufficiently documented
24	Unrelated Evaluation and Management Service by the Same Physician or Other Qualified Health Care Professional During a Postoperative Period	Allows payment
25	Significant, Separately Identifiable Evaluation and Management Service by the Same Physician or Other Qualified Health Care Professional on the Same Day of the Procedure or Other Service	Allows payment
50	Bilateral Procedures	Second side reimbursed at 50%
51	Multiple Procedure	Secondary procedures reimbursed using the multiple procedure payment reduction formula (100% paid for the first code, 50% paid for subsequent stand-alone codes)
52	Reduced Services	By report
53	Discontinued Procedure	By report

continues

Table 11–17. *continued*

CPT Modifier	CPT Description	Medicare Payment Implication
57	Decision for Surgery	Allows payment
58	Staged or Related Procedure or Service by the Same Physician or Other Qualified Health Care Professional During the Postoperative Period	Paid the usual amount; global period resets
59	Distinct Procedural Service	Allows payment; any multiple or bilateral procedure reduction also applies
62	Two Surgeons	62.5% of the allowable
63	Procedure Performed on Infants less than 4 kg	By report; usually an additional amount reimbursed
66	Surgical Team	By report
76	Repeat Procedure or Service by Same Physician or Other Qualified Health Care Professional	When used as a global period modifier, the payment is typically for the intraoperative service only and a new global period does not apply. When used as a same day modifier, it allows payment. Many Medicare carriers do not recognize this modifier on surgery or E/M codes.
77	Repeat Procedure by Another Physician or Other Qualified Health Care Professional	When used as a global period modifier by a different otolaryngologist in the same practice, the payment is typically for the intraoperative service only and a new global period does not apply. When used as a same-day modifier, it allows payment. Many Medicare carriers do not recognize this modifier on surgery or E/M codes.
78	Unplanned Return to the Operating/Procedure Room by the Same Physician or Other Qualified Health Care Professional Following Initial Procedure for a Related Procedure During the Postoperative Period	Allows payment; payment is typically for the intraoperative service only and a new global period does not apply
79	Unrelated Procedure or Service by the Same Physician or Other Qualified Health Care Professional During the Postoperative Period	Allows payment; a new global period begins
80	Assistant Surgeon	Payment is at 16% of the MPFS; bilateral and multiple procedure adjustments also apply
81	Minimum Assistant Surgeon	By report
82	Assistant Surgeon (when qualified resident surgeon not available)	Payment is at 16% of the MPFS; bilateral and multiple procedure adjustments also apply

Resources

1. OIG report. Use of Modifier 25. http://oig.hhs.gov/oei/reports/oei-07-03-00470.pdf. Accessed March 22, 2015.
2. OIG report. Use of Modifier 59 to Bypass Medicare's National Correct Coding Initiative Edits. http://oig.hhs.gov/oei/reports/oei-03-02-00771.pdf. Accessed March 22, 2015.
3. Medicare Physician Fee Schedule (PFS) files showing CPT and HCPCS Level II codes and other important information such as relative value units, modifier applicability (eg, whether code is paid with modifier 50), postoperative global period. http://www.cms.gov/Medicare/Medicare-Fee-for-Service-Payment/PhysicianFeeSched/PFS-Relative-Value-Files.html.
4. Grider, Deborah J. *Coding with Modifiers: A Guide to Correct CPT® and HCPCS Level II Modifier Usage*, 5th ed. Chicago, IL: American Medical Association; 2014.
5. Medicare Claims Processing Manual, Internet Manual, Chapter 12—Physicians/Nonphysician Practitioners for Medicare's guidelines on physician and nonphysician practitioner services including global surgery, modifier adjustments, assistant-at-surgery, audiology billing, and teaching physician guidelines. http://www.cms.gov/Regulations-and-Guidance/Guidance/Manuals/downloads/clm104c12.pdf.
6. American Academy of Otolaryngology-Head and Neck Surgery Clinical Indicators. http://www.entnet.org/content/clinical-indicators.

SECTION II

Office-Based Otolaryngology

CHAPTER 12

Office Rhinology

Seth M. Brown

Introduction

This chapter describes rhinologic procedures done in the office. All *Current Procedural Terminology* (CPT®) codes, when billed in the physician office setting (place of service 11), include the use of the facility and equipment in the office. This is reflected in Medicare's nonfacility Relative Value Units (RVUs) and ultimately, reimbursement. Medicare reduces the reimbursement to the physician when the service is performed in a facility setting such as a hospital outpatient department (place of service 22), because the facility is paid a separate fee for its use, equipment, support staff, etc. The RVUs often change yearly and can be found in various places including various American Medical Association (AMA) publications and the Centers for Medicare and Medicaid Services (CMS) website, or obtained through the American Academy of Otolaryngology-Head and Neck Surgery (AAO-HNS). Procedures must be done for proper indications and be separate from the evaluation and management (E/M) component of the visit if billed separately.

Sample Nasal Endoscopy Note

Procedure: Nasal endoscopy, bilateral

Indications: Chronic sinusitis refractory to treatment

Discussion: Risks, benefits, and alternatives of the procedure were discussed with the patient including the risks of mucosal trauma, nasal bleeding, and infection.

Anesthesia: Oxymetazoline topically

Technique: Rigid endoscopy, 30-degree scope

Findings:

Nasal mucosa—congested and boggy

Septum—deviated to right with 80% obstruction

Inferior turbinates—enlarged and boggy bilaterally

Nasopharynx—1+ residual adenoids, no drainage

Middle meatus—no purulence or polyps seen, moderate edema on left

Sinuses—clear accessory ostium of maxillary on left, remainder of sinuses not visualized

Sphenoid recess—clear bilaterally without purulence or polyps seen

Olfactory cleft—free of polyps on left, not visualized on right

Patient status: tolerated procedure well

Complications: no complications

The AAO-HNS Clinical Indicators are a good resource for proper indications. All office-based procedures should also include a separate procedure note that is distinct from the body of the E/M note. The procedure note should include indications, discussion of risks/benefits, anesthesia, if a scope was used, description of the procedure, findings, and any complications encountered.

Key Points

- Endoscopy includes evaluation of one or both sides of the nose and cannot be billed twice.
- Endoscopic surgical codes (including debridement, biopsy, and control of epistaxis) are unilateral codes and can be billed for each side.
- If you use the endoscope, then report an endoscopic code and not an open code. Be sure to document use of the endoscope.
- CMS assigns most endoscopic procedure codes a 0-day postoperative global period, and most nonendoscopic office nasal codes have a 10-day postoperative global period.

Key Procedure Codes

Incision and Drainage Codes

30000 Drainage abscess or hematoma, nasal, internal approach
wRVU 1.48; Global 10

30020 Drainage abscess or hematoma, nasal septum
wRVU 1.48; Global 10

Nonendoscopic Biopsy and Excision Codes

These codes are nonendoscopic codes. If polyps are removed with an endoscope then choose the proper sinus code or CPT 31237. Polyp removal is included with all the endoscopic sinus codes.

30100 Biopsy, intranasal
wRVU 0.94; Global 0

30110 Excision, nasal polyp(s), simple
wRVU 1.68; Global 10

30115 Excision, nasal polyp(s), extensive
wRVU 4.44; Global 90

30117 Excision or destruction (eg, laser), intranasal lesion; internal approach
wRVU 3.26; Global 90

Other Nonendoscopic Codes

The lavage codes cannot be added to a balloon dilation code.

30220 Insertion, nasal septal prosthesis (button)
wRVU 1.59; Global 10

30300 Removal foreign body, intranasal; office type procedure
wRVU 1.09; Global 10

31000 Lavage by cannulation; maxillary sinus (antrum puncture or natural ostium)
wRVU 1.20; Global 10

    31002 sphenoid sinus
wRVU 1.96; Global 10

Office Turbinate Codes

30200 Injection into turbinate(s), therapeutic
wRVU 0.78; Global 0

30801 Ablation, soft tissue of inferior turbinates, unilateral or bilateral, any method (eg, electrocautery, radiofrequency ablation, or tissue volume reduction); superficial
wRVU 1.14; Global 10

    30802 intramural (ie, submucosal)
wRVU 2.08; Global 10

Epistaxis Codes

30901 Control nasal hemorrhage, anterior, simple (limited cautery and/or packing) any method
wRVU 1.10; Global 0

30903 Control nasal hemorrhage, anterior, complex (extensive cautery and/or packing) any method
wRVU 1.54; Global 0

30905 Control nasal hemorrhage, posterior, with posterior nasal packs and/or cautery, any method; initial
wRVU 1.97; Global 0

> **30906** subsequent
> *wRVU 2.45; Global 0*

31238 Nasal/sinus endoscopy, surgical; with control of nasal hemorrhage
wRVU 2.74; Global 0

Endoscopic Codes

31231 Nasal endoscopy, diagnostic unilateral or bilateral (separate procedure)
wRVU 1.10; Global 0

31237 Nasal/sinus endoscopy, surgical; with biopsy, polypectomy or debridement (separate procedure)
wRVU 2.60; Global 0

Balloon Dilation Codes

31295 Nasal/sinus endoscopy, surgical; with dilation of maxillary sinus ostium (eg, balloon dilation), transnasal or via canine fossa
wRVU 2.70; Global 0

> **31296** with dilation of frontal sinus ostium (eg, balloon dilation)
> *wRVU 3.29; Global 0*

> **31297** with dilation of sphenoid sinus ostium (eg, balloon dilation)
> *wRVU 2.64; Global 0*

Other Unlisted

92700 Unlisted otorhinolaryngological service or procedure
wRVU 0.00; Global XXX

Stent Placement

These category III codes can be used in the office or operating room setting. They are intended to be used for stent placement or placement with debridement in the ethmoid cavity. Although they can be used with some of the other endoscopic codes, many of them cannot be billed at the same time, specifically the ethmoidectomy and diagnostic codes. These codes are effective January 1, 2016, and thus further information was not available about these codes at the time of publication.

0406T Nasal endoscopy, surgical, ethmoid sinus; placement of drug eluting implant

> **0407T** with biopsy, polypectomy or debridement

Key Modifiers

25 Significant, Separately Identifiable Evaluation and Management Service by the Same Physician or Other Qualified Health Care Professional on the Same Day of the Procedure or Other Service
This code can be added to an E/M code when a procedure is done. This implies that the office visit is above and beyond the work that was traditionally done as part of the procedure. Often this means a separate diagnosis has been used and the problem can stand alone as a billable service. The key components of the E/M service need to be done and documented.

50 Bilateral Procedure
Most therapeutic codes are unilateral. Therefore, when done on both sides a 50 modifier is added to inform the payer that this was done twice. This is often used with the debridement code (31237) following sinus surgery.

76   Repeat Procedure or Service by Same Physician or Other Qualified Health Care Professional
Used to report that the same procedure was done following the initial procedure. Can be used on procedures such as epistaxis control that may have to be repeated several days later should the initial intervention be unsuccessful.

79   Unrelated Procedure or Service by the Same Physician or Other Qualified Health Care Professional During the Postoperative Period
This is used when a procedure has to be done during a global period that is unrelated to the global period. This is often used for debridement or endoscopy that is done to evaluate a sinus surgery cavity following a sinus surgery along with a septoplasty. Because the septoplasty has a 90-day global period, the procedure can be billed with the 79 modifier when the procedure is done for the sinus portion of the procedure.

Key ICD-9-CM/ICD-10-CM Codes

For sinonasal disorders most *International Classification of Diseases, Tenth Revision, Clinical Modification* (ICD-10-CM) codes are converted one to one (eg, 473.0 chronic maxillary sinusitis becomes J32.0). What is different is that there are often more descriptions of each code and additional language. For instance there will now be 2 codes for acute maxillary sinusitis—461.0 can become: J01.00 Acute maxillary sinusitis, unspecified or J01.01 Acute recurrent maxillary sinusitis. Most codes in ICD-10-CM will have laterality (left or right). This is not true with sinus codes, as laterality is not specified.

In *International Classification of Diseases, Ninth Revision, Clinical Modification* (ICD-9-CM) chronic pansinusitis was coded under an "other" code (473.8). In ICD-10-CM, chronic pansinusitis has its own code (J32.4). Another important change in ICD-10-CM is how to code sinusitis when involving 2 or 3 sinuses but not pansinusitis (all 4 sinuses). In ICD-9-CM each sinus involved was coded separately unless it was pansinusitis. However, in ICD 10 CM, if 2 or 3 sinuses are infected then the "other" sinusitis code will be used rather than

coding each sinus separately (J32.8 Other chronic sinusitis or J01.80 Other acute sinusitis). See Chapter 3, "Transition to ICD-10-CM," for more details.

Below is a list of some of the commonly used codes in the office with a description of the code. Certain codes have more than one description:

239.1/D49.1   Neoplasm of unspecified behavior of respiratory system

461.0/J01.00   Acute maxillary sinusitis, unspecified

461.0/J01.01   Acute recurrent maxillary sinusitis

461.1/J01.10   Acute frontal sinusitis, unspecified

461.1/J01.11   Acute recurrent frontal sinusitis

461.2/J01.20   Acute ethmoidal sinusitis, unspecified

461.2/J01.21   Acute recurrent ethmoidal sinusitis

461.3/J01.30   Acute sphenoidal sinusitis, unspecified

461.3/J01.31   Acute recurrent sphenoidal sinusitis

461.8/J01.40   Acute pansinusitis, unspecified

461.8/J01.41   Acute recurrent pansinusitis

--/J01.80   Other acute sinusitis

--/J01.81   Other acute recurrent sinusitis

461.9/J01.90   Acute sinusitis unspecified

461.9/J01.91   Acute recurrent sinusitis, unspecified

470/J34.2   Deviated nasal septum

471.0/J33.0   Polyp of nasal cavity

471.0/J33.1   Polypoid sinus degeneration

471.0/J33.8   Other polyp of sinus

471.0/J33.9   Nasal polyp, unspecified

473.0/J32.0   Chronic maxillary sinusitis

473.1/J32.1   Chronic frontal sinusitis

473.2/J32.2 Chronic ethmoidal sinusitis

473.3/J32.3 Chronic sphenoidal sinusitis

473.8/J32.4 Chronic pansinusitis

--/J32.8 Other chronic sinusitis

473.9/J32.9 Chronic sinusitis, unspecified

477.9/J30.9 Allergic rhinitis, unspecified

478.0/J34.3 Hypertrophy of nasal turbinates

478.19/J34.0 Abscess, furuncle and carbuncle of nose

478.19/J34.1 Cyst and mucocele of nose and nasal sinus

478.19/J34.89 Other specified disorders of nose and nasal sinuses

781.1/R43.0 Anosmia

781.1/R43.1 Parosmia

781.1/R43.2 Parageusia

784.7/R04.0 Epistaxis

Definition of Codes

1. Diagnostic Endoscopy (31231)
   a. *Indications*—this should be performed only if the practitioner is unable to adequately evaluate the nose with anterior rhinoscopy and the patient has disease or symptoms that need to be further assessed. This can include sinusitis that is refractory to medical treatment, surveillance of polyposis, evaluation of postsurgical patency or epistaxis without an anterior source or suspicion of a mass. Inability to see on anterior rhinoscopy could include anatomic reasons that prohibit visualization, posterior nasal pathology or an inability to adequately evaluate the area of interest.
   b. *Definition*—evaluation of the nose and sinus passages with an endoscope, whether rigid or flexible. This is a diagnostic procedure and cannot be billed with a surgical endoscopic procedure code. Common ana-

tomic areas that should be evaluated and documented include the nasal septum, the middle turbinate, middle meatus, sphenoethmoid recess, quality of the secretions, and choana. Inclusion of the paranasal sinus cavities is indicated in postoperative patients. For practical purposes, examination of the nasopharynx is also routinely included in the procedure findings.
   c. *Key points*—this includes evaluation of both sides of the nose and cannot be reported twice or with modifier 50. Anesthesia and equipment is included in this code, even if recording equipment is used. If the patient's symptoms are nasopharyngeal or laryngeal in nature, the nasopharyngoscopy or laryngoscopy should be performed and billed instead, even though the nose is transversed and often evaluated as part of the exam.
   d. Performing a laryngoscopy at same visit. This is an area of coding controversy. If you report both 31231 and 31575, be sure certain requirements are met. However, reimbursement for both procedures is inconsistent.
      i. There must be indications to evaluate both areas independently.
      ii. A separate scope must be used for the larynx and the nose.

2. Surgical Endoscopy (31237)
   a. *Indications*—obstructing polyps, nasal lesion/mass, extensive crusting, and debris postsurgical, as well as other unusual circumstances as discussed below.
      i. Biopsy—this is usually done if there is a unilateral lesion or if a polyp looks suspicious for a malignancy. This can be performed bilaterally and reported with modifier 50 if indicated. If two separate areas on the same side of the nose are biopsied, this should be only reported once. The biopsy must be done with the endoscope because the lesion is not accessible with a headlight alone. The diagnostic endoscopy and hemostasis are included in this code and should not be billed separately. If

the endoscope is used to evaluate the nose and the lesion is then biopsied with a headlight, report only the open biopsy code (30100).

ii. Debridement—this is usually done in the immediate postoperative period but may be performed in other unusual nonsurgical circumstances such as for postradiation necrosis. This is a unilateral code and can be reported with modifier 50 if both sides are debrided. This should be used if tissue and debris are removed using endoscopic guidance and is not used for simply suctioning of mucus. Under most circumstances this will only be performed with the first month of surgery. Prolonged debridement might be necessary in unusual circumstances including tumors, advanced disease, allergic fungal sinusitis, and postoperative infections. Often a septoplasty is done at the same time as a sinus surgery. Although the endoscopic sinus surgery codes have a 0-day global period, the septoplasty code has a 90-day global period. If a debridement is thus done after the endoscopic sinus procedure and for the purpose of the sinus surgery, not the septoplasty, then modifier 79 should be added to 31237 to let the payer know that the debridement is not related to postop care of the septoplasty.

b. *Key points*—A separate procedure note must be included for this code. Diagnostic endoscopy (31231) is included in debridement. CPT 31237 is a unilateral code and can be reported with modifier 50 if appropriate. Many payers monitor this code, thus avoid overutilizing this code.

3. Abscess/Hematoma Drainage
   a. Nasal (30000)
      This is used for drainage of an abscess or hematoma in the nasal mucosa. This involves an intranasal approach.
   b. Septal (30020)
      This is used for drainage of an abscess or hematoma of the nasal septum. Often this

requires an incision, a hemostat, and packing or a drain.

4. Epistaxis
   a. Anterior (30901, 30903)
      This is used for control of epistaxis using a headlight. An example would be controlling the bleeding using silver nitrate. 30901 is defined as "simple" and 30902 is "complex". There is no description of what is simple and complex. Simple would be best used for straightforward cautery or packing. If multiple attempts are required, or additional time, or extensive packing is required it would thus be appropriate to use the complex code. Multiple sites on the same side can only be billed using one code. If bleeding is controlled on both sides then modifier 50 can be used to let the payer know that this was done on each side.
   b. Posterior (30905, 30906)
      This is used to control posterior epistaxis without needing an endoscope. Modifier 50 (bilateral procedure) does not apply since the posterior nasal cavity is a single entity. An example of this is the placement of a posterior pack. CPT 30906 is used for subsequent control and includes removing the existing pack and placing a new pack at the same session. There is not a separate surgical CPT code for removing a posterior nasal pack as this activity is included in the placement code. If you did not place the original pack then the removal is included in your E/M code or in 31231 if you do a diagnostic endoscopy.
   c. Endoscopic (31238)
      This is used for control of epistaxis requiring the use of an endoscope. An endoscope is thus used to perform the procedure and is placed parallel to the instrument(s) used to control the bleeding. An example would be using an endoscope to control posterior nasal bleeding with silver nitrate as this is unable to be visualized with a headlight. If, however, the endoscope is used for the diagnostic procedure and then the bleeding is controlled using a headlight, the proper code to report is the appropriate nonendoscopic control code such as 30901-30906.

5. In-Office Turbinate Procedures
   a. Turbinate injection (30200)
      This can be steroids or a sclerosing agent and can only be reported once. This is normally injected into the submucosa of the turbinate. The HCPCS II J code for the medication injected may also be separately reported if performed in the physician office setting (place of service 11).
   b. Superficial (30801)
      This code can be used for radiofrequency ablation, cautery, or coblation as well.
   c. Intramural (30802)
      This code can be used for radiofrequency ablation, cautery, or coblation as well.

6. Nonendoscopic Codes
   a. Biopsy (30100)
      This procedure involves removing mucosa or a lesion from inside the nose using a headlight. Surrounding mucosa may be included. The surrounding tissue can be left to granulate in or closed with a suture.
   b. Excision or destruction (30117)
      This involves destruction of an intranasal lesion using a laser, cryosurgery, or a chemical application via an intranasal approach.
   c. Nasal polyp excision (30110)
      This code is a unilateral procedure for polyp removal using a headlight. Modifier 50 may be appended when performed bilaterally. If an endoscope is used, report code 31237 instead.
   d. Nasal polyp excision, extensive (30115)
      This code is a unilateral procedure for polyp removal using a headlight. This is deemed extensive and is usually performed in the operating room. There is not an official definitive of "extensive" so the surgeon's impression and documentation are important. The code may be reported with modifier 50 when performed bilaterally.
   e. Nasal button (30220)
      A physician inserts a septal prosthesis into a perforation.
   f. Foreign body (30300)
      A physician removes a foreign body from inside the nasal cavity. If general anesthesia is required, code 30310 is used instead.
   g. Sinus lavage (31000, 31002)

These codes are used to puncture the maxillary (31000) or sphenoid (31002) sinus using a headlight. Through the puncture the sinuses are irrigated out. These codes are included in the endoscopic balloon sinus ostia catheterization codes (31295–31297) and should not be separately reported when performed on the same sinus.

7. Office-Based Balloon Surgery
   a. Balloon surgery basics—Diagnostic nasal endoscopy (31231) is included in all the balloon codes. All these codes require visualization of the sinus passages with the endoscope. Anesthesia and equipment costs are included in the codes. Each sinus is reported separately, as these are unilateral codes. Append modifier 50 for bilateral procedures. An operative report or a procedure note should be documented including the indications. Removal of tissue from the sinuses is not included, and this requires the use of a traditional endoscopic code (31254–31288) instead of the balloon code. An endoscopic sinus code and the balloon code cannot be reported together for procedures on the same sinus. An endoscopic ethmoidectomy, however, can be billed as a separate procedure.
   b. Maxillary (31295)
      This is dilation of the maxillary sinus ostium either transnasally or via the canine fossa with endoscopic guidance without removal of tissue. It includes sinus lavage (31000) when performed.
   c. Frontal (31296)
      This is dilation of the natural frontal sinus ostium with endoscopic guidance without removal of tissue.
   d. Sphenoid (31296)
      This is dilation of the sphenoid sinus ostium with endoscopic guidance without removal of tissue. It includes sinus lavage (31002) when performed.

8. Smell Testing
   There is currently not a CPT code for this service. If the medical assistant or nurse is administering the test, then it would likely be included in the physician E/M code billed and

not separately billed (and the cost incurred by the practice) OR one could potentially use an unlisted code, 92700. If the physician administered the test, then reporting 92700 is again a possibility. Other centers do not bill this service and the patient incurs the expense.

Controversial Areas

Use of the 25 Modifier

This is commonly used when performing rhinologic procedures. Often patients come to the otolaryngologist for several different complaints and a procedure, such as a nasal endoscopy is done in the same setting. When this occurs, modifier 25 is appended to the E/M code to show that the E/M is a separate, identifiable service and was performed in addition to the procedure. The hallmark of this modifier is that the office visit should stand apart from the procedure. In many cases this means there are separate diagnosis codes for the office visit and the procedure, though this is not a requirement by CPT or Medicare. Both the E/M service (appended with modifier 25) and procedure codes should be billed in many cases where additional management decisions are made, multiple diagnosis codes are used, and significant time is spent with the patient outside the standard procedure time (which includes both preprocedure and postprocedure time). In 2013 CMS reviewed 31231 and reduced the postprocedure time to 3 min. This should be separate from the E/M visit, should the E/M visit be billed at the same setting. Please consult your professional coder for individual circumstances.

Debridement After Sinus Surgery

It is common to debride the sinus cavity following endoscopic sinus surgery. This is a unilateral code and can be billed with modifier 50 should it be performed on both sides. Debridement includes nasal endoscopy (31231) and cannot be billed separately. Debridement is described as removing crusts, lysing scar tissue, and cleansing the sinus cavity; however, simply suctioning the nose and sinuses is not adequate to bill this code. Like all procedures, a separate procedure note should be generated describing indications, anesthetic used, procedure performed, findings, and complications. The AAO-HNS has written statements on the appropriate use of debridement, and it is standard to perform between 1 and 3 debridements after sinus surgery. There are times when more debridements may be necessary, and this can be found on the AAO-HNS website. A *CPT Assistant* article in the December 2011 issue is also a good resource.

Balloon Ostial Dilation Reimbursement

Many payers continue to deny claims for balloon ostial dilation procedures claiming this is experimental. To date, significant literature exists which supports the use of the balloon both as an adjunct to traditional endoscopic sinus surgery as well as a stand-alone procedure. The American Academy of Otolaryngology-Head and Neck Surgery and The American Rhinologic Society have produced a position statement regarding balloon ostial dilation. This reads as follows:

> Sinus ostial dilation (eg, balloon ostial dilation) is an appropriate therapeutic option for selected patients with sinusitis. This approach may be used alone to dilate a sinus ostium (frontal, maxillary, or sphenoid) or in conjunction with other instruments (eg, microdebrider, forceps). The final decision regarding use of techniques or instrumentation for sinus surgery is the responsibility of the attending surgeon (http://www.entnet.org/?q=node/542)

It is important to get preauthorization for these procedures and when payment is denied to appeal these rulings to the highest level. Please see Chapter 6, "Successful Navigation of the Appeals Process," for further information.

CHAPTER 13

Otolaryngic Allergy

Gavin Setzen and Michelle M. Mesley-Netoskie

Introduction

Otolaryngic allergy care is an integral part of providing comprehensive diagnosis and treatment for patients with a wide variety of otolaryngologic conditions in both children and adults. Whether one is just starting an allergy practice, or has an established allergy practice, it is important to continuously maintain a dialogue with insurance carriers and payers in one's region to ensure the ability to provide allergy care (initial and ongoing) and to derive appropriate reimbursement for the care you provide to their beneficiaries.

Key Points

- Allergy testing *Current Procedural Terminology* (CPT®) codes (CPT 95004, 95024, 95027, 95028) include test interpretation and report by a physician or other qualified health care professional. Provision of test results by the nurse or medical assistant is included in the allergy testing codes as well. An evaluation and management (E/M) code may be separately reported, and appended with modifier 25, if a significant separately identifiable E/M service is performed. For example, the provider's service involves more than just giving testing results (eg, discussing treatment options).

- Allergy testing must specify the number of tests (antigens) being performed. These data are required for CPT coding and should be documented in the patient record and on the insurance claim form in the "unit" field.
- Intradermal dilutional testing (IDT) (CPT code 95027) coverage varies by insurer, with caps on the number of antigens allowed, frequency of IDT testing, and length of immunotherapy coverage. Bill the code per dilution tested which is the same as "per stick."
- Skin tests and controls are billed "per stick" (CPT 95004).
- Titration skin tests are billed per antigen (CPT 95024) which is the same as "per stick."
- CPT 95028 requires reading the test result on a different day. The reading service is included in 95028 and is not separately billable with an E/M code on the second day.

Key Procedure Codes

Allergy Testing

Allergy testing is typically performed in the office by scratch, puncture, prick, or intradermal testing. Coding is based on the type of test, specifying the number of tests. Codes are broken out based on whether extracts or drugs are used and

129

immediate- or delayed-type reactions. There are also additional codes for ingestion challenges. For an ingestion challenge, if the total testing time is less than 61 minutes (eg, positive challenge resulting in cessation of testing), report an E/M service, instead of a testing code.

95004   Percutaneous tests (scratch, puncture, prick) with allergenic extracts, immediate type reaction, including test interpretation and report, specify number of tests
wRVU 0.01; Global XXX

95018   Allergy testing, any combination of percutaneous (scratch, puncture, prick) and intracutaneous (intradermal), sequential and incremental, with drugs or biologicals, immediate type reaction, including test interpretation and report, specify number of tests
wRVU 0.14; Global XXX

95024   Intracutaneous (intradermal) tests with allergenic extracts, immediate type reaction, including test interpretation and report, specify number of tests
wRVU 0.01; Global XXX

95027   Intracutaneous (intradermal) tests, sequential and incremental, with allergenic extracts for airborne allergens, immediate type reaction, including test interpretation and report, specify number of tests
wRVU 0.01; Global XXX

95028   Intracutaneous (intradermal) tests with allergenic extracts, delayed type reaction, including reading, specify number of tests
wRVU 0.00; Global XXX

95044   Patch or application test(s) (specify number of tests)
wRVU 0.00; Global XXX

95076   Ingestion challenge test (sequential and incremental ingestion of test items, eg, food, drug or other substance); initial 120 minutes of testing
wRVU 1.50; Global XXX

+95079   each additional 60 minutes of testing (List separately in addition to code for primary procedure)
wRVU 1.38; Global ZZZ

Treatment

Allergy immunotherapy codes are billed based on whether one or more injections are given. Only one unit of each allergy immunotherapy code is billed regardless of the number of injections. Furthermore, separate codes exist if the service includes preparation of the extract.

95115   Professional services for allergen immunotherapy not including provision of allergenic extracts; single injection
wRVU 0.00; Global XXX

95117   2 or more injections
wRVU 0.00; Global XXX

95120   Professional services for allergen immunotherapy in office of institution of the prescribing physician or other qualified health care professional, including provision of allergenic extract; single injection
wRVU 0.00; Global XXX

95125   2 or more injections
wRVU 0.00; Global XXX

Preparation/Provision of Vial

95144   Professional services for the supervision of preparation and provision of antigens for allergen immunotherapy, single dose vial(s) (specify number of vials)
wRVU 0.06; Global XXX

95165   Professional services for the supervision of preparation and provision of antigens for allergen immunotherapy; single or multiple antigens (specify number of doses)
wRVU 0.06; Global XXX

Unlisted

An unlisted code is currently used for services such as sublingual immunotherapy drops (SLIT), tests; taste tests; and a simple sip, spit, and rinse test.

95199 Unlisted allergy/clinical immunologic service or procedure.
wRVU 0.00; Global XXX

Key Modifiers

25 Significant, Separately Identifiable Evaluation and Management Service by the Same Physician or Other Qualified Health Care Professional on the Same Day of the Procedure or Other Service
Used when an office visit is done in addition to an allergy procedure on the same day. This must meet the criteria for a separate visit.

Key ICD-9-CM/ICD-10-CM Codes

Comment: Below is a list of commonly used codes for allergy testing and treatment in the office with a description of the code (understand that certain codes may have more than one description). *International Classification of Diseases, Tenth Revision, Clinical Modification* (ICD-10-CM) has provided more specificity for otitis media, asthma, and allergies than *International Classification of Diseases, Ninth Revision, Clinical Modification* (ICD-9-CM), such as left, right, bilateral, controlled, and uncontrolled. For example, all ear codes have specificity for right, left, and bilateral. The unspecified ear code is thus generally inappropriate but used here for example purposes.

372.05/H10.1X   Acute atopic conjunctivitis

372.13/H10.44   Vernal conjunctivitis

372.14/H10.45   Other chronic allergic conjunctivitis

381.00/H65.199   Other acute nonsuppurative otitis media, unspecified ear

381.01/H65.00   Acute serous otitis media, unspecified ear

--/H65.11   Acute and subacute allergic otitis media (mucoid) (sanguinous) (serous)

381.10/H65.20   Chronic serous otitis media, unspecified ear

471.0/J33.0   Polyp of nasal cavity

471.8/J33.8   Other polyp of sinus

472.0/J31.0   Chronic rhinitis

473.0/J32.0   Chronic maxillary sinusitis

473.1/J32.1   Chronic frontal sinusitis

473.2/J32.2   Chronic ethmoidal sinusitis

473.3/J32.3   Chronic sphenoidal sinusitis

473.8/J32.4   Chronic pansinusitis

473.8/J32.8   Other chronic sinusitis

473.9/J32.9   Chronic sinusitis, unspecified

477.0/J30.1   Allergic rhinitis due to pollen

477.8/J30.2   Other seasonal allergic rhinitis

477.8/J30.89   Other allergic rhinitis

477.9/J30.0   Vasomotor rhinitis

477.9/J30.9   Allergic rhinitis, unspecified

--/J45.2   Mild intermittent asthma

--/J44   Other chronic obstructive pulmonary disease

493.90/J45.909   Unspecified asthma, uncomplicated

493.90/J45.998   Other asthma

493.91/J45.902   Unspecified asthma with status asthmaticus

493.92/J45.901   Unspecified asthma with (acute) exacerbation

691.8/L20.0   Besnier's prurigo

691.8/L20.81   Atopic neurodermatitis

691.8/L20.82   Flexural eczema

691.8/L20.84   Intrinsic (allergic) eczema

691.8/L20.89   Other atopic dermatitis

692.0/L24.0   Irritant contact dermatitis due to detergents

692.1/L24.1   Irritant contact dermatitis due to oils and grease

692.2/L24.2   Irritant contact dermatitis due to solvents

692.3/L25.1   Unspecified contact dermatitis due to drugs in contact with skin

692.4/L25.3   Unspecified contact dermatitis due to other chemical products

692.5/L25.4   Unspecified contact dermatitis due to food in contact with skin

692.6/L25.5   Unspecified contact dermatitis due to plants, except food

692.81/L25.0   Unspecified contact dermatitis due to cosmetics

692.83/L23.0   Allergic contact dermatitis due to metals

692.83/L24.81   Irritant contact dermatitis due to metals

692.84/L23.81   Allergic contact dermatitis due to animal (cat) (dog) dander

692.89/L25.2   Unspecified contact dermatitis due to dyes

692.89/L25.8   Unspecified contact dermatitis due to other agents

692.9/L25.9   Unspecified contact dermatitis, unspecified cause

693.1/L27.2   Dermatitis due to ingested food

698.9/L29.9   Pruritus, unspecified

708.0/L50.0   Allergic urticaria

708.1/L50.1   Idiopathic urticaria

708.8/L50.6   Contact urticarial

708.8/L50.8   Other urticaria

786.07/R06.2   Wheezing

786.2/R05   Cough

995.0/T78.2XXA   Anaphylactic shock, unspecified, initial encounter

995.1/T78.3XXA   Angioneurotic edema, initial encounter

995.27/T50.995A   Adverse effect of other drugs, medicaments and biological substances,   initial encounter

995.3/T78.40XA   Allergy, unspecified, initial encounter

V14.0/Z88.0   Allergy status to penicillin

V14.1/Z88.1   Allergy status to other antibiotic agents status

V14.2/Z88.2   Allergy status to sulfonamides status

V14.3/Z88.3   Allergy status to other anti-infective agents status

V15.01/Z91.010   Allergy to peanuts

V15.02/Z91.011   Allergy to milk products

V15.03/Z91.012   Allergy to eggs

V15.04/Z91.013   Allergy to seafood

V15.05/Z91.018   Allergy to other foods

V15.07/Z91.040   Latex allergy status

Definition of Procedure Codes

Office Testing to Confirm IgE-Mediated Allergy

InVitro Allergy Testing (IVAT; RAST or ELISA)

Due to the overhead associated with establishing and maintaining an in vitro serological allergy testing laboratory in the office (RAST or ELISA), as well as the burdensome regulatory standards that need to be adhered to (CLIA certification and other federal/state specific regulations), most physician practices send patients to an outside reference laboratory for IVAT (allergy lab test CPT 86000-86999).

Skin Testing

- Intradermal testing, 95024
- Intradermal dilutional titration testing (IDT), 95027
- Prick testing, 95004
- Allergy testing, drugs (eg, penicillin), 95018
- Intradermal testing with delayed reading, 95028

Immunotherapy

- Typically we do not bill the bundled vial preparation and shot code (95120, 95125). For the most part, payers (including Medicare) prefer billing the "unbundled" codes—one code for the injection (95115, 95117) and a second code for the vial (usually 95165).
- Avoid overtesting (in vivo and in vitro for the same antigen). Repeat testing for the same antigen by different techniques does not necessarily increase diagnostic yield but does add cost.
- Nurse practitioners and physician assistants can perform testing on their own but cannot supervise anyone (eg, nurse, medical assistant, allergy tech) performing testing. Physician extenders can, however, supervise someone giving immunotherapy injections.

Example of Billing for Typical Allergy Skin Test Patient

A clinician orders allergy testing on a patient. The patient is tested for 15 allergens.

The billing for the testing is

CPT 95004 × 15 units (prick testing of 15 separate allergens)

or

CPT 95024 × 15 units (intradermal testing of 15 allergens with a single concentration of each allergen)

or

CPT 95027 × 45 units (IDT test of 15 allergens with 3 concentrations of each allergen)

The example of 95027 assumes an average of 3 sticks or dilutional tests per antigen (eg, dilution #6, #4, and #2)

A clinician then prepares a 10-dose multidose vial for a patient. At that same encounter, one dose from the vial is administered by one injection to the patient. The encounter is billed as CPT 95165 × 10 in the unit box and one injection CPT 95115. In this scenario when the patient returns for the next injection this would be billed as 95115 until the vial is depleted.

Controversial Areas

1. Preparation of vial (CPT code 95165). Medicare does not follow the CPT definition. Medicare defines a billable dose (or unit on the claim form) as 1cc aliquot from a single multidose vial containing 10cc—maximum 10 doses per vial. Do not bill Medicare for dilution from concentrate. The physician should report a maximum of 10 doses per vial, even if more or less than 10 injections are obtained from that 10cc vial. For example, a physician may provide 20, 0.5cc doses but still may only report to Medicare 10, 1cc doses.

2. Medicare, and good practice, requires direct physician supervision in the office/allergy suite during testing, but the physician does not need to be in the room. Medicare's "incident to" provisions apply when therapeutic service(s) are provided such as immunotherapy injections CPT 95115, 95117, as well as, preparation of antigens for immunotherapy CPT codes 95144 and 95165.

Allergy testing CPT codes 95004, 95024, 95027, 95028 are covered under Medicare's physician supervision for diagnostic testing guidelines and require direct physician supervision. There are three levels of supervision:

a. General Supervision: the procedure is performed under the physician's overall direction and control, but the physician's presence is not required during the performance of the procedure. The physician is, however, responsible for the training of the nonphysician personnel actually performing the test, and also the maintenance of supplies and equipment necessary for performing that procedure. Currently, there are no allergy testing codes that require general supervision.

b. Direct Supervision: the physician must be present in the office and must be immediately available to provide assistance and direction throughout the performance of the procedure. The allergy testing codes (95004, 95024, 95027, 95028) all require direct physician supervision at this time.

c. Personal Supervision: the physician must be present in the room during the performance of the procedure. There are no allergy-related CPT codes requiring personal supervision currently.

Medicare guidelines allow Physician Assistants (PA) and Nurse Practitioners (NP) to bill for supervised immunotherapy services. However, Medicare does not allow PAs and NPs to bill for supervised testing because diagnostic testing is required to be supervised by a physician.

3. Commercial payers may have limits on the number of tests and how often a patient can be tested.

4. Sublingual Immunotherapy (SLIT)
   a. SLIT is not currently FDA approved and therefore constitutes "off-label" treatment and may not be covered by insurance carriers.
   b. There is no designated CPT code for SLIT; therefore, when submitting a CPT code one has to use CPT code 95199, Unlisted allergy/clinical immunologic service or procedure.
   c. If SLIT is not covered, notification should be given to the patient and a written agreement to pay for drops should be signed by the patient prior to starting treatment.
   d. Do not use CPT code 95165 for SLIT unless you (and the patient) have a written policy from the carrier that this an appropriate code to use.
   e. Patient education regarding practice policy and payer policy regarding SLIT coverage and payment should be performed and clearly documented prior to starting therapy.

Allergy Evaluation and Management (E/M) Services

- Accurate diagnosis coding and documentation is essential; demonstrate medical necessity for initial diagnostic testing, implementation of treatment (eg, immunotherapy), and comment on clinical status, improvement (or lack thereof) at follow-up visits, and justification for continued treatment.
- Use a diagnosis code other than allergic rhinitis for a visit occurring on the same day of an allergy shot, if for a different problem (sinusitis, hoarseness, hearing loss, etc) to facilitate payment for both services.

American Medical Association (AMA) CPT and ICD-9-CM/ICD-10-CM guidelines should always be adhered to. Guidelines with respect to documentation, coding and billing are subject to change. Insurance carrier interpretation, adoption, and implementation of guidelines with respect to coverage and reimbursement may vary, both by carrier and by region. Otolaryngologists should remain well informed and vigilant of these issues to ensure optimal patient outcomes and fair reimbursement.

CHAPTER 14

Office Laryngology

John W. Ingle and Clark A. Rosen

Introduction

Advances in office-based procedures in laryngology present a unique opportunity to provide patients advanced, safe, comfortable, and cost-effective care of laryngeal conditions.[1] The procedures are well tolerated with a high completion rate and high level of patient satisfaction.[2] The rise in the number of office-based laryngology procedures necessitates the need for a practical guide on how to consider the most appropriate coding and billing for these procedures. The billing and coding process for office-based laryngology procedures is in flux, as new codes for vocal fold injection and office-based laser treatments are in the developmental phase.

The process can be quite challenging when one is establishing a laryngology practice in a region where insurance companies are unfamiliar with advances in the field of laryngology. This often requires persistence and patience with prior authorizations, denied claims, and education of the payers. It is helpful to provide coverage policies from other major insurance companies for procedures such as vocal fold injection. Providing appropriate journal articles can also be very helpful, especially during peer-to-peer reviews of prior authorizations and appeals for denied claims. Most issues can be resolved in peer-to-peer reviews; specifically requesting a review by an otolaryngologist can be helpful. Including the medical director of the insurance company in these communications can also reduce or eliminate a duplicative process.

This chapter and the medical literature will often refer to procedures as "office-based." Despite the term "office-based," these laryngology procedures can be performed in a variety of settings. These settings include an exam room, a clinic procedure room, or a procedure room at an outpatient surgery center. "Office-based" procedures refer to procedures typically performed under local anesthesia only, with the patient in an upright and seated position, without sedation, and without an anesthesia practitioner. Some surgeons choose to incorporate sedation along with local anesthesia for select patients and select procedures in the appropriate setting. It is important to know your site of service and if you are billing office-based laryngology procedures from a facility/hospital-based setting/clinic (eg, place of service code 11) versus a non-facility-/non-hospital-based setting/clinic (eg, place of service code 22). Site of service has important implications for reimbursement for supplies, medications, laser fibers, and vocal fold injection implant materials. Whether the equipment, such as the electromyography machine, is hospital owned or department owned can have some implications for billing as well.

Healthcare Common Procedure Coding System (HCPCS) Level II J codes are supply codes used to report injectable drugs that ordinarily cannot be self-administered (eg, botulinum toxin, cidofovir, or injectable steroid). Facility-/hospital-based settings allow the billing of a separate facility fee, with the use of J codes and other HCPCS Level II codes for certain implant materials, supplies, medications, and disposables. The reimbursement for these items in non-facility-/

135

non-hospital-based clinic settings is included in the reimbursement for the billed *Current Procedural Terminology* (CPT) codes or alternatively paid by the patient if allowed by the payer. The cost of laser fibers, implant materials, and disposables may make one setting for performing the procedure more appropriate than the other for different practices, clinical situations, insurances, and locations.

Linking of *International Classification of Diseases, Ninth Revision, Clinical Modification* (ICD-9-CM) and *International Classification of Diseases, Tenth Revision, Clinical Modification* (ICD-10-CM) diagnoses codes to appropriate CPT procedural codes is essential to ensure timely and adequate reimbursement for the care delivered and the procedures performed. Properly linking codes will help to ensure reimbursement especially when multiple diagnostics or therapeutic procedures are performed at the same clinical visit. One must also consider appropriate linking of speech pathology CPT codes with appropriate ICD-9-CM/ICD-10-CM codes when speech pathology procedures are billed in association with a clinical visit. Please refer to Chapter 15, "Speech Pathology," for more information.

Key Points

- Many laryngeal codes are for use in the operating room only, as these assume general anesthesia is used. It is not appropriate to use these particular codes in the office setting.
- Do not use the flexible esophagoscopy code (43200) for transnasal esophagoscopy, as new transnasal esophagoscopy codes were added in 2014 (43197, 43198).
- Botox codes changed in 2013. CPT 64617 was added for percutaneous injection, and 64613 was deleted.
- When performing Botox it is helpful to understand the HCPC code (J0585) for the units used and the HCPCS Level II modifier (JW) for the units wasted.

- Office-based laryngology procedures are a vital part of a robust laryngology practice, and proper billing and coding is essential to the success of the practice and to the professional integrity of the field of laryngology.

Key Procedure Codes

Therapeutic Vocal Fold Injection Procedures

The unlisted code should be used for flexible laryngoscopy with injection into vocal cord when performed transorally or through the working channel of the flexible scope. This also includes when done through the mouth using a rigid 70-degree scope. Vocal cord injections are one or both cords; however, chemodenervation is a unilateral code and may be reported twice by using modifier 50.

31570 Laryngoscopy, direct, with injection into vocal cord(s), therapeutic;
wRVU 3.86; Global 0

> **31571** with operating microscope or telescope
> *wRVU 4.26; Global 0*

31599 Unlisted procedure, larynx
wRVU 0.00; Global YYY

64617 Chemodenervation of muscle(s); larynx, unilateral, percutaneous (eg, for spasmodic dysphonia), includes guidance by needle electromyography, when performed
wRVU 1.90; Global 10

CPT 64617 includes all laryngeal botulinum toxin injections performed **percutaneously**, despite method for guidance; electromyography (EMG), flexible laryngoscopy, point-touch technique.[3] Do not include 95874 for needle electromyography guidance as this is already included in 64617.

Vocal Fold/Larynx Laser-Based Procedures

31540 Laryngoscopy, direct, operative, with excision of tumor and/or stripping of vocal cords or epiglottis;
wRVU 4.12; Global 0

> **31541** with operating microscope or telescope
> *wRVU 4.52; Global 0*

Botulinum Toxin Injection of Salivary Gland, Facial Muscles, Oral Muscles, Neck Muscles (excluding muscles of the larynx)

For 64611, append modifier 52 if fewer than 4 salivary glands are injected. Report 95874 for needle electromyography guidance when used, noting that absence of the EMG signal confirms placement in salivary gland. For 64612 and 64616 append modifier 50 for bilateral procedures, and report 95874 for needle electromyography guidance when used.

64611 Chemodenervation of parotid and submandibular salivary glands, bilateral
wRVU 1.03; Global 10

64612 Chemodenervation of muscle(s); muscle(s) innervated by facial nerve, unilateral (eg, for blepharospasm, hemifacial spasm)
wRVU 1.41; Global 10

> **64616** neck muscle(s), excluding muscles of the larynx, unilateral (eg, for cervical dystonia, spasmodic torticollis)
> *wRVU 1.53; Global 10*

+95874 Needle electromyography for guidance in conjunction with chemodenervation (List separately in addition to code for primary procedure)
wRVU 0.37; Global ZZZ

HCPCS Codes

These codes do not have relative value units (RVUs) because they are codes for supplies, not physician work.

C1878 Material for vocal cord medialization, synthetic (implantable)

J0585 Injection, onabotulinumtoxinA, 1 unit Botulinum toxin type A (Botox®, Dysport®, Xeomin®) per unit

J0587 Injection, rimabotulinumtoxinB, 100 units Botulinum toxin type B (Myobloc®), per 100 units

J3590 Unclassified biologics

Q2026 Radiesse®, injectable, 0.1 cc

Q4112 Cymetra®, injectable, 1 cc

Flexible Laryngoscopy and Stroboscopy

31575 Laryngoscopy, flexible fiberoptic; diagnostic
wRVU 1.10; Global 0

> **31576** with biopsy
> *wRVU 1.97; Global 0*

> **31577** with removal of foreign body
> *wRVU 2.47; Global 0*

> **31578** with removal of lesion
> *wRVU 2.84; Global 0*

> **31579** Laryngoscopy, flexible or rigid fiberoptic, with stroboscopy
> *wRVU 2.26; Global 0*

Instrumental Swallowing Tests and Laryngeal Sensory Testing

All codes listed below include the flexible fiberoptic laryngoscopy so do not separately report 31575. Also, all recording codes listed below require permanent images be saved.

92611 Motion fluoroscopic evaluation of swallowing function by cine or video recording
wRVU 1.34; Global XXX

This is also known as videofluoroscopic swallowing study (VFSS) or modified barium swallow (MBS) study. For radiologic supervision and interpretation, only use 74230.

92612 Flexible fiberoptic endoscopic evaluation of swallowing by cine or video recording;
wRVU 1.27; Global XXX

Commonly referred to as FEES.

> **92613** interpretation and report only
> *wRVU 0.71; Global XXX*

This code is typically reported by the physician.

92614 Flexible fiberoptic endoscopic evaluation, laryngeal sensory testing by cine or video recording;
wRVU 1.27; Global XXX

This code is for laryngeal sensory testing only.

> **92615** interpretation and report only
> *wRVU 0.63; Global XXX*

This code is typically reported by the physician.

92616 Flexible fiberoptic endoscopic evaluation of swallowing and laryngeal sensory testing by cine or video recording;
wRVU 1.88; Global XXX

Commonly referred to as FEESST.

> **92617** interpretation and report only
> *wRVU 0.79; Global XXX*

This code is typically reported by the physician.

Transnasal Esophagoscopy

Transnasal esophagoscopy codes were added in 2014. A code exists for diagnosis as well as a separate code for when a biopsy is performed. There is also a code for performing a tracheoesophageal fistula. Some otolaryngologists and laryngologists perform creation of the tracheoesophageal fistula for placement of a laryngeal speech prosthesis/

tracheoesophageal prosthesis (TEP valve) under local anesthesia in the office-based setting.[4,5] The procedure is safe and effective for secondary TEP placement in patients who underwent laryngectomy. The procedure requires a channeled transnasal esophagoscopy (TNE) scope with insufflation. Use 31611 when this is done. The transnasal esophagoscopy should not be billed separately when this is done, even if used for visualization.

43197 Esophagoscopy, flexible, transnasal; diagnostic, including collection of specimen(s) by brushing or washing, when performed (separate procedure)
wRVU 1.52; Global 0

> **43198** with biopsy, single or multiple
> *wRVU 1.82; Global 0*

31611 Construction of tracheoesophageal fistula and subsequent insertion of an alaryngeal speech prosthesis (eg, voice button, Blom-Singer prosthesis)
wRVU 6.00; Global 90

Flexible Bronchoscopy

31615 Tracheobronchoscopy through established tracheostomy incision
wRVU 2.09; Global 0

31622 Bronchoscopy, rigid or flexible, including fluoroscopic guidance, when performed; diagnostic, with cell washing, when performed (separate procedure)
wRVU 2.78; Global 0

> **31623** with brushing or protected brushings
> *wRVU 2.88; Global 0*

Key Modifiers

JW Drug amount discarded/not administered to any patient
This is a HCPCS Level II modifier that can be used to indicate when botulinum toxin was wasted and the entire vial was not used on the patient.

50 Bilateral Procedure

Used for unilateral procedures when done on both sides. For example use in 64617 when both sides are injected.

52 Reduced Services

Used when the procedure requires less work or is reduced in nature. For example, use on 64611 when less than 4 glands are injected.

Key ICD-9-CM/ICD-10-CM Codes

212.1/D14.1   Benign neoplasm of larynx
(eg, recurrent respiratory papillomatosis of larynx, adenomatous polyps)

333.1/G25.0   Essential tremor
(includes benign essential tremor and essential voice tremor)

333.81/G24.5   Blepharospasm

333.82/G24.4   Idiopathic orofacial dystonia
(includes oromandibular dystonia,
Meige syndrome—blepharospasm with oromandibular dystonia)

333.83/G24.3   Spasmodic torticollis

351.8/G51.2   Melkersson syndrome

351.8/G51.4   Facial myokymia

351.8/G51.8   Other disorders of facial nerve
(eg, Hemifacial spasm)

356.9/G60.9   Hereditary and idiopathic neuropathy, unspecified

438.82/I69.991   Dysphagia following unspecified cerebrovascular disease

464.0/J04.0   Acute laryngitis
(eg, not otherwise specified, edematous, *Haemophilus influenzae*, pneumococcal, septic, supportive, ulcerative)

464.10/J04.10   Acute tracheitis without obstruction

464.11/J04.11   Acute tracheitis with obstruction

476.0/J37.0   Chronic laryngitis
(eg, catarrhal, hypertrophic, sicca)

478.30/J38.00   Paralysis of vocal cords and larynx, unspecified

478.31/J38.01   Paralysis of vocal cords and larynx, unilateral

478.32/J38.01   Paralysis of vocal cords and larynx, unilateral
(used to be partial or complete)

478.33/J38.02   Paralysis of vocal cords and larynx, bilateral

478.34/J38.02   Paralysis of vocal cords and larynx, bilateral
(used to be partial or complete)

478.4/J38.1   Polyp of vocal cord and larynx

478.5/J38.3   Other diseases of vocal cords
(includes glottic insufficiency, vocal fold scar, sulcus vocalis, granuloma, chorditis-fibrinous, nodosa, tuberosa, singer's nodes)

478.6/J38.4   Edema of the larynx

478.71/J38.7   Other disease of larynx

478.74/J38.6   Stenosis of larynx

478.75/J38.5   Laryngeal spasm
(definition involuntary muscle contraction of the larynx) (some otolaryngologists uses code for spasmodic dysphonia)

478.79/J38.7   Other disease of larynx
(some otolaryngologists use this code for spasmodic dysphonia and laryngopharyngeal reflux)

490/J40   Bronchitis, not specified as acute or chronic

519.19/J39.8   Other specified diseases of upper respiratory tract

519.19/J98.09   Other diseases of bronchus, not elsewhere classified
(eg, tracheal stenosis, tracheomalacia, bronchomalacia)

527.7/K11.7   Disturbances of salivary secretion
(including sialorrhea, ptyalism)

530.0/K22.0 Achalasia of cardia
(eg, Cricopharyngeal achalasia)

530.11/K21.0 Gastro-esophageal reflux
disease with esophagitis

786.09/R06.00 Dyspnea, unspecified

786.09/R06.09 Other forms of dyspnea

786.09/R06.3 Periodic breathing

786.09/R06.83 Snoring

786.09/R06.89 Other abnormalities of
breathing

748.2/Q31.0 Web of larynx

748.3/Q31.1 Congenital subglottic stenosis

748.3/Q31.3 Laryngocele

748.3/Q31.8 Other congenital malformation
of larynx

748.3/Q32.1 Other congenital malformations
of trachea

748.3/Q32.4 Other congenital malformations
of bronchus

786.1/R06.1 Stridor

787.2/-- Dysphagia

787.20/R13.0 Aphagia

787.20/R13.10 Dysphagia, unspecified

787.21/R13.11 Dysphagia, oral phase

787.22/R13.12 Dysphagia, oropharyngeal
phase

787.23/R13.13 Dysphagia, pharyngeal phase

787.24/R13.14 Dysphagia,
pharyngoesophageal phase
(includes cricopharyngeal dysphagia)

787.29/R13.19 Other dysphagia
(eg, cervical dysphagia, neurogenic dysphagia,
cricopharyngeal hypertrophy, cricopharyngeal
spasm)

Definition of Codes

Diagnostic Office-Based Laryngology Procedures

1. Diagnostic procedures
   a. *Definitions*—diagnostic office-based laryngology procedures are the most frequently billed procedures for many laryngologists and otolaryngologists. Adequate documentation of these procedures as essential in order to justify the reimbursement for the work done, the resources and equipment used, and the expert interpretation and diagnoses made related to the findings.
   b. *Key Points*—stroboscopy reports should contain adequate documentation describing the essential features of the mucosal wave of musculomembranous true vocal fold and the vocal fold closure pattern at minimum. Other common reported aspects include presence of masses, symmetry, and phase of vibration. Using commonly held standards for interpretation of stroboscopy exams is a good guide to performing adequate documentation. There has been a favorable rise in the number of office-based biopsies of laryngeal and pharyngeal lesions, assisted by advancements in smaller flexible endoscopes with working channels to pass biopsy forceps. Office-based biopsy can offer cost-effective and expedited time to treatment for many appropriately selected patients.[6,7]

Therapeutic Office-Based Procedures

1. Vocal fold/larynx injection procedures with flexible laryngoscopes:
   a. *Definitions*—vocal fold/larynx injection procedures can be divided into therapeutic or augmentation. Common procedures of the former include vocal fold/larynx injection of any therapeutic substance such as steroid injections or medications such as bevacizumab or cidofovir. The most com

mon vocal fold injection procedure is injection augmentation with a filler substance; sometimes referred to as injection laryngoplasty or injection medialization laryngoplasty. Some of the commonly injected materials include carboxymethylcellulose, calcium hydroxyapatite,[8] micronized human dermis, collagen, and hyaluronic acid. The procedure is used to treat glottic insufficiency from conditions such as vocal fold immobility, hypomobility, paralysis, paresis, vocal fold atrophy, or vocal fold scar. The traditional injection augmentation procedure is performed under general anesthesia, with direct visualization of the vocal folds through a laryngoscope, or visualization through the laryngoscopy with a microscope or telescope (CPT codes 31570 or 31571). In contrast, the "office-based" procedure is performed with visualization of the vocal folds with a flexible transnasal laryngoscope or rigid 70-degree transoral laryngoscope in an awake and upright patient under local anesthesia.[9] The injection needle can be passed through the working channel of the flexible scope, through the mouth, or through the neck.[10] Office-based vocal fold injection augmentation is both clinically and financially effective.[11]

b. *Key Points*—existing CPT codes for laryngoscopy with vocal fold injection such as 31570 and 31571 were created for injections performed under general anesthesia, and are exclusively operative billing codes. Operative billing codes indicate that the vocal fold injection procedure was performed when the patient is under general anesthesia, with visualization of the true vocal folds either directly (31570) or with telescope or microscopic visualization (31571). These billing codes do not describe vocal fold injection procedures performed with a flexible laryngoscope or transoral rigid 70-degree laryngoscope and in an awake or a sedated patient. As a result, 31599 (Unlisted procedure, larynx) should be submitted and can be compared

to an existing code (ie, 31570, 31571) with supporting documentation. Some payers have been rejecting the use of the unlisted code and thus appealing this may be necessary (see Chapter 6, "Successful Navigation of the Appeals Process").

2. Vocal fold/larynx laser treatments with flexible laryngoscopes
   a. *Definitions*—office-based laser treatments of laryngeal conditions have expanded as flexible laser technology has been developed and subsequently applied as a treatment for a variety of laryngeal conditions.[12,13] Benign laryngeal neoplasms such as recurrent respiratory papillomatosis are increasingly being treated with office-based KTP laser treatments. Specific benign vocal fold lesions are sometimes preferentially and successfully treated with office-based KTP laser.[14,15]
   b. *Key Points*—CPT 31599 is the appropriate code for laser treatments of the larynx performed with flexible laryngoscopes and transoral 70-degree rigid laryngoscopes, in awake or sedated patient. Operative codes such as 31540 and 31541 describe the use of a laser for laryngeal conditions performed under direct laryngoscopy or laryngoscopy with a telescope or microscope, in patients under general anesthesia. Office-based laser laryngeal surgery is safe and cost-effective for payers. However, in a non-facility-based office, there are often net financial losses.[16] An appropriate new CPT code for office-based laser laryngeal procedures is expected in the future to address this problem.

3. Botulinum toxin injections of the larynx, neck muscles, and salivary glands
   a. *Definitions*—laryngeal botulinum toxin (Botox) injections for spasmodic dysphonia and essential voice tremor are a routine part of an office-based laryngeal practice. The CPT code used for laryngeal Botox injections can differ based on whether or not the injection is performed percutane-

ously, transorally, or through the working channel of the flexible laryngoscope. The codes also differ significantly if the botulinum toxin injection is performed operatively under general anesthesia. The CPT code used for office-based percutaneous botulinum toxin changed in 2013. The most appropriate CPT code for percutaneous laryngeal Botox injections is 64617. Older codes that are no longer used for the procedure include 64613, which was deleted in 2013.

b. *Key Points*—adding the CPT code 95873 or 95874 for electrical stimulation needle or electromyography guidance in conjunction with chemodenervation is no longer accurate and neither code should be reported with 64617. The work of the electromyography and/or needle guidance is now bundled with the work of the injection and the new RVUs reflect this change. Insurance companies have different policies for coverage of the botulinum toxin used for laryngeal injections; some companies prefer to pay for an entire bottle for each patient; however, most reimburse for units used. Check with your local companies to understand policy for the setting that you practice in. Many otolaryngologists bill for the number of units used for each patient, including those used to prime the syringe and needle. The appropriate J code is J0585 onabotulinumtoxinA, 1 unit (report the number of units used). Medicare will reimburse for unused ("waste") botulinum toxin that is wasted during the procedure, if the remainder of the vial is discarded; in this situation you must code with a JW modifier and you must report the number of units in the vial wasted. You can refer to CMS transmittal 1248 for more information (https://www.cms.gov/Regulations-and-Guidance/Guidance/Transmittals/downloads/R1248CP.pdf). Accurate documentation of botulinum toxin injected, the location(s), amount of botulinum toxin wasted should be maintained for each patient in a separate procedure note.

Accurate electronic and/or paper logs are essential.

Instrumental Swallowing and Laryngeal Sensory Tests

1. Swallowing evaluation
   a. *Definitions*—office-based evaluation of swallowing can provide timely evaluation[17] and patient guidance for appropriate liquid and food consistencies to facilitate swallowing rehabilitation and reduce the risk of aspiration. Compensatory strategies can be trialed during the exam. The studies are typically performed by speech-language pathologists in many settings. Some otolaryngologist and laryngologist physicians with special training perform radiologic and endoscopic instrumental swallowing tests; others only interpret the tests and write reports based on their interpretation.
   b. *Key Points*—the CPT codes are different based on whether or not the physician actually performed the exam or just interpreted the exam. The CPT codes billed by physicians are different from those used by speech-language pathologists. Some practices decide to have the physician perform these procedures in conjunction with speech pathology. The physician may bill for the actual procedure or may only bill the interpretation code. Both the physician and the speech pathologist cannot bill for performing the procedure. Please refer to Chapter 15 on billing for speech-language pathology for speech pathology billing codes.

Office-Based Transnasal Esophagoscopy

1. Transnasal esophagoscopy
   a. *Definitions*—office-based transnasal esophagoscopy and gastroscopy (TNE) is a safe, well-tolerated and cost-effective procedure that is typically performed under local

anesthesia.[18,19] The procedure is indicated in patients with significant laryngopharyngeal reflux and/or gastroesophageal reflux where endoscopic evaluation of the esophagus and stomach would be helpful. Typically, patients with biliary colic symptoms, pancreatitis symptoms, or lower gastrointestinal symptoms are best of evaluated by gastroenterology with an esophagogastroduodenoscopy (EGD) procedure in lieu of performing transnasal esophagoscopy.

b. *Key Points*—CPT codes for TNE were added in 2014 and thus older flexible esophagoscopy codes (eg, 43200) should not be used for TNE. The specific codes for TNE must be used if the flexible scope is passed through the nasal cavity to visualize the esophagus and or gastric cavity. A complete exam includes retroflexion of the scope to visualize the gastroesophageal junction. If the flexible scope is passed through the oral cavity or if a rigid esophagoscope was used, an entirely different set of CPT codes are applicable.

Office-Based Flexible Bronchoscopy

1. Flexible bronchoscopy
   a. *Definitions*—flexible bronchoscopy performed entirely under local anesthesia is a useful diagnostic tool for patients with airway stenosis and unknown sources of stridor or dyspnea.[20] The most commonly billed CPT is 31622. It provides an awake dynamic airway examination prior to any possible operative intervention. It can often identify membranous airway stenoses that are thin and otherwise missed by standard wide cut CT scans of the chest. It is very useful in patients with multilevel airway stenosis. It can be more useful and safer than sedated bronchoscopy at identifying patients with tracheomalacia and/or bronchomalacia. It is more cost-effective than sedated bronchoscopy and can be safely performed by otolaryngologists and laryngologists who are skilled in deliver-

ing local anesthesia to the nasal cavity, larynx, and lower airway.
   b. *Key Points*—a complete exam includes passing the tip of the flexible bronchoscope beyond the carina to evaluate the bronchi and to rule out bronchial pathology. If the larynx and trachea are evaluated but the tip of the scope is not passed beyond the carina to evaluate the bronchial airways, then the correct CPT is 31575 (Laryngoscopy, flexible fiberoptic, diagnostic). The office-based tracheal airway exam performed in nonsedated pediatric patients[21] is typically billed with CPT 31575 because the scope is typically not passed beyond the carina to evaluate the distal bronchial airways. These pediatric patients typically receive topical anesthesia of the nasal cavity only. Adult patients typically receive direct topical anesthesia of the larynx and lower airway. Topical anesthesia of the larynx and lower airway often involves nebulization and drip catheter delivery of local anesthetics with additional time, effort, and equipment such as channeled bronchoscopes and anesthesia drip catheters.

Controversial Areas

Use of 31599 Unlisted procedure, larynx

CPT 31599, Unlisted procedure, larynx is the most appropriate code at this time for laser procedures and vocal fold injection procedures assisted with flexible laryngoscopy. This will likely only be a temporary measure until the new CPT codes are released for use.

Office-based balloon dilation procedures of the esophagus, larynx, and airway under local anesthesia are being performed in small numbers in select clinical settings.[20,22,23] Some centers are performing office-based transnasal esophagoscope-guided botulinum toxin injection of the esophagus.[24] The billing and coding for this procedure was not included in this chapter because it is typically performed by gastroenterologists.

Multidose Botox Bottle

There is controversy with the concept of a multidose bottle for multiple patients versus a single-dose bottle. Many otolaryngology providers utilize a 100-unit botulinum toxin bottle as multidose bottle. Each patient typically requires a small amount of botulinum toxin for each laryngeal injection (general range of less than 1 unit up to 10 units). Although dosing regimens range widely between patients and practicing otolaryngologists, the amount of botulinum toxin used per patient is relatively small in comparison to the size of the bottle. Patients require individualized dosing regimens in order to maximize voice functional outcomes and minimize the side effects of therapy.[25] Controversy also exists on the shelf life of the botulinum toxin after it has been mixed. There is a discrepancy between manufacturer recommendations and studies that have demonstrated full efficacy and safety of the botulinum toxin used in a multiple patient fashion, even weeks after it was mixed and properly stored in refrigeration.[26]

Conclusion

Billing and coding for office-based laryngology procedures is a moving target as new codes are being developed for office-based vocal fold injection procedures and office-based laser procedures. Adequate documentation of procedures is essential in order to convey the work performed, resources, equipment utilized, and the expert interpretation of these exams for accurate diagnosis.

References

1. Rosen CA, Amin MR, Sulica L, et al. Advances in office-based diagnosis and treatment in laryngology. *Laryngoscope.* 2009;119 (suppl) 2:S185–212. doi:10.1002/lary.20712.
2. Young VN, Smith LJ, Sulica L, Krishna P, Rosen CA. Patient tolerance of awake, in-office laryngeal pro-cedures: a multi-institutional perspective. *Laryngoscope.* 2012;122(2):315–321. doi:10.1002/lary.22185.
3. Morzaria S, Damrose EJ. The point-touch technique for botulinum toxin injection in adductor spasmodic dysphonia: quality of life assessment. *J Laryngol Otol.* 2011;125(7):714–718. doi:10.1017/S0022215111000739.
4. LeBert B, McWhorter AJ, Kunduk M, et al. Secondary tracheoesophageal puncture with in-office transnasal esophagoscopy. *Arch Otolaryngol Head Neck Surg.* 2009;135(12):1190–1194. doi:10.1001/archoto.2009.166.
5. Britt CJ, Lippert D, Kammer R, et al. Secondary tracheoesophageal puncture in-office using Seldinger technique. *Otolaryngol Head Neck Surg.* 2014;150(5):808–812. doi:10.1177/0194599814521570.
6. Lippert D, Hoffman MR, Dang P, McCulloch TM, Hartig GK, Dailey SH. In-office biopsy of upper airway lesions: safety, tolerance, and effect on time to treatment. *Laryngoscope.* 2014. doi:10.1002/lary.25007.
7. Richards AL, Sugumaran M, Aviv JE, Woo P, Altman KW. The utility of office-based biopsy for laryngopharyngeal lesions: comparison with surgical evaluation. *Laryngoscope.* 2014. doi:10.1002/lary.25005.
8. Rosen CA, Gartner-Schmidt J, Casiano R, et al. Vocal fold augmentation with calcium hydroxylapatite: twelve-month report. *Laryngoscope.* 2009; 119(5):1033–1041. doi:10.1002/lary.20126.
9. Mallur PS, Rosen CA. Office-based laryngeal injections. *Otolaryngol Clin North Am.* 2013;46(1):85–100. doi:10.1016/j.otc.2012.08.020.
10. Zeitler DM, Amin MR. The thyrohyoid approach to in-office injection augmentation of the vocal fold. *Curr Opin Otolaryngol Head Neck Surg.* 2007;15(6):412–416. doi:10.1097/MOO.0b013e3282f033ec.
11. Bové MJ, Jabbour N, Krishna P, et al. Operating room versus office-based injection laryngoplasty: a comparative analysis of reimbursement. *Laryngoscope.* 2007;117(2):226–230. doi:10.1097/01.mlg.0000250898.82268.39.
12. Zeitels SM, Burns JA. Office-based laryngeal laser surgery with the 532-nm pulsed-potassium-titanyl-phosphate laser. *Curr Opin Otolaryngol Head Neck Surg.* 2007;15(6):394–400. doi:10.1097/MOO.0b013e3282f1fbb2.
13. Franco RA. In-office laryngeal surgery with the 585-nm pulsed dye laser. *Curr Opin Otolaryngol Head Neck Surg.* 2007;15(6):387–393. doi:10.1097/MOO.0b013e3282f19ef2.
14. Sheu M, Sridharan S, Kuhn M, et al. Multi-institutional experience with the in-office potassium tit-

anyl phosphate laser for laryngeal lesions. *J Voice.* 2012;26(6):806–810. doi:10.1016/j.jvoice.2012.04.003.

15. Mallur PS, Tajudeen BA, Aaronson N, Branski RC, Amin MR. Quantification of benign lesion regression as a function of 532-nm pulsed potassium titanyl phosphate laser parameter selection. *Laryngoscope.* 2011;121(3):590–595. doi:10.1002/lary.21354.

16. Kuo CY, Halum SL. Office-based laser surgery of the larynx: cost-effective treatment at the office's expense. *Otolaryngol Head Neck Surg.* 2012;146(5):769–773. doi:10.1177/0194599811434896.

17. Merati AL. In-office evaluation of swallowing: FEES, pharyngeal squeeze maneuver, and FEESST. *Otolaryngol Clin North Am.* 2013;46(1):31–39. doi:10.1016/j.otc.2012.08.015.

18. Amin MR, Postma GN, Setzen M, Koufman JA. Transnasal esophagoscopy: a position statement from the American Bronchoesophagological Association (ABEA). *Otolaryngol Head Neck Surg.* 2008;138(4):411–414. doi:10.1016/j.otohns.2007.12.032.

19. Bush CM, Postma GN. Transnasal esophagoscopy. *Otolaryngol Clin North Am.* 2013;46(1):41–52. doi:10.1016/j.otc.2012.08.016.

20. Belafsky PC, Kuhn MA. Office airway surgery. *Otolaryngol Clin North Am.* 2013;46(1):63–74. doi:10.1016/j.otc.2012.08.018.

21. Eshaq M, Chun RE, Martin T, Link TR, Kerschner JE. Office-based lower airway endoscopy (OLAE) in pediatric patients: a high-value procedure. *Int J Pediatr Otorhinolaryngol.* 2014;78(3):489–492. doi:10.1016/j.ijporl.2013.12.026.

22. Rees CJ, Fordham T, Belafsky PC. Transnasal balloon dilation of the esophagus. *Arch Otolaryngol Head Neck Surg.* 2009;135(8):781–783. doi:10.1001/archoto.2009.115.

23. Rees CJ. In-office unsedated transnasal balloon dilation of the esophagus and trachea. *Curr Opin Otolaryngol Head Neck Surg.* 2007;15(6):401–404. doi:10.1097/MOO.0b013e3282f1a92c.

24. Rees CJ. In-office transnasal esophagoscope-guided botulinum toxin injection of the lower esophageal sphincter. *Curr Opin Otolaryngol Head Neck Surg.* 2007;15(6):409–411. doi:10.1097/MOO.0b013e3282f1bf39.

25. Novakovic D, Waters HH, D'Elia JB, Blitzer A. Botulinum toxin treatment of adductor spasmodic dysphonia: longitudinal functional outcomes. *Laryngoscope.* 2011;121(3):606–612. doi:10.1002/lary.21395.

26. Barrow EM, Rosen CA, Hapner ER, et al. Safety and efficacy of multiuse botulinum toxin vials for intralaryngeal injection. *Laryngoscope.* 2014. doi:10.1002/lary.25068.

CHAPTER 15

Speech Pathology

Manderly A. Cohen and Michael Setzen

Introduction

This chapter describes coding and billing for evaluations and treatments that speech-language pathologists (SLPs) routinely perform in an otolaryngology practice. SLP *Current Procedural Terminology* (CPT®) codes are primarily service based. There are also CPT codes that are reported by SLPs that are time based. All other codes are procedure based. That is, the CPT code is reported once regardless of the length of the appointment.

Medicare Improvements for Patients and Providers Act of 2007 (MIPPA), which came into effect July 1, 2009, granted SLPs independent billing. Medicare changed the status of SLPs with the Centers for Medicare and Medicaid Services (CMS) to a Medicare Provider, thereby recognizing SLPs as professionals rather than technical assistants.

Key Points

- CPT 92506 was deleted as of January 1, 2014, and replaced with 4 new evaluation codes related to speech sound production, language, fluency, and voice and resonance (92521–92524).
- Effective October 1, 2011, diagnostic laryngoscopy with stroboscopy (31579) and nasopharyngoscopy (92511) can be billed by independent SLPs without supervision, unless supervision is required by state law or regional

Medicare Administrative Contractors. Laryngoscopy, flexible fiberoptic; diagnostic (31575) cannot be billed by an SLP.

- CMS previously instructed providers to use 92506 for non-speech-generating augmentative and alternative communication device (SGD) evaluation and treatment; this code was deleted as of January 2014. Non-SGD services are considered bundled and should be billed under 92523 or 92507 according to CMS.

Key Procedure Codes

31579 Laryngoscopy, flexible or rigid fiberoptic, with stroboscopy
wRVU 2.26; Global 0

74230 Swallowing function, with cineradiography/videoradiography
wRVU 0.53; Global XXX

92507 Treatment of speech, language, voice, communication, and/or auditory processing disorder; individual
wRVU 1.30; Global XXX

92508 group, 2 or more individuals
wRVU 0.33; Global XXX

92511 Nasopharyngoscopy with endoscope (separate procedure)
wRVU 0.61; Global 0

147

92520   Laryngeal function studies (ie, aerodynamic testing and acoustic testing)
wRVU 0.75; Global XXX

Use modifier 52 if only one test is performed (ie, aerodynamic testing only, acoustic testing only).

92521   Evaluation of speech fluency (eg, stuttering, cluttering)
wRVU 1.75; Global XXX

92522   Evaluation of speech sound production (eg, articulation, phonological process, apraxia, dysarthria)
wRVU 1.50; Global XXX

   92523   with evaluation of language comprehension and expression (eg, receptive and expressive language)
wRVU 3.00; Global XXX

For evaluation of language only, apply a modifier 52.

92524   Behavioral and qualitative analysis of voice and resonance
wRVU 1.50; Global XXX

92526   Treatment of swallowing dysfunction and/or oral function for feeding
wRVU 1.34; Global XXX

There is no dysphagia group therapy code. Medicare payers may accept 97150 based on section 15/230.A of the Medicare Benefit Policy Manual or 92508 for dysphagia group therapy.

92597   Evaluation for use and/or fitting of voice prosthetic device to supplement oral speech
wRVU 1.26; Global XXX

Under Medicare, applies to tracheoesophageal prostheses (eg, Passy-Muir Valve), artificial larynges, as well as voice amplifiers. Use 92507 for training and modification of voice prostheses.

92605   Evaluation for prescription of non-speech-generating augmentative and alternative communication device, face-to-face with the patient; first hour
wRVU 1.75; Global XXX

A communication board that uses pictures, words or symbols is an example of a non-SGD. CMS previ-

ously instructed SLPs to use 92506 for this service. Because 92506 has been deleted, CMS officials state that non-SGD services (evaluation and treatment) are considered "bundled" (ie, not separately billable) and are captured under any other service the SLP provided that day (eg, 92523 or 92507). Currently, this would not be billable under CMS' interpretation.

   #+92618   each additional 30 minutes (List separately in addition to code for primary procedure)
wRVU 0.65; Global ZZZ

92606   Therapeutic service(s) for use of non-speech-generating device, including programming and modification
wRVU 1.40; Global XXX

92607   Evaluation for prescription for speech-generating augmentative and alternative communication device, face-to-face with the patient; first hour
wRVU 1.85; Global XXX

SGDs generate synthesized or digital speech. Include modifier 52 if less than 1 hour.

   +92608   each additional 30 minutes (List separately in addition to code for primary procedure)
wRVU 0.70; Global ZZZ

92609   Therapeutic services for the use of speech-generating device, including programming and modification
wRVU 1.50; Global XXX

92610   Evaluation of oral and pharyngeal swallowing function
wRVU 1.30; Global XXX

92612   Flexible fiberoptic endoscopic evaluation of swallowing by cine or video recording;
wRVU 1.27; Global XXX

FEES. This is the complete endoscopic procedure for evaluation of swallowing. It encompasses both the technical and interpretation aspects of the procedure. Level of physician supervision varies by state. Use 92700 if performed without cine or video recording. 92612 can be billed together with 74230 (Swallowing function, with cineradiography/videoradiography) on the same day. 92612 can be billed by a SLP but 74230 must be billed by a physician.

92613 interpretation and report only
wRVU 0.71; Global XXX

May be appropriate if SLP does not pass the scope but provides interpretation and report. The SLP should not bill 92613 in addition to 92612.

92614 Flexible fiberoptic endoscopic evaluation, laryngeal sensory testing by cine or video recording;
wRVU 1.27; Global XXX

This is not a swallow evaluation; sensory testing only. It encompasses both the technical and interpretation aspects of the procedure.

92615 interpretation and report only
wRVU 0.63; Global XXX

May be appropriate if SLP does not pass the scope but provides interpretation and report. The SLP should not bill in addition to 92614.

92616 Flexible fiberoptic endoscopic evaluation of swallowing and laryngeal sensory testing by cine or video recording;
wRVU 1.88; Global XXX

(FEESST). This is the complete endoscopic procedure for swallowing and sensory testing combined. It encompasses both the technical and interpretation aspects of the procedure. Level of physician supervision varies by state and/or MAC. 92616 can be billed together with 74230 (Swallowing function, with cineradiography/ videoradiography) on the same day. 92616 can be billed by a SLP but 74230 must be billed by a physician.

92617 interpretation and report only
wRVU 0.79; Global XXX

This may be appropriate if SLP does not pass the scope but provides interpretation and report. The SLP should not bill in addition to 92616.

92626 Evaluation of auditory rehabilitation status; first hour
wRVU 1.40; Global XXX

+92627 each additional 15 minutes (List separately in addition to code for primary procedure)
wRVU 0.33; Global ZZZ

92700 Unlisted otorhinolaryngological service or procedure
wRVU 0.00; Global XXX

96105 Assessment of aphasia (includes assessment of expressive and receptive speech and language function, language comprehension, speech production ability, reading, spelling, writing, eg, by Boston Diagnostic Aphasia Examination) with interpretation and report, per hour
wRVU 1.75; Global XXX

96125 Standardized cognitive performance testing (eg, Ross Information Processing Assessment) per hour of a qualified health care professional's time, both face-to-face time administering tests to the patient and time interpreting these test results and preparing the report
wRVU 1.70; Global XXX

97150 Therapeutic procedure(s), group (2 or more individuals)
wRVU 0.29; Global XXX

97532 Development of cognitive skills to improve attention, memory, problem solving (includes compensatory training), direct (one-to-one) patient contact, each 15 minutes
wRVU 0.44; Global XXX

97533 Sensory integrative techniques to enhance sensory processing and promote adaptive responses to environmental demands, direct (one-on-one) patient contact, each 15 minutes
wRVU 0.44; Global XXX

Key Modifiers

Modifiers are used to provide more information about who used the code, or special circumstances regarding the code use.

22 Increased Procedural Services
Indicates a much longer than usual procedure on a non-time-based code. This code should not be used frequently as the Medicare contractor could make the determination that the procedure reflects typical service delivery. A description of

the need for extended services should accompany the claim.

52   Reduced Services
Indicates an abbreviated procedure. Rarely applies in speech-related procedures.

59   Distinct Procedural Service
Is the only modifier used with edits for 2 procedures not ordinarily performed on the same day by the same practitioner, but which, under certain circumstances, may be appropriate to perform and therefore code on the same day.

This includes but is not limited to

CPT 31579 (Laryngeal videostroboscopy) and
CPT 92520 (Laryngeal function studies)

CPT 92526 (Dysphagia therapy) and
CPT 92520 (Laryngeal function studies)

CPT 92507 (Individual therapy) and
CPT 92508 (Group therapy)

GN: Medicare's therapy modifier GN is required to indicate the therapy service provided by the SLP. The GN modifier is also required for all of the CPT therapy codes (92xxx) and Medicare's G-codes reported on a claim.

Key ICD-9-CM/ICD-10-CM Codes

Voice Disorders

784.40/R49.9   Unspecified voice and resonance disorder

784.41/R49.1   Aphonia

784.42/R49.0   Dysphonia

784.43/R49.21   Hypernasality

784.44/R49.22   Hyponasality

784.49/R49.8   Other voice and resonance disorder

Swallowing Disorders

787.20/R13.0   Aphagia

787.20/R13.10   Dysphagia, unspecified

787.21/R13.11   Dysphagia, oral phase

787.22/R13.12   Dysphagia, oropharyngeal phase

787.23/R13.13   Dysphagia, pharyngeal phase

787.29/R13.19   Other dysphagia
(eg, cervical or neurogenic dysphagia)

783.3/R63.3   Feeding difficulties

Definition of Codes

Medicare's G-Codes and Severity Modifiers for Claims-Based Outcomes Reporting

CMS established nonpayable G-Codes for reporting on claims for Medicare Part B beneficiaries receiving therapy services. Each nonpayable G-Code listed on the claim form must be accompanied with a severity/complexity modifier at the time of the initial evaluation, the 10th visit, and at discharge. The modifier represents the functional impairment on a 7-point severity/complexity scale. This was implemented on January 1, 2013, with a 6-month testing period. As of July 1, 2013, claims that do not comply with the data reporting requirements will be returned unpaid. The G-Codes related to SLP services and severity modifiers are listed below and appear on the American Speech-Language-Hearing Association (ASHA) website (http://www.asha.org/Practice/reimbursement/medicare/G-Codes-and-Severity-Modifiers-for-Outcomes-Reporting/)

CMS does not require Medicare's G-Codes or severity modifiers on the videostroboscopy code, 31579, because it is a surgical CPT code. Furthermore, CMS billing requirements do not mandate a GN (speech pathology) modifier on 31579 so G-Coding is not required. CMS's G-Codes are only used for therapy CPT codes, 92xxx, that require a GN modifier on the bill.

Speech-Language Pathology Related G-Codes

There are three sets of G-Codes for functional limitation and status for the following areas: Swallowing, Motor Speech, Spoken Language Comprehension, Spoken Language Expression, Attention, Memory, Voice, and other SLP Functional Limitation. The first G-Code in each area describes functional limitation, current status at time of initial therapy treatment/episode outset and reporting invervals. The second G-Code describes functional limitation, projected goal status at initial therapy treatment/outset and at discharge from therapy. The third G-Code describes functional limitation, discharge status at discharge from therapy/end of reporting on limitation. The following G-Codes related to SLP services should be used:

- Swallowing: G8996, G8997, G8998
- Motor Speech: G8999, G9186, G9158 (the codes for Motor Speech are not sequentially numbered)
- Spoken Language Comprehension: G9159, G9160, G9161

- Spoken Language Expression: G9162, G9163, G9164
- Attention: G9165, G9166, G9167
- Memory: G9168, G9169, G9170
- Voice: G9171, G9172, G9173
- Other SLP Functional Limitation: G9174, G9175, G9176

All three G-Codes should be used when your interaction will not be an ongoing process. An example of this is if a patient is seen for a FEES (Flexible fiberoptic endoscopic evaluation of swallowing by cine or video recording; [92612]) or a FEESST (Flexible fiberoptic endoscopic evaluation of swallowing and laryngeal sensory testing by cine or video recording [92616]). All three G-Codes would be applied in this case. Individual G-Codes are used when it is an ongoing process.

Severity Modifiers

Note: Modifiers are required by CMS with use of all G-Codes. Corresponding National Outcomes Measurement System (NOMS) Functional Communication Measures levels are also listed in Table 15–1. Use of NOMS can assist with G-code and severity modifier selection but is not required by CMS.

Table 15–1. Medicare's Impairment Limitation Restriction Modifiers

Modifier	Impairment Limitation Restriction	FCM Level
CH	0% impaired, limited, or restricted	7
CI	At least 1% but less than 20% impaired, limited, or restricted	6
CJ	At least 20% but less than 40% impaired, limited, or restricted	5
CK	At least 40% but less than 60% impaired, limited, or restricted	4
CL	At least 60% but less than 80% impaired, limited, or restricted	3
CM	At least 80% but less than 100% impaired, limited, or restricted	2
CN	100% impaired, limited, or restricted	1

Time-Based Codes

1. *Indications:* Speech pathologist can bill based on time for a limited number of codes.
2. *Definition:* Most SLP sessions are billed for 1 hour. CPT states: For reporting purposes, a unit of time is attained when the midpoint is passed when billing for 1 hour. For example, an hour is attained when 31 minutes have elapsed (more than midway between 0 and 60 minutes). (*CPT Assistant*, October 2013, p. 7). Medicare has established specific minimum and maximum times for 15-minute codes which would apply to 97532 (Cognitive skills development) and 97533 (Sensory integration). The minimum time for one 15-minute code is 8 minutes. Two units would be a minimum of 15 + 8 minutes = 23 minutes. This rule continues for each additional 15 minutes.
3. *Key Points:* Codes for SLP were historically not assigned time units as a whole. It is difficult to revise descriptors because of the way codes are developed and established. Most SLP codes are not time based and do not have time units assigned to them. Each code counts as one session if no time is noted in the descriptor.

Frequently Used Time-Based Codes by Speech Pathologists

- Nonspeech device codes (92605, 92618)
- Speech-generating device codes (92607, 92608)
- Auditory rehabilitation (92626, 92627)
- Aphasia (96105)
- Cognitive (96125, 97532)
- Sensory (97533)

Resources

1. American Speech-Language-Hearing Association (ASHA). Medicare coding rules for SLP services. http://www.asha.org/Practice/reimbursement/medicare/SLP_coding_rules.htm. Accessed QQAugust 5, 2015.
2. Centers for Disease Control and Prevention. *International Classification of Diseases, Ninth Revision, Clinical Modification* (ICD-9-CM). http://www.cdc.gov/nchs/icd/icd9cm.htm. Accessed August 5, 2015.
3. Setzen M, Cohen M, Minton J. Coding update: new CMS G-Code/modifier requirements for therapy services. *American Academy of Otolaryngology-Head and Neck Surgery Bulletin.* 2014;33(5).
4. American Speech-Language-Hearing Association (ASHA). G-Codes and severity modifiers for claims-based outcomes reporting: Medicare Part B therapy services. http://www.asha.org/Practice/reimbursement/medicare/G-Codes-and-Severity-Modifiers-for-Outcomes-Reporting/. Accessed August 5, 2015.
5. Centers for Medicare and Medicaid Services. ICD-9-CM diagnosis and procedure codes: abbreviated and full code titles. https://www.cms.gov/Medicare/Coding/ICD9ProviderDiagnosticCodes/codes.html. Accessed August 5, 2015.
6. Centers for Disease Control and Prevention. *International Classification of Diseases, Tenth Revision, Clinical Modification* (ICD-10-CM). http://www.cdc.gov/nchs/icd/icd10cm.htm. Accessed August 5, 2015.
7. American Speech-Language-Hearing Association (ASHA). ICD-10-CM diagnosis codes for audiology and speech-language pathology. http://www.asha.org/Practice/reimbursement/coding/ICD-10/. Accessed August 6, 2015.
8. Centers for Medicare and Medicaid Services. ICD-10. http://www.cms.gov/ICD10/. Accessed August 6, 2015.

CHAPTER 16

Office Otology

Benjamin J. Wycherly

Introduction

This chapter describes coding for otologic office procedures. All office codes billed by physicians with a place of service 11 (physician office) include the use of the facility and equipment, both of which are factored into the relative value units (RVUs). Office services billed by physicians with a place of service 22 (hospital outpatient department) do not include the facility payment, according to Medicare, which is separately billed by the facility. All office-based procedures should include a separate procedure note, distinct from the body of the office visit note. The procedure note should include the indications, a discussion of the risks and benefits, the type of anesthesia (if any), the use of the microscope (if applicable), a description of the procedure including types of instruments used, the findings, and any complications that may have occurred.

Sample Procedure Note for an Intratympanic Steroid Injection

Procedure: Intratympanic steroid injection, right ear, 69801 with dexamethasone, J1100

Indications: Active Ménière's disease, cochleovestibular

Discussion: Risks, benefits, and alternatives of the procedure for the right ear were discussed with the patient, including the risks of vertigo and tympanic membrane perforation.

Anesthesia: Topical phenol was placed over a small area of the anterior superior tympanic membrane.

Technique: The patient was placed in the supine position with the head turned 45 degrees to the left. Using the binocular operating microscope, a transtympanic injection with a 27-gauge needle was performed through the anesthetized tympanic membrane to instill 10 mg/mL dexamethasone into the middle ear.

Findings: The middle ear was filled with approximately 0.5 cc of dexamethasone. The steroid was still present in the middle ear after 20 minutes.

Patient status: The patient tolerated procedure well and complained of only mild vertigo lasting approximately 30 seconds.

Complications: None.

Key Points

The following are key points to keep in mind when coding for in-office otologic procedures:

- Almost all otologic office procedure codes have a 0- or 10-day global period.
- Almost all otologic office procedures may be reported as a bilateral procedure with modifier 50.
- Almost all *Current Procedural Terminology* (CPT) codes include the use of the binocular microscope; only in specific instances may the use of the microscope be reported in addition to the primary procedure code.
- Use of the microscope may be reported for diagnostic purposes when there is no code for an ear procedure (eg, wick placement, debridement or topical treatment of the ear canal).
- All office procedure codes include use of local anesthesia.
- In 2015, all eustachian tube codes were deleted from the CPT code set.
- Centers for Medicare and Medicaid Services' (CMS's) intent of a 10-day postoperative global period is that the first postoperative visit to assess the surgical site is included in the payment for the procedure rendered and billed whether the provider chooses to see the patient within the 10 days following surgery or a short time afterward.

Key Procedure Codes

69000 Drainage external ear, abscess or hematoma; simple
wRVU 1.50; Global 10

    69005 complicated
wRVU 2.16; Global 10

69020 Drainage external auditory canal, abscess
wRVU 1.53; Global 10

69090 Ear piercing
wRVU 0.00; Global XXX

69100 Biopsy external ear
wRVU 0.81; Global 0

69105 Biopsy external auditory canal
wRVU 0.85; Global 0

69110 Excision external ear; partial, simple repair
wRVU 3.53; Global 90

69145 Excision soft tissue lesion, external auditory canal
wRVU 2.70; Global 90

69200 Removal foreign body from external auditory canal; without general anesthesia
wRVU 0.77; Global 0

69210 Removal of impacted cerumen requiring instrumentation, unilateral
wRVU 0.61; Global 0

69220 Debridement, mastoidectomy cavity, simple (eg, routine cleaning)
wRVU 0.83; Global 0

69222 Debridement, mastoidectomy cavity, complex (eg, with anesthesia or more than routine cleaning)
wRVU 1.45; Global 10

69420 Myringotomy including aspiration and/or eustachian tube inflation
wRVU 1.38; Global 10

69433 Tympanostomy (requiring insertion of a ventilating tube), local or topical anesthesia
wRVU 1.57; Global 10

69540 Excision aural polyp
wRVU 1.25; Global 10

69610 Tympanic membrane repair, with or without site preparation of perforation for closure, with or without patch
wRVU 4.47; Global 10

69620 Myringoplasty (surgery confined to drumhead and donor area)
wRVU 6.03; Global 90

69799 Unlisted procedure, middle ear
wRVU 0.00; Global YYY

69801 Labyrinthotomy, with perfusion of vestibuloactive drug(s); transcanal
wRVU 2.06; Global 0

92504 Binocular microscopy (separate diagnostic procedure)
wRVU 0.18; Global XXX

92511 Nasopharyngoscopy with endoscope (separate procedure)
wRVU 0.61; Global 0

95992 Canalith repositioning procedure(s) (eg, Epley maneuver, Semont maneuver), per day
wRVU 0.75; Global XXX

HCPCS Level II Codes

J0696 Injection, ceftriaxone sodium, per 250 mg

J1020 Injection, methylprednisolone acetate, 20 mg

J1094 Injection, dexamethasone acetate, 1 mg

J1100 Injection, dexamethasone sodium phosphate, 1 mg

J1580 Injection, Garamycin, gentamicin, up to 80 mg

J2930 Injection, methylprednisolone sodium succinate, up to 125 mg

Key Modifiers

25   Significant, Separately Identifiable Evaluation and Management Service by the Same Physician or Other Qualified Health Care Professional on the Same Day of the Procedure or Other Service
Placed on office visit code when doing a separate identifiable procedure. For instance, if a patient comes in for sudden hearing loss and needs to have a steroid injection; the 25 modifier would be placed on the evaluation and management (E/M) code.

50   Bilateral Procedure
Placed on most procedures that are performed bilaterally. For example, if an ear tube is placed bilaterally then modifier 50 will be appended to 69433.

79   Unrelated Procedure or Service by the Same Physician or Other Qualified Health Care Professional During the Postoperative Period
Placed on a procedure when performed during the global period of another procedure or surgery. For instance, if the patient has a 90-day global period for a major surgery and then comes in with a separate complaint that requires a procedure. This could occur if a patient had a tonsillectomy and then comes in requiring an ear tube during the global period.

Key ICD-9-CM/ICD-10-CM Codes

For otologic disorders, *International Classification of Diseases, Tenth Revision, Clinical Modification* (ICD-10-CM) codes are typically more descriptive than *International Classification of Diseases, Ninth Revision, Clinical Modification* (ICD-9-CM) codes. For example, with ICD-10-CM, there will be 4 codes for cholesteatoma of the external ear (H60.4), as follows:

1. Cholesteatoma of an unspecified external ear H60.40
2. Cholesteatoma of the right external ear H60.41
3. Cholesteatoma of the left external ear H60.42
4. Cholesteatoma of bilateral external ears H60.43.

The ICD-9-CM and ICD-10-CM codes listed below are commonly used diagnostic codes in otology. The ICD-10-CM codes are listed without the last digit for simplicity; however, they may not be reported as listed below without additional digits because they will not be complete diagnostic codes. Typically ICD-10-CM uses the last digit of "0" for an unspecified ear, "1" for the right ear, "2" for the left ear, and "3" for bilateral; however, this is not always the case. The laterality space is marked below as a "-". Some ICD-10-CM codes are new and do not have an ICD-9-CM equivalent; the absence of an ICD-9-CM code will be indicated below by "—".

External Ear

054.73/B00.1   Herpesviral vesicular dermatitis

112.82/B37.84   Candidal otitis externa

173.20/C44.201-   Unspecified malignant neoplasm of skin of ear and external auditory canal

216.2/D23.2-   Other benign neoplasm of skin of ear and external auditory canal

232.2/D04.20-   Carcinoma in situ of skin of ear and external auditory canal

380.01/H61.01-   Acute perichondritis of external ear

380.02/H61.02-   Chronic perichondritis of external ear

380.10/H60.0-   Abscess of external ear

380.10/H60.1-   Cellulitis of external ear

380.10/H60.31-   Diffuse otitis externa

380.10/H60.32-   Hemorrhagic otitis externa

380.10/H60.39-   Other infective otitis externa

380.12/H60.33-   Swimmer's ear

380.14/H60.2-   Malignant otitis externa

380.21/H60.4-   Cholesteatoma of external ear

380.22/H60.50-   Unspecified acute noninfective otitis externa

380.22/H60.51-   Acute actinic otitis externa

380.22/H60.52-   Acute chemical otitis externa

380.22/H60.53-   Acute contact otitis externa

380.22/H60.54-   Acute eczematoid otitis externa

380.22/H60.55-   Acute reactive otitis externa

380.22/H60.59   Other noninfective acute otitis externa

380.23/H60.6-   Unspecified chronic otitis externa

380.23/H60.8X-   Other otitis externa

380.23/H60.9-   Unspecified otitis externa

380.31/H61.12-   Hematoma of pinna

380.4/H61.2-   Impacted cerumen

380.50/H61.30-   Acquired stenosis of external ear canal, unspecified

380.50/H61.39-   Other acquired stenosis of external ear canal

380.52/H61.39-   Other acquired stenosis of external ear canal

380.81/H61.81-   Exostosis of external canal

Middle Ear

381.01/H65.00   Acute serous otitis media, unspecified ear (*right ear H65.01, left ear H65.02, bilateral H65.03*)

—/H65.0-   Acute serous otitis media, recurrent (*right ear H65.04, left ear H65.05, bilateral H65.06, unspecified ear H65.07*)

381.4/H65.9-   Unspecified nonsuppurative otitis media

381.10/H65.2-   Chronic serous otitis media

381.20/H65.3-   Chronic mucoid otitis media

382.00/H66.00-   Acute suppurative otitis media with spontaneous rupture of ear drum (*right ear H66.001, left ear H66.002, bilateral H66.003, unspecified ear H66.009*)

—/H66.00-   Acute suppurative otitis media without spontaneous rupture of the tympanic membrane, recurrent (*right ear H66.004, left ear H66.005, bilateral H66.006, unspecified ear H66.009*)

382.01/H66.01-   Acute suppurative otitis media with spontaneous rupture of ear drum (*right ear H66.011, left ear H66.012, bilateral H66.013, unspecified ear H66.019*)

/H66.01   Acute suppurative otitis media with spontaneous rupture of the ear drum, recurrent (*right ear H66.014, left ear H66.015, bilateral H66.016, unspecified ear H66.017*)

382.1/H66.1-   Chronic tubotympanic suppurative otitis media

382.2/H66.2-   Chronic atticoantral suppurative otitis media

382.9/H66.9   Otitis media, unspecified

385.10/H74.1-   Adhesive middle ear disease

385.30/H71.9-   Unspecified cholesteatoma

385.31/H71.0-   Cholesteatoma of attic

385.32/H71.1-   Cholesteatoma of tympanum

385.32/H74.4-   Polyp of middle ear

Mastoid

383.1/H70.1-   Chronic mastoiditis

383.32/H95.0-   Recurrent cholesteatoma of postmastoidectomy cavity

383.33/H95.12-   Granulations of postmastoidectomy cavity

383.81/H70.81-   Postauricular fistula

385.33/H71.2-   Cholesteatoma of mastoid

Tympanic Membrane

384.1/H73.1-   Chronic myringitis

384.20/H72.9-   Unspecified perforation of tympanic membrane

384.21/H72.0-   Central perforation of tympanic membrane

384.22/H72.1-   Attic perforation of tympanic membrane

384.23/H72.2X-   Other marginal perforations of tympanic membrane

384.24/H72.81-   Multiple perforations of tympanic membrane

384.25/H72.82-   Total perforations of tympanic membrane

—/S09.21XA   Traumatic rupture of the right ear drum, initial encounter

—/S09.21XD   Traumatic rupture of the right ear drum, subsequent encounter

—/S09.21XS   Traumatic rupture of the right ear drum, sequela

—/S09.22XA   Traumatic rupture of the left ear drum, initial encounter

—/S09.22XD   Traumatic rupture of the left ear drum, subsequent encounter

—/S09.22XS   Traumatic rupture of the left ear drum, sequela

Vestibular Disorders

386.01/H81.0-   Ménière's disease

386.11/H81.1-   Benign paroxysmal vertigo

386.40/H83.1-   Labyrinthine fistula

386.51/H83.2X-   Labyrinthine dysfunction

386.53/ H83.2X-   Labyrinthine dysfunction

780.4/R42   Dizziness and giddiness

Auditory Disorders

387.0/H80.0-   Otosclerosis involving oval window, nonobliterative

387.1/H80.1-   Otosclerosis involving oval window, obliterative

—/H80.2-   Cochlear otosclerosis

387.9/H80.9-   Unspecified otosclerosis

388.01/H91.1-   Presbycusis

388.10/H83.3X-   Noise effects on inner ear

388.12/ H83.3X-   Noise effects on inner ear

388.2/H91.2-   Sudden idiopathic hearing loss

388.30/H93.1-   Tinnitus

388.31/H93.1-   Tinnitus

388.40/H93.24-   Temporary auditory threshold shift

388.40/H93.29-   Other abnormal auditory perceptions

389.00/H90.2   Conductive hearing loss, unspecified

389.05/H90.1-   Conductive hearing loss, unilateral with unrestricted hearing on the contralateral side

389.06/H90.0   Conductive hearing loss, bilateral

389.10/H90.5   Unspecified sensorineural hearing loss

389.15/H90.4-   Sensorineural hearing loss, unilateral, with unrestricted hearing on the contralateral side

389.18/H90.3   Sensorineural hearing loss, bilateral

389.20/H90.8   Mixed conductive and sensorineural hearing loss, unspecified

389.21/H90.7-   Mixed conductive and sensorineural hearing loss, unilateral, with unrestricted hearing on the contralateral side

389.22/H90.6   Mixed conductive and sensorineural hearing loss, bilateral

389.9/H91.9-   Unspecified hearing loss

Facial Nerve

351.0/G51.0   Bell's palsy

351.8/G51.2   Melkersson syndrome

351.8/G51.4   Facial myokymia

351.8/G51.8   Other disorders of the facial nerve

767.5/P11.3   Birth injury to facial nerve

951.4/S04.50XA   Injury of facial nerve, unspecified side, initial encounter

Eustachian Tube/Nasopharynx

381.60/H68.10-   Unspecified obstruction of Eustachian tube

381.7/H69.0-   Patulous Eustachian tube

381.81/H69.8-   Other specified disorders of Eustachian tube

474.01/J35.02   Chronic adenoiditis

474.12/J35.2   Hypertrophy of adenoids

472.2/J31.1   Chronic nasopharyngitis

Other

388.70/H92.0-   Otalgia

931/T16.1XXA   Foreign body in right ear, initial encounter

—/T16.1XXD   Foreign body in right ear, subsequent encounter

—/T16.1XXS   Foreign body in right ear, sequela

931/T16.2XXA   Foreign body in left ear, initial encounter

—/T16.2XXD   Foreign body in left ear, subsequent encounter

—/T16.2XXS   Foreign body in left ear, sequela

V72.11/Z01.110   Encounter for hearing examination following failed hearing screening

V72.19/Z01.10   Encounter for examination of ears and hearing without abnormal findings

V72.19/Z01.118   Encounter for examination of ears and hearing with other abnormal findings

Definition of Codes

1. Drainage external ear, abscess or hematoma (69000, 69005)
   a. *Indications*—Hematoma or abscess of the auricle.
   b. *Definition*—An incision is created to drain an abscess or hematoma. A complicated procedure (69005) is reported if a drain, packing, or bolster is placed or if additional time is spent cleaning the hematoma or abscess cavity.
   c. *Key points*—It is important to document precisely whether the procedure was sim-

ple or complex. The procedure note should explain the rationale behind the placement of a drain, packing, or bolster to justify reporting the complex code.

2. Drainage of an abscess of the external ear canal (69020)
   a. *Indications*—Examples include abscess, otitis externa.
   b. *Definition*—An incision is made in the external auditory canal to drain an abscess; packing may be inserted.
   c. *Key points*—Use of the operating microscope (92504) is considered part of the procedure and should not be coded separately.

3. Biopsy of the external ear (69100) and external auditory canal (69105)
   a. *Indications*—Examples include benign and malignant neoplasms, perichondritis, cholesteatoma of the ear canal, granulation tissue.
   b. *Definition*—A scalpel or punch forcep is used to remove a portion of a lesion of the auricle or external ear canal for diagnostic purposes. For a biopsy of the auricle, a suture may or may not be necessary.
   c. *Key points*—The code for a biopsy of the external ear (69100) includes simple closure, if required. Use of the operating microscope (92504) is considered part of both procedures and should not be coded separately.

4. Excision of the external ear, partial, simple repair (69110) or excision of a soft tissue lesion of the external ear canal (69145)
   a. *Indications*—Examples include benign or malignant neoplasms, open wound of the auricle, cholesteatoma of the external ear canal, granulation tissue.
   b. *Definition*—For 69110, a full-thickness section of the external ear is removed with a small area of surrounding normal tissue; usually, the wound is closed in layers. For 69145, a lesion of the external ear canal is removed along with a small amount of normal tissue from the surrounding area.
   c. *Key points*—Excising a lesion of the external ear canal, such as a cholesteatoma of the

external ear canal, may require drilling and is more likely to be performed in the operating room. If the area of excision is large, a skin graft may be required. The skin graft is reported in addition to the excision code. Use of the operating microscope (92504) is considered part of the procedure and should not be coded separately.

5. Foreign body removal (69200)
   a. *Indications*—Foreign body in the ear canal.
   b. *Definition*—Removal of a foreign body (eg, insect, toy) but does not include cerumen, purulence, ventilation tubes, or debridement of a mastoid cavity.
   c. *Key points*—69200 should not be reported when removing a ventilation tube in the office. Because there is no code for the removal of a ventilation tube in the office, the removal of a ventilation tube is reported only when performed under general anesthesia (69424, ventilating tube removal from the external auditory canal with general anesthesia). Use of the operating microscope (92504) is considered part of the procedure when removing a foreign body and should not be coded separately. The procedure note should describe the foreign body and the instrumentation that was required to remove it.

6. Removal of impacted cerumen requiring instrumentation, unilateral (69210)
   a. *Indications*—Impacted cerumen in the ear canal.
   b. *Definition*—As defined by the American Academy of Otolaryngology-Head and Neck Surgery (AAO-HNS) and CPT, cerumen is considered to be impacted if it meets any of the following criteria:
      - Impairs the examination of the clinically significant portions of the external auditory canal, tympanic membrane, or middle ear.
      - Is extremely hard, dry, or irritating and causes pain, itching, hearing loss, etc.
      - Is associated with foul odor, infection, or dermatitis.

- Is obstructive or copious and cannot be removed without magnification and multiple instruments that require the skills of a physician.[1]

c. *Key points*—Simple, nonimpacted cerumen removal (with lavage or irrigation) should not be reported separately from an evaluation and management (E/M) code; it is considered part of the E/M service.

In order to report code 69210 and an E/M visit code on the same day of service, all of the following criteria must be met:

- The reason for the patient visit should not be for cerumen removal.
- An otoscopic examination of the tympanic membrane is not possible.
- Removal of the cerumen requires the expertise of a physician or nonphysician practitioner and is performed by him or her.
- The procedure requires a significant amount of time and effort.

Each of the above criteria should be clearly documented in the medical record, making it clear that the E/M code and code 69210 are separate services.

If the operating microscope is used to remove cerumen, you may also use code 92504 (binocular microscopy-separate diagnostic procedure). The add-on code 69990 (microsurgical techniques, requiring use of operating microscope) should not be used. However, while CPT allows reporting 92504 with 69210, many payers bundle this diagnostic service (92504) into the definitive surgical procedure (69210).

Removal of impacted cerumen requiring instrumentation, unilateral (69210) requires the use of instrumentation to code for the procedure. The AAO-HNS defines instrumentation as the use of an otoscope and other instruments such as curettes, wire loops, or suction plus specific ear instruments (eg, cup forceps, right angled hook). The procedure note should include the instruments required to complete the procedure.

For Medicare patients who have cerumen removal on the same day as a diagnostic test performed by an audiologist, the physician reports 69210 on his or her claim while the audiologist reports the audiologic diagnostic testing on his or her own separate claim. Audiologists must bill Medicare using their own national provider identifier (NPI) for any diagnostic services provided. Code 69210 billed by a physician will never be on the same Medicare claim as an audiologic diagnostic test code; therefore, code G0268 should never be billed to Medicare. Refer to Chapter 17, "Audiology," for more information.

If a physician removes cerumen on a non-Medicare patient on the same day that an audiologist within the same practice performs audiology testing, some payers may not reimburse 69210 for the physician because the cerumen removal is bundled into the audiologic diagnostic testing code. In those situations, use the Healthcare Common Procedure Coding System Level II (HCPCS II) code G0268 instead. HCPCS Level II codes represent items, supplies, and nonphysician services not covered by CPT codes. HCPCS code G0268 is defined as the following: removal of impacted cerumen (one or both ears) by physicians on same date of service as audiologic function testing. Practices should determine the policies of local commercial carriers as some carriers may adopt this code. If an audiologist from outside the physician's practice refers a patient for cerumen removal, use code 69210, not G0268. G0268 is a bilateral code and should not be coded with modifier 50. CMS will not reimburse audiologists for codes 69210 or G0268 as audiologists are only allowed to be paid for diagnostic services.

Although 69210 is a unilateral code, it is not reimbursed by Medicare as a bilateral procedure and should not be reported with modifier 50 to Medicare; however, some private payers do reimburse when billed bilaterally (see Controversial Areas section)

7. Mastoid debridement (69220, 69222)
   a. *Indications*—Examples include acute and chronic mastoiditis, granulations of post-mastoidectomy cavity, cholesteatoma.
   b. *Definition*—Skin, cerumen, and other accumulated debris is debrided from an open mastoid cavity and may be required every 3 to 6 months. A mastoid debridement is usually performed using binocular microscopy.
   c. *Key points*—More extensive cleaning is reported as a complex debridement (69222). A complex debridement may be reported only when there is more than routine cleaning with a difficult cavity (small meatus, canal stenosis, or high facial ridge), severe pain, an uncooperative patient, the presence of a labyrinthine fistula, severe vertigo during debridement, significant granulation tissue, infection, or bleeding or with anesthesia. The reason for coding for a complex debridement should be clearly documented in the procedure note.

      Mastoid debridement codes are unilateral procedures, so modifier 50 should be used if a bilateral mastoid debridement is performed. Local anesthesia is included in the service of these codes. All mastoid surgeries have 90 day global periods, so any debridement performed in the surgical global period is included and not separately reported.

8. Myringotomy including aspiration and/or eustachian tube inflation (69420)
   a. *Indications*—Examples include eustachian tube dysfunction, otitis media.
   b. *Definition*—An incision is made in the tympanic membrane. Fluid may be aspirated from the middle ear space and may be sent for diagnostic analysis.
   c. *Key points*—A myringotomy is a unilateral procedure. If performed bilaterally, a myringotomy should be reported with modifier 50. Use of the operating microscope (92504) is considered part of the procedure and should not be coded separately. Do not separately report a myringotomy

when placing a ventilation tube as this is included in the tube placement codes.

9. Tympanostomy (requiring the insertion of a ventilating tube), local or topical anesthesia (69433)
   a. *Indications*—Examples include eustachian tube dysfunction, otitis media.
   b. *Definition*—Ventilation tubes are inserted after performing a myringotomy under direct visualization with a microscope or endoscope.
   c. *Key points*—Bilateral ear tube placement may be performed and should be coded with modifier 50. Do not code for a myringotomy (69420) when coding for a ventilation tube placement. For the ventilation tube, you may choose to report code 99070, which is defined as supplies and materials, provided by the physician or other qualified health professional over and above those usually included with the procedure rendered. Code 99070 is unlikely to be reimbursed because a tympanostomy tube is inherent to the CPT code for placement of it.

10. Excision of an aural polyp (69540)
    a. *Indications*—Examples include polyp of the external ear canal, cholesteatoma.
    b. *Definition*—An aural polyp is removed with cup forceps or another instrument through the ear canal. Bleeding may need to be controlled and, often, topical medications are applied to the ear canal.
    c. *Key points*—Use of the operating microscope (92504) is considered part of the procedure and should not be coded separately. Removing an aural polyp during another procedure (tympanic membrane repair or removing a ventilation tube in the operating room) is included in the primary procedure code and not separately reported.

11. Tympanic membrane repair, with or without site preparation of perforation for closure, with or without patch (69610)
    a. *Indications*—Examples include central tympanic membrane perforation.

b. *Definition*—This code is used when freshening the edges of a perforation with or without the placement of a nontissue graft (eg, paper patch, hyaluronic acid disc).

c. *Key points*—The middle ear is not entered in this procedure. This code may be reported with modifier 50 when performed bilaterally.

12. Myringoplasty (surgery confined to drumhead and donor area) (69620)
    a. *Indications*—Examples include central tympanic membrane perforation.
    b. *Definition*—After preparing the edges of a tympanic membrane perforation, an autologous tissue graft is used to fill the perforation. A tissue graft is used to improve the likelihood of closing the perforation.
    c. *Key points*—The middle ear is usually not, but may be, entered in this procedure. This code includes harvesting of the donor graft, therefore, a code such as 20926 (Tissue grafts, other [eg, paratenon, fat, dermis]) should not be reported separately. Code 69620 may be reported with modifier 50 when performed bilaterally.

13. Intratympanic therapy (69801)
    a. *Indications*—Examples include Ménière's disease, sudden hearing loss, labyrinthitis.
    b. *Definition*—Administration of drugs into the middle ear through the tympanic membrane to treat inner ear conditions.
    c. *Key points*—There is a 0-day global period for this procedure; however, it may not be reported more than once a day. Do not also code for a myringotomy (69240), tympanostomy with ventilation tube (69433), or binocular microscopy (92504) when coding for intratympanic therapy.
    HCPCS Level II codes represent items, supplies, and nonphysician services not covered by CPT codes. If the practice incurs an expense for certain medications, an HCPCS Level II J code should be billed in addition to the CPT code. A J code is used for injectable drugs that ordinarily may not be self-administered.

The following are several J codes that may be used for intratympanic therapy:

- J1580 gentamicin, up to 80 mg
- J1020 methylprednisolone sodium succinate, up to 40 mg
- J2930 methylprednisolone sodium succinate, up to 125 mg
- J1100 dexamethasone sodium phosphate, 1 mg
- J1094 dexamethasone acetate, 1 mg
- J0696 ceftriaxone sodium, per 250 mg

Supplies such as needles and syringes are included in the CPT code reported and should not be separately billed.

14. Binocular microscopy (separate diagnostic procedure) (92504)
    a. *Indications*—Examples include exostoses, otitis externa, eczema of the external ear canal, myringitis, tympanic membrane perforations, conductive or mixed hearing loss, pulsatile tinnitus.
    b. *Definition*—A physician uses an operating binocular microscope to examine the ear for a detailed, high-magnification examination. This procedure is performed when a detailed examination of the ear canal, tympanic membrane, and/or middle ear is required and handheld otoscopy is inconclusive.
    c. *Key points*—Binocular microscopy (92504) is a separate diagnostic procedure code and is not reported when coding for other otology codes (except when used for cerumen removal, see the *CPT Assistant* October 2013). It is important to document the need for the binocular microscope to demonstrate why an otoscope was insufficient for diagnostic purposes.

15. Nasopharyngoscopy (92511)
    a. *Indications*—Examples include dysfunction of the eustachian tube, adenoid hypertrophy, nasopharyngitis, otitis media, nasopharyngeal neoplasm.
    b. *Definition*—A flexible or rigid endoscope is advanced through the nose to examine the

eustachian tube orifices, soft palate, choanae, and posterior pharyngeal wall.

c. *Key points*—If the patient's symptoms are nasopharyngeal in nature, a nasopharyngoscopy (92511), not a nasal endoscopy (31231), should be reported. (This is in spite of the fact that the nose is transversed and often evaluated as part of the exam.) A nasopharyngoscopy code (92511) may not be reported with a flexible fiberoptic laryngoscopy (31575) code as the services overlap.

16. Canalith repositioning procedure(s) (eg, Epley maneuver, Semont maneuver), per day (95992)
   a. *Indication*—Examples include benign paroxysmal positional vertigo.
   b. *Definition*—95992 may be used as a single treatment or in a treatment series to reposition displaced otoliths.
   c. *Key points*—This code may be used once a day for each day of treatment and may be used for any repositioning maneuver (Epley, Semont, etc). This code may be reported by audiologists and physical therapists; however, Medicare's payment guidelines do not allow reimbursement to audiologists. Other payer policies may vary.

17. Wick placement
   • There is no CPT code for placing an ear wick. Placement of an ear wick for external otitis is included in the E/M service. If the ear was examined with the binocular microscope to make a diagnosis or to place a wick, code 92504 (binocular microscopy, separate diagnostic procedure) may be used. If a wick was placed after draining an abscess from the external auditory canal, it is considered part of the code for drainage of an abscess of the external auditory canal (69020).

18. Debridement of the external ear canal
   • There is no code for debriding an ear canal. Removal of impacted cerumen

requiring instrumentation, unilateral (69210) may be reported if the ear was cleaned of impacted cerumen. If the ear was examined with the binocular microscope to make a diagnosis, code 92504 (binocular microscopy, separate diagnostic procedure) may be used.

19. Topical treatment of the ear canal
   • There is no code for treating the ear canal with topical medications (eg, silver nitrate, gentian violet). If the ear was cleaned of impacted cerumen, removal of impacted cerumen requiring instrumentation, unilateral (69210) may be reported. If the ear was examined with the binocular microscope to make a diagnosis, code 92504 (binocular microscopy, separate diagnostic procedure) may be used.

Controversial Areas

Removal of Impacted Cerumen as a Unilateral or Bilateral Procedure

It has been debated recently as to whether to code a unilateral or bilateral procedure when removing cerumen. Although CPT defines the code as a unilateral procedure, CMS issued a policy in 2014 that refused to acknowledge the use of modifier 50 when removing cerumen bilaterally. Most claims for 69210-50 are denied as most private payers are following the CMS guidelines, though not all payers follow this incorrect policy. The American Academy of Otolaryngology-Head and Neck Surgery is making efforts to change this policy.[1]

Eustachian Tube Codes

In 2015, three eustachian tube codes were deleted from the CPT code set:

   • 69400—Eustachian tube inflation, transnasal with catheterization

- 69401—Eustachian tube inflation, transnasal without catheterization
- 69405—Eustachian tube catheterization, transtympanic

These codes were rarely used and are considered to be outmoded. This change was supported by the AAO-HNS.[2] If reporting the three procedures listed above, Eustachian tube inflation, transnasal without catheterization (69401) is captured in the E/M encounter and should not be reported separately. Eustachian tube inflation, transnasal with catheterization (69400) and Eustachian tube catheterization, transtympanic (69405) should be reported using unlisted procedure, middle ear (69799). If performed with endoscopy and reported as an unlisted procedure (69799), nasal endoscopy (31231) or nasopharyngoscopy (92511) should not be reported separately as endoscopy is considered an integral part of the procedure.

There is no CPT code for balloon dilation of the eustachian tube because it is a new technology and does not have the approval of the U.S. Food and Drug Administration. If performed, it should be reported as unlisted procedure, middle ear (69799). If performed with nasal endoscopy (31231) or nasopharyngoscopy (92511), these should not be reported separately because endoscopy is considered an integral part of the procedure.

References

1. CPT for ENT: cerumen removal. http://www.ent net.org/content/cpt-ent-cerumen-removal. *Revised November 2013.* Accessed October 20, 2014.
2. CPT for ENT: deletion of eustachian tube codes for 2015. http://www.entnet.org/content/cpt-ent-deletion-eustachian-tube-codes-2015. Accessed October 20, 2014.

CHAPTER 17

Audiology

Debra Abel

Introduction

For many years, the most common place of employment for an audiologist was within an otolaryngology practice, offering audiologic support for the diagnosis and treatment of hearing loss, disequilibrium, and tinnitus. As the profession has changed, so too has the delivery of health care. This chapter will review Medicare regulations pertaining to audiology, the codes utilized by audiologists, contracting with commercial payers, and the use of technicians within an otolaryngology practice.

Embedded in the history of audiologists working as employees or contractors in otolaryngology offices, a fallacy prevailed: if diagnostic audiologic services were provided in an otolaryngology office, they were to be filed under the physician's Medicare Provider Identification Number (PIN) as "incident to" services. The major contributing factor to this misconception was that audiologists were reimbursed less, but in reality, have been reimbursed at the same allowable rate as physicians by way of the same Medicare Physician Fee Schedule. For audiologic services, Medicare has the most stringent regulations pertaining to audiologists, and as a result, commercial payers may follow the same guidelines. To understand the foundation of the regulations, the Centers for Medicare and Medicaid Services (CMS) Program Memorandum AB-02-080 states, "diagnostic testing, including hearing and balance assessment services, performed by a qualified audiologist is

paid for as 'other diagnostic tests' under §1861 (s) (3) of the Social Security Act (the Act) when a physician orders testing to obtain information as part of his or her diagnostic evaluation or to determine the appropriate medical or surgical treatment of a hearing deficit or related medical problem" (CMS, 2002).

Diagnostic audiologic services provided under the "other diagnostic test" category in section 1861(s)(3) of the Social Security Act are not considered acceptable to be billed as "incident to" services to Medicare. In 2008, the CMS issued Transmittal 84, which required all audiologists to bill services supplied to Medicare Part B beneficiaries under their own national provider identifier (NPI) and not the NPI of a physician. Unfortunately, this practice of billing audiology services performed by an audiologist and billed by an otolaryngologist continues, and if discovered, Medicare may seek repayments as well as penalties and interest.

At the time of this publication, Medicare recognizes audiologists only as diagnosticians, not as providers of treatment of hearing and balance disorders such as the rehabilitation of hearing loss, tinnitus management, and management of those experiencing balance disorders. Many third-party payers with whom audiologists contract establish their policies based on these Medicare-imposed requirements. Although these restrictions are in opposition to state licensure laws, which define a provider's scope of practice allowing diagnosis and treatment, some payers do recognize and reimburse for all professional services that audiologists are licensed to provide. It behooves a practice to be aware of the differences in requirements for audiological services.

Key Points

- Audiologic services should be billed to Medicare under the providing audiologists NPI number, not that of the associated physician.
- Currently, Medicare recognizes audiologists as diagnosticians only and not as providers of treatment or therapy services such as cerumen removal.
- Use as specific a diagnostic code as possible and minimize the use of unspecified codes to decrease the chance of denials.
- A comprehensive audiogram (92557) includes the combination of 92553 (pure tone threshold, air and bone) as well as 92556 (speech audiometry threshold with speech recognition).
- The basic electronystagmography testing (92540) includes 4 component tests: spontaneous nystagmus (92541), positional nystagmus (92542), optokinetic nystagmus (92544), and oscillating tracking test (92545). However, caloric testing may be separately reported, and beginning on January 1, 2016, there will be 2 caloric testing codes, one for bithermal and bilateral and the other, bithermal and monaural. The *Current Procedural Terminology* (CPT) codes for these procedures were unknown at the time of publication.
- All audiology diagnostic testing codes assume bilateral testing—do not append modifier 50 for testing of both ears. In fact, modifier 52 (reduced services) should be appended if only one ear is tested (does not apply to audiology time-based codes).
- All audiological services require a written report; diagnostic testing services should also include a printout or **diagram** of the results.

Key Procedure Codes

As with any provider of health care services, audiologists utilize CPT, International Classification of Diseases (ICD), and Healthcare Common Procedure Coding System, Level II (HCPCS Level II) codes. Specific HCPCS Level II codes include the L section for osseointegrated devices and the V section related to hearing aid technology, dispensing fees, assistive listening devices, and a few hearing aid–related procedures. Under the Medicine/Special Otorhinolaryngological Services section of CPT, the codes utilized by audiologists include the following categories:

- Vestibular function
- Audiologic function
- Evaluation/assessment services

All CPT codes utilized by audiologists are for both ears unless a modifier is utilized (eg, 52, RT, LT as indicated by the payer).

Vestibular Function Tests

92540   Basic vestibular evaluation, includes spontaneous nystagmus test with eccentric gaze fixation nystagmus, with recording, positional nystagmus test, minimum of 4 positions, with recording, optokinetic nystagmus test, bidirectional foveal and peripheral stimulation, with recording, and oscillating tracking test, with recording
wRVU 1.50; Global XXX

92541   Spontaneous nystagmus test, including gaze and fixation nystagmus, with recording
wRVU 0.40; Global XXX

92542   Positional nystagmus test, minimum of 4 positions, with recording
wRVU 0.48; Global XXX

92543   Caloric vestibular test, each irrigation (binaural, bithermal stimulation constitutes 4 tests), with recording
wRVU 0.10; Global XXX

92544 Optokinetic nystagmus test, bidirectional, foveal or peripheral stimulation, with recording
wRVU 0.27; Global XXX

92545 Oscillating tracking test, with recording
wRVU 0.25; Global XXX

92546 Sinusoidal vertical axis rotational testing
wRVU 0.29; Global XXX

+92547 Use of vertical electrodes (List separately in addition to code for primary procedure)
wRVU 0.00; Global ZZZ

92548 Computerized dynamic posturography
wRVU 0.50; Global XXX

Audiological Tests

92550 Tympanometry and reflex threshold measurements
wRVU 0.35; Global XXX

92552 Pure tone audiometry (threshold); air only
wRVU 0.00; Global XXX

    92553 air and bone
wRVU 0.00; Global XXX

92555 Speech audiometry threshold;
wRVU 0.00; Global XXX

    92556 with speech recognition
wRVU 0.00; Global XXX

92557 Comprehensive audiometry threshold evaluation and speech recognition (92553 and 92556 combined)
wRVU 0.60; Global XXX

92558 Evoked otoacoustic emissions, screening (qualitative measurement of distortion product or transient evoked otoacoustic emissions), automated analysis
wRVU 0.00; Global XXX

92567 Tympanometry (impedance testing)
wRVU 0.20; Global XXX

92570 Acoustic immittance testing, includes tympanometry (impedance testing), acoustic reflex threshold testing, and acoustic reflex decay testing
wRVU 0.55; Global XXX

92579 Visual reinforcement audiometry (VRA)
wRVU 0.70; Global XXX

92582 Conditioning play audiometry
wRVU 0.00; Global XXX

92584 Electrocochleography
wRVU 0.00; Global XXX

92585 Auditory evoked potentials for evoked response audiometry and/or testing of the central nervous system; comprehensive
wRVU 0.50; Global XXX

92587 Distortion product evoked otoacoustic emissions; limited evaluation (to confirm the presence or absence of hearing disorder, 3-6 frequencies) or transient evoked otoacoustic emissions, with interpretation and report
wRVU 0.35; Global XXX

    92588 comprehensive diagnostic evaluation (quantitative analysis of outer hair cell function by cochlear mapping, minimum of 12 frequencies), with interpretation and report
wRVU 0.55; Global XXX

92590 Hearing aid examination and selection: monaural
wRVU 0.00; Global XXX

    92591 binaural
wRVU 0.00; Global XXX

92592 Hearing aid check; monaural
wRVU 0.00; Global XXX

    92593 binaural
wRVU 0.00; Global XXX

Evaluation and Therapeutic Services

92601 Diagnostic analysis of cochlear implant, patient younger than 7 years of age; with programming
wRVU 2.30; Global XXX

92602   subsequent reprogramming
wRVU 1.30; Global XXX

92603   Diagnostic analysis of cochlear implant, age 7 years or older; with programming
wRVU 2.25; Global XXX

92604   subsequent reprogramming
wRVU 1.25; Global XXX

92620   Evaluation of central auditory function, with report; initial 60 minutes
wRVU 1.50; Global XXX

+92621   each additional 15 minutes (List separately in addition to code for primary procedure)
wRVU 0.35; Global ZZZ

92625   Assessment of tinnitus (includes pitch, loudness matching, and masking)
wRVU 1.15; Global XXX

92626   Evaluation of auditory rehabilitation status; first hour
wRVU 1.40; Global XXX

+92627   each additional 15 minutes (List separately in addition to codes for primary procedure)
wRVU 0.33; Global ZZZ

92700   Unlisted otorhinolaryngological service or procedure
wRVU 0.00; Global XXX

Healthcare Common Procedure Coding System Level II (HCPCS II) Codes

The Healthcare Common Procedure Coding System Level II (HCPCS II) V codes are for hearing and vision services. The hearing services codes (V5000-V5299) include a few procedures, but the remainder of these codes are for the type, style, and technology of the hearing aid and the professional services associated with each of those styles or technology. The HCPCS Level II L codes are for "Orthotic/Prosthetic Procedures" which include the auditory osseointegrated devices. Typically the physician bills the surgical code; however, most often the device is supplied and billed by the facility where the surgical implan-

tation occurs. The L codes are utilized by audiologists for cochlear implant and osseointegrated devices, repairs, and/or supplies. The HCPCS Level II codes also include S0618 for "Audiometry for hearing aid evaluation to determine the level and degree of hearing loss" to determine the level and degree of hearing loss and S1001 for "Deluxe item, patient aware (list in addition to code for basic item)" which can be used for a hearing aid upgrade beyond which the patient's benefit plan allows. The S codes are usually recognized by some private payers such as Blue Cross Blue Shield.

V5008   Hearing screening

V5010   Assessment for hearing aid

V5020   Conformity evaluation

L7510   Repair of prosthetic device, repair or replace minor parts

L7520   Repair prosthetic device, labor component, per 15 minutes

L8690   Auditory osseointegrated device, includes all internal and external components

L8691   Auditory osseointegrated device, external sound processor, replacement

L8692   Auditory osseointegrated device, external sound processor, used without osseointegration, body worn, includes headband or other means of external attachment

L8693   Auditory osseointegrated device abutment, any length, replacement only

L9900   Orthotic and prosthetic supply, accessory, and/or service component of another HCPCS "L" code

Key Modifiers

22   Increased Procedural Services
This can be used during an evaluation that requires additional testing such as when a child

or an adult with dementia is distracted during the testing and needs to be reminded of how and when to respond, resulting in an increase of time and complexity of the procedure.

26 Professional Component

This can be used when only the interpretation and report is performed for a code that has both professional and technical components (eg, 92540-92546, 92548, 92585, 92587, and 92588). For example, the audiologist provides only the professional component (interpretation and report) of a basic vestibular evaluation (92540-26).

TC Technical Component

This is used when only the technical aspects are performed for a code that has both technical and professional components (eg, 92540-92546, 92548, 92585, 92587, and 92588). For example, the audiologist provides only the technical component of a basic vestibular evaluation (92540-TC).

52 Reduced Services

This is used when only one ear is tested or if not all of a test was completed.

59 Distinct Procedure Service

This is used to indicate when two or more procedures not typically performed on the same date of service are appropriate to be billed due to the National Correct Coding Initiative (NCCI) edits. An explanation can be found at the CMS website: http://www.cms.gov/Medicare/Coding/National CorrectCodInitEd/Downloads/modifier59.pdf.

Key ICD-9-CM/ICD-10-CM Codes

In the *International Classification of Diseases, Ninth Revision, Clinical Modification* ICD-9-CM coding system, the most frequent disease codes utilized by audiologists fall under the hearing loss codes, 389–389.9. These are to be selected based on the outcome of the test results or the reason for the tests, which may also include signs or symptoms. This must be a part of the documentation in the patient's medical record. The more specific the

code is, the less the chance for denial; therefore, it is preferred that in the ICD-9-CM system that unspecified codes are not billed.

Specificity is more critical in the *International Classification of Diseases, Tenth Revision, Clinical Modification* (ICD-10-CM) system, as is the detail in the documentation supporting the choice of disease codes. The hearing loss codes are H90.0–H91.23. There are exceptions within this coding system, so it is imperative for offices to have an updated resource, especially during the transition. Some examples of those exceptions with ICD-10-CM include the following:

- Unilateral hearing loss codes suggest normal or near-normal hearing thresholds in the opposite ear when the description includes "with unrestricted hearing on the contralateral side."
- There is no distinction between sensory hearing loss or neural hearing loss; both are categorized as sensorineural hearing loss.
- In the ICD-9-CM system, the middle ear hearing loss codes were classified by their location in the ear (eg, tympanic membrane, middle ear). This is not specified in the ICD-10-CM system.
- Tinnitus is not classified as subjective or objective in the ICD-10-CM codes as it is in ICD-9-CM.
- When a patient has a different type of hearing loss in each ear, the unspecified ICD-10-CM code for each will need to be utilized until new codes are introduced. For example, if the left ear has a sensorineural hearing loss and the right a conductive hearing loss, utilize H90.5 for the left ear and H90.2 for the right ear.

In the ICD-10-CM coding system, laterality is addressed with the following ear indicators, with some exceptions:

- 1 = right ear
- 2 = left ear
- 3 = bilateral
- 0 or 9 = unspecified

Examples of commonly used codes are as follows:

386.00/H81.0-   Ménière's disease

386.11/H81.1-   Benign paroxysmal vertigo

386.12/H81.2-   Vestibular neuronitis

386.30/H83.0-   Labyrinthitis

388.01/H91.1-   Presbycusis

388.10/H83.3X-   Noise effects on inner ear

388.12/H83.3X-   Noise effects on inner ear

388.2/H91.2-   Sudden idiopathic hearing loss

388.30/H93.1-   Tinnitus

388.31/—   Subjective tinnitus

388.32/—   Objective tinnitus

388.40/H93.24-   Temporary auditory threshold shift

388.70/H92.0-   Otalgia

389.00/H90.2   Conductive hearing loss, unspecified

389.05/H90.11   Conductive hearing loss, unilateral, right ear, with unrestricted hearing on the contralateral side

389.06/H90.0   Conductive hearing loss, bilateral

389.10/H90.5   Unspecified sensorineural hearing loss

389.15/H90.41   Sensorineural hearing loss, unilateral, right ear, with unrestricted hearing on the contralateral side

389.18/H90.3   Sensorineural hearing loss, bilateral

389.20/H90.8   Mixed conductive and sensorineural hearing loss, unspecified

389.21/H90.71   Mixed conductive and sensorineural hearing loss, unilateral, right ear, with unrestricted hearing on the contralateral side

389.22/H90.6   Mixed conductive and sensorineural hearing loss, bilateral

389.9/H91.90   Unspecified hearing loss, unspecified ear

780.4/R42   Dizziness and giddiness

Definition of Codes

Vestibular Function Tests (92540–92546, 92548)

Introduction—CPT codes 92540–92546 and 92548 have separate technical and professional components. Medicare requires the testing to be billed under the NPI of the performing audiologist, and the code is reported without any modifiers; this is called global billing. A technician may perform the technical component of the test and the physician providing direct supervision will bill the code with modifier TC to Medicare. Either the audiologist or the physician may perform the interpretation and report and would bill the code with modifier 26 for the professional component. For all tests, a printout and the interpretation of the test results should be included in the patient's medical record.

1. Basic vestibular evaluation (92540)
   a. *Definition*—CPT 92540 includes 92541, 92542, 92544, and 92545. For electronystagmography (ENG), vertical electrodes (+92547) are applied and are billed as one unit per date of service. Eye movements are tracked with a light stimulus, and eye movement is evaluated, upward, downward, and side to side, looking for the presence of nystagmus.
   b. *Key points*—Do not report 92540 with any of the 4 tests listed above. If only 1 to 3 of these are performed on the same date of service, use modifier 59 (distinct procedural service) on the lower-valued separate codes and include in the documentation why the tests were performed.

2. Calorics (92543)
   a. *Definition*—The caloric vestibular test is performed by irrigating the ear canal with

either water or air for a period of 30 to 60 seconds, then recording the eye movement response (nystagmus) for approximately 2 minutes following the irrigation.

b. *Key points*—Report the code once per test performed. For example, binaural (both ears) and bithermal (two temperatures, usually warm and cool) are considered 4 tests which is 4 units on the claim form. This will change after January 1, 2016, when there will be 2 caloric codes (bithermal/unilateral and bithermal/bilateral) and only 1 unit will be filed.

3. Rotary Chair (92546)
   a. For CPT 92546 the use of a computer-controlled rotary chair is used to evaluate nystagmus with the patient, wearing electrodes, seated with their head bent forward at 30° in the vertical axis position with their eyes closed, stimulating the horizontal vestibular canal.
   b. Some payers are requesting the serial number of the chair in order to ensure that correct billing by the appropriate provider has occurred.

4. Computerized Dynamic Posturography (92548)
   a. *Definition*—For CPT 92548, the patient stands on a computer-controlled platform equipped with sensors that examines body sway as well as utilizing abrupt movements, to evaluate posture in differentiating between motor, sensory, and central impairments used for balance control.
   b. *Key points*—Test protocols include the Sensory Organization Test (SOT), an Adaptation Test (ADT), Motor Control Test (MCT), and the Limits of Stability (LOS) test.

Audiologic Function Tests

Introduction—The following audiological tests do not have separate professional and technical components; therefore, they may not be performed by a technician and billed to Medicare under a supervising physician or audiologist NPI. As with all testing, a printout and the interpretation of the test results should be included in the patient's medical record.

1. Tympanometry and reflex threshold measurements (92550)
   a. *Definition*—CPT 92550 includes tympanometry and acoustic reflexes, ipsilaterally and contralaterally. The CPT code descriptor notes 500, 1000, 2000, and 4000 Hz for right and left contralateral stimulations and 500, 1000, and 2000 for right and left ipsilateral stimulations, for a total of 14 frequencies, performed at the maximum pressure compliance of the tympanic membrane, the equipment typically defaulting to this pressure setting.
   b. *Key points*—if performing only ipsilateral or only contralateral reflexes, use modifier 52 to indicate that the entire procedure was not completed.

2. Comprehensive audiometry threshold evaluation and speech recognition (92557)
   a. *Definition*—This includes otoscopy, pure tone air and bone conduction, speech reception thresholds, and word recognition scores.
   b. *Key points*—This code includes 92553 and 92556 and should not be billed separately.

3. Screening evoked otoacoustic emissions (92558)
   a. *Definition*—This is often utilized for newborn infant hearing screening, typically with automated equipment at one decibel level, resulting in a pass or refer. An otoscopic exam is performed and a probe tip is inserted into the ear canal. The test begins with automated otoacoustic emissions presented and evaluated, to determine if the responses are present (a "pass") or not (a "refer").
   b. *Key points*—This code has 0 wRVUs and is a noncovered service by Medicare.

4. Tympanometry (92567)
   a. *Definition*—This is a test of middle ear pressure and is performed by inserting a probe tip into the ear canal, securing a seal,

and once that is obtained, differing types of air pressure are automatically placed into the ear canal resulting in varying tympanic membrane movement. This determines normal versus pathologic conditions often described by Jerger Type (A, B, C, and As and Ad).

b. *Key points*—There is no definitive coding guidance if a seal cannot be obtained or maintained, but proof of attempts in the documentation should be noted; modifier 52 is suggested when this occurs.

5. Acoustic immittance testing (92570)
   a. *Definition*—This includes tympanometry and acoustic reflex thresholds, ipsilaterally and contralaterally, and acoustic reflex decay as described above at 500 and 1000 Hz, bilaterally, 10 dB higher than the acoustic reflex threshold at those specific frequencies. The CPT code descriptor for acoustic reflex thresholds notes 500, 1000, 2000, and 4000 Hz for right and left contralateral stimulations and 500, 1000, and 2000 for right and left ipsilateral stimulations, for a total of 14 frequencies, performed at the maximum pressure compliance of the tympanic membrane.
   b. *Key points*—If performing only ipsilateral or only contralateral reflexes, append modifier 52 to indicate that the entire procedure was not completed. Acoustic reflex decay may indicate further testing or consultations with other health care professionals.

6. Visual reinforcement audiometry (92579)
   a. *Definition*—This test includes obtaining both tonal or speech information using speakers or earphones, with the head-turning response reinforced by the use of moving toys, flashing lights, and/or video.
   b. *Key Points*—This is typically utilized with the pediatric, cognitively impaired, and/or nonverbal populations.

7. Conditioning play audiometry (92582)
   a. *Definition*—This too is typically utilized with the pediatric population; they are taught and conditioned to drop a block or

a toy in a box when they hear a sound, usually presented via earphones.
   b. *Key points*—Speech detection or reception thresholds can be filed separately (eg, 92555) as speech testing is not included in this code.

Audiology Function Tests With Separate Technical and Professional Components

Introduction—Unlike the audiologic function tests in the previous section, codes 92585 and 92587–92588, do have separate technical and professional components. Medicare allows a technician to perform the test, and the physician providing direct supervision may bill the code with modifier TC. Either the audiologist or the physician may perform the interpretation and report and would bill the code with modifier 26 for the professional component. If the audiologist performed the test, the interpretation, and the report, then the claim is filed with the global code (no modifiers) under the NPI of the audiologist. As with the other tests discussed, a printout and the interpretation of the test results should be included in the patient's medical record.

1. Auditory Evoked Potentials (92585)
   a. *Definition*—This is a neurophysiological test is used as a site of lesion testing for acoustic neuromas, effects of toxins that can impact the central auditory pathway, for auditory neuropathy as well as threshold detection. A series of waveforms are produced and classified based on wave morphology, time, intensity, and latencies.
   b. *Key points*—Electrodes are required and are part of the test protocol, with no separate reporting of 92547.

2. Transient or Distortion Product Otoacoustic Emissions (OAEs), Limited Evaluation (92587)
   a. *Definition*—This test is typically used to evaluate cochlear status in infants, toddlers, those who are difficult to test, and/or malingerers; also utilized to differentiate cochlear vs retrocochlear function in those with asymmetric hearing loss and for ototoxicity monitoring.

b. *Key points*—If using distortion product otoacoustic emissions (DPOAEs), 3 to 6 frequencies must be tested in each ear, with interpretation and report.

3. Distortion Production Otoacoustic Emissions, Comprehensive (92588)
   a. *Definition*—A minimum of 12 frequencies each ear are tested.
   b. *Key points*—This is typically performed for tinnitus and/or ototoxicity monitoring, pediatric testing, and cochlear vs retrocochlear lesion differential diagnosis to determine outer hair cell function.

Evaluative and Therapeutic Services

Introduction—The following codes are for common evaluation and assessment services performed by audiologists.

1. Evaluation of central auditory function (92620)
   a. *Definition*—This is a battery of tests that include auditory figure-ground tests, tonal pattern recognition, competing words, speech in noise and tonal duration.
   b. *Key points* The beginning and end times of the face-to-face evaluation should be included in the chart documentation, as this is a test for the initial 60 minutes. If additional time is required, each 15-minute block can be billed with CPT 92621. The reduced services modifier, 52, does not apply to time-based codes.

2. Assessment of Tinnitus (92625)
   a. *Definition*—This code requires 3 procedures when evaluating patients with tinnitus (self-perceived sounds). This includes pitch, loudness matching, and masking. The patient is to match the type of tinnitus when stimuli are offered in a bracketing method as well as for the intensity of their tinnitus. Once established, minimum masking levels are introduced for 1 minute to determine if the patient experienced a change in his or her tinnitus.

3. Evaluation of Auditory Rehabilitation Status (92626)
   a. *Definition*—this assesses the effectiveness of a patient's residual hearing either prior to or after receiving hearing aid(s), cochlear implant(s), osseointegrated device(s), and/or a brainstem implant. The audiologist determines auditory rehabilitation status with a series of speech-perception (speech awareness, speech recognition, sound discrimination, and speech in noise) and communication outcome measures, prior to any therapeutic intervention, to determine the need for any therapies and to monitor progress.
   b. *Key Points*—This is not a counseling code and it does not include hearing aid examination and selection, hearing aid fitting, or the cochlear implant programming (see 92601–92604). The times when the face-to-face evaluation began and ended should be included in the chart documentation. CPT code 92626 should not be used if the procedure lasted less than 31 minutes. If the procedure was 30 minutes or less, CPT code 92700 (unlisted otorhinolaryngological service or procedure) may be utilized, likely requiring supporting documentation. The reduced services modifier, 52, does not apply to time-based codes and thus cannot be used. If this requires more than an hour of time, then 92627 can be billed for each additional 15-minute time period.

4. Cochlear Implant Codes (92601–92604)
   a. *Definition*—Also included in the Evaluative and Therapeutic Services section are the four cochlear implant codes (92601–92604) which are age and function based.
   b. *Key Points*—CPT codes 92601 and 92602 are utilized for those cochlear implant patients younger than 7 years of age. For the initial stimulation of the implant(s), for those younger than 7, use 92601 and for subsequent reprogramming/mapping for the same aged patient, 92602. For those age 7 or older, the initial stimulation of the implant(s) is 92603 and for subsequent reprogramming/mapping, 92604.

5. Unlisted Procedures (92700)
   a. *Definition*—When there is not a dedicated CPT code describing a service provided, as in the example of vestibular evoked myogenic potentials (VEMPs), an unlisted code may be reported as instructed in the March 2011 *CPT Assistant*.
   b. *Key points*—A narrative describing the procedure and accompanying literature demonstrating its validity should be submitted for a denial.

Specific Audiology Issues

Evaluation and Management Codes (99201–99205, 99211–99215)

An area of controversy is whether an audiologist may report an E/M code as these are not recognized by Medicare when reported by an audiologist, and as a result, other payers have followed this guidance. Check with your local payers as well as state licensure laws.

Billing Provider Guidelines

As previously discussed, Medicare will allow a technician to perform the technical component of tests that have separate technical and professional components (eg, ENG, rotary chair, platform posturography, otoacoustic emissions, auditory brainstem response) if the billing/supervising physician provides general supervision. The technical services performed by the technician are billed under the supervising physician's NPI with modifier TC. General supervision means the procedure is furnished under the physician's overall direction and control, but the physician's presence is not required during the performance of the procedure. Under general supervision, the training of the nonphysician personnel who actually performs the diagnostic procedure and the maintenance of the necessary equipment and supplies are the continuing responsibility of the physician. Technicians can only perform the test and not any interpretive services.

Audiologists may also perform the test if someone else (eg, physician, nonphysician practitioner) is providing the interpretation and report. The audiologist would report the appropriate code(s) with modifier TC. When an audiologist only performs the interpretation and report, that test is then billed by the audiologist with modifier 26. If the same audiologist performs the test as well as completes the interpretation and report, it is reported as a global code, without any modifiers. The reimbursement is the same when the TC and PC components are filed separately as the reimbursement for filing the global code(s).

Four scenarios to describe the different providers performing the test and billing for them are discussed below:

- Scenario 1: The audiologist performs the technical and professional components of the test. The code, without a modifier, is billed by the audiologist.
- Scenario 2: The technician performs the test under general physician supervising, and the audiologist performs the report and interpretation. The physician reports the code with modifier TC (technical component), and the audiologist reports the same code with modifier 26 (professional component).
- Scenario 3: The technician performs the test under general physician supervision, and the same physician performs the interpretation and report. The physician reports the code without a modifier.
- Scenario 4: The audiologist performs the test while the physician (or nonphysician provider) performs the interpretation and report. The audiologist reports the code with modifier TC and the physician/nonphysician provider reports the code with modifier 26.

Check with your private payers for their guidelines. Many will separately credential audiologists as a billing provider that will keep their charges, collections, and other measures of productivity consistently aligned with the provider performing the service rather than a supervising physician.

National Correct Coding Initiative (NCCI) Edits

There are several audiology procedures that Medicare considers bundled when performed on the same date of service. For example, a comprehensive audiometry (92557) and cochlear implant mapping (92601–92604) billed together would not be allowed according to Medicare's National Correct Coding Initiative (NCCI) edits. The NCCI edits also include Medically Unlikely Edits (MUEs) that are specific to the number of allowed code units in a day.

NCCI edits either disallow specific code combinations from being billed on the same date of service or allow the code combination indicating if a modifier may be utilized to bypass the denial edit. NCCI edits are updated quarterly and can be found on the CMS website: http://www.cms.gov/Medicare/Coding/NationalCorrectCodInitEd/index.html.

Medicare

Medicare is the largest insurer and stringent rules apply to all participating providers including audiologists, who must enroll in Medicare unless all diagnostic audiology services are given to each patient at no charge. Although physicians, including otolaryngologists, are allowed to opt out of Medicare, audiologists are not. In an otolaryngology office with audiologist employees, this could be problematic if an otolaryngologist chooses to opt out of Medicare but the practice audiologist cannot. It is imperative for every practice manager to read Chapter 15, sections 80.3, Audiology Services and section 80.6.1, definitions in the *Medicare Benefits Policy Manual*, addressing the definition of a qualified audiologist, audiology services, physician orders, coverage, individuals who furnish audiology tests, documentation, treatment, and opting out.

"Incident to" Versus Physician Supervision of Diagnostic Tests

As previously noted, diagnostic audiology services are never to be billed "incident to," including CPT

code 92557, basic comprehensive audiometry, because these services reside in the "other diagnostic test" Medicare category and are excluded from the "incident to" requirements. Check with your Medicare Administrative Contractor (MAC) for guidance on the recognition and use of automated audiometry using Category III CPT codes (0208T, 0209T, 0210T, 0211T, and 0212T) if this testing method is utilized in your office, because Medicare does not pay for these services. Many payers do not reimburse for automated audiometry.

Currently audiologists have 2 requirements in the provision of diagnostic services to a Medicare beneficiary: medical necessity and a physician order. Medical necessity is defined as "reasonable and necessary for the diagnosis or treatment of illness or injury or to improve the functioning of a malformed body member." Medicare requires a physician order to ensure the information is needed for the diagnosis and treatment of the patient. Change in hearing acuity, balance function, and/or tinnitus must meet medical necessity, and the order should indicate the reason for the referral. If specific CPT codes are ordered, the Medicare policy states that the audiologist can only perform the tests that were specifically ordered. So if another test is necessary for differential diagnosis, another order will need to be obtained.

If no CPT codes are specified on the physician order, the audiologist is able to perform the evaluation utilizing the appropriate medically necessary tests to determine the patient's diagnosis and treatment. Medicare will pay for an audiologic evaluation if the only diagnosis is sensorineural hearing loss; however, they will deny the evaluation if the outcome is already known to the physician or the test was ordered for the specific purpose of modifying or fitting a hearing aid. The case history and the performed audiologic services must clearly be documented in the chart and signed and dated by the provider. The physician order may be from any Medicare-recognized provider assuming the order is within the provider's state scope of practice.

Medicare's Advanced Beneficiary Notice

The Advanced Beneficiary Notice (ABN), a notice of the patient's financial responsibility, is a component of the Beneficiary Notices Initiative (BNI). The ABN is designed for the patient to understand that not all of the services or procedures provided may be a covered service and informs the patient of any expected out-of-pocket payment.

For many services and procedures, there is a mandatory and voluntary use of the ABN. The mandatory ABN informs the patient that the service may not be covered, that it will be filed to Medicare, but if it denied as "Medicare does not pay for everything, even some care that you or your health care provider have good reason to think you need" (CMS, 2012), then the patient is responsible. One of the four Medicare specific modifiers, GA, is used to alert Medicare that the ABN was provided to the patient and the patient was made aware that the procedure may not be covered. If an ABN is not issued to the patient and the service is denied, the provider is liable and cannot pursue payment from the Medicare beneficiary. A signed and dated ABN must be on file in order to bill the patient if a denial is issued by Medicare.

Contact your Medicare carrier as local policies differ and therefore contractors may differ in their guidance. The ABN forms and directions can be located on the CMS website (https://www.cms.gov/BNI/02_ABN.asp#TopOfPage).

Medicare ABN Modifiers

There are 4 Medicare modifiers that are used to indicate an ABN situation: GA, GY, GX, and GZ. The Medicare modifiers are described below and include examples of when they are used with audiology procedures and services.

- GA: "Waiver of Liability Statement issued as Required by Payer Policy," is utilized when a required/mandatory ABN is given to the patient when the audiologist is not certain if the procedures will be covered by Medicare to be medically necessary or reasonable. If a denial is issued then the patient can then be billed for these procedures because the patient signed the ABN prior to the service. Without an ABN and signature, the patient cannot be billed,

and the practice will have to write off the claim amount.
- GY: "Item or service statutorily excluded or does not meet the definition of any Medicare benefit," is utilized when the procedure is statutorily excluded and does not meet the definition of a Medicare benefit, such as hearing aids. Many commercial payers require a denial from Medicare in order for the patient to access the hearing aid benefit provided by the secondary payer. In addition, indicate in box 19 of the CMS claim for that the denial by Medicare is necessary in order for the secondary to pay for the hearing aid(s). This will prompt an automatic denial. The GY modifier can be appended with modifier GX modifier for the same purpose.
- GX modifier: "Notice of Liability Issued, Voluntary Under Payer Policy," indicates a nonrequired/voluntary ABN, and was issued for noncovered services such as a routine audiologic evaluation that is not based on medical necessity, hearing aids, tinnitus treatment, or aural rehabilitation. Patients may be given the voluntary ABN, attesting to understanding of fiscal responsibility by way of a signature, in case the claim is contested at a later date.
- GZ modifier: "Item or Service Expected To Be Denied As Not Reasonable and Necessary" is utilized when an ABN is not on file, often occurring in an emergent situation. When claims are submitted with this modifier, billing the patient for those services is disallowed and they must be written off. This is the least common Medicare modifier utilized by audiologists.

Medicaid

Medicaid programs are administered by the state in which the practice resides. If your office is a Medicaid provider, familiarize yourself with the fee schedule, covered services, and applicable otolaryngology and audiology policies, especially for hearing aids. Many states no longer reimburse for hearing aids or for hearing aid evaluations for adults. Due to the Early and Periodic Screening, Diagnostic and Treatment (EPSDT) program responsible for child health, services including hearing aids that meet medical necessity, such as for those at risk for hearing loss, are a required covered service for Medicaid beneficiaries from birth to age 21. To find your state's requirements, go to http://www.hearingloss.org/sites/default/files/docs/MEDICAID_REGULATIONS.pdf.

Commercial Payers

Accepting commercial insurance is a critical practice decision; each contract should be weighed for its advantages and disadvantages. Some combination otolaryngology and audiology practices have found a separate corporation for hearing aids to be helpful when contracted for otolaryngology services, but consultation with legal counsel familiar with federal and state health care laws is imperative to see if this is a viable and legal option. Many joint profession contracts require the discount of services be applied to hearing aids, something that will have a substantial impact on the financial health of a practice. It is critical to read each contract, and some practices even have them reviewed by legal counsel.

At the time of publication approximately 19 states mandate commercial payers to have hearing aid coverage for children and several states mandate coverage for both children and adults.

Itemization of Hearing Aid Fees

Some payers prefer the itemization of all the fees associated with the dispensing of a hearing aid, including the acquisition of the device as well as the professional fees, while others prefer all the fees to be bundled, filing one fee for all hearing aid–related services, including professional services. Private pay patients should be billed the same way, with the same codes and the same fees. By itemizing fees, each service performed

is listed individually including the dispensing, orientation, and verification of the hearing aid(s), earmold(s), earmold impression(s), batteries, and follow-up visits. These are listed separately with the corresponding HCPCS Level II code.

The hearing aid codes are listed by style, including the following:

- CIC [completely in the canal]
- ITE [in the ear]
- ITC [in the canal]
- BTE [behind the ear]
- Body

The codes are also listed whether monaural or binaural, and by technology (analog, programmable, and digital). There are codes for combinations of all these types of hearing aids. By itemizing, the practice's potential is optimized to be paid not only for the device but for professional fees. These are lost in a bundled model and may not allow for the total reimbursement capture. A practice should know the hourly rate to have a sustainable and viable hearing aid fee schedule.

Verification of Hearing Aid Services

Every practice must know how hearing aids are to be paid at the time the devices are ordered. Payment for every hearing aid covered by a third party, in whole or in part, should be discussed with the patient and listed on the purchase agreement, requiring the patient's signature as well as the date the hearing aids were ordered, the date they were dispensed, and the patient's financial responsibility. The patient should receive a copy of this signed agreement. This should also lessen any misunderstanding of what the third-party coverage will be as that will be verified at the appointment that includes the purchase agreement; a contract specifying payment; the make, model, and serial numbers of the device(s); and any state licensure law requirements that are to be included. For private cash pay patients, the patient's fiscal responsibility should be itemized, and the patient needs to sign a statement attesting to his or her understanding of what is owed and when it needs to be paid.

Conclusion

This chapter has attempted to offer detailed guidance on many facets of billing and coding of audiologic services when offered in an otolaryngology office. There are many nuances, especially those required by Medicare, that are not experienced by other health care providers but are specific to audiologists. It is the hope that this chapter enlightens the staff of an otolaryngology practice in creating successful patient services provided by audiologists.

Resources

1. American Academy of Audiology. Audiology superbill template. http://www.audiology.org/practice_management/coding/international-classification-diseases-10th-edition. Published 2015. Accessed January 11, 2016.
2. Centers for Medicare and Medicaid Services. Advanced Beneficiary Notice. http://www.cms.gov/Medicare/Medicare-General-Information/BNI/ABN.html. Published 2013. Accessed February 2, 2013.
3. Centers for Medicare and Medicaid Services. Program memorandum AB-02-080, Audiologists—payment for services furnished. http://www.noridianmedicare.com/cgibin/coranto/viewnews.cgi?id. Published 2001. Accessed August 11, 2014.
4. Centers for Medicare and Medicaid Services. Transmittal 84. https://www.cms.gov/transmittals/downloads/R84BP.pdf. Published 2008. Accessed March 2, 2008.
5. Centers for Medicare and Medicaid Services. MLN Matters Number SE 0908. http://www.cms.gov/Outreach-and-Education/Medicare-Learning-Network-MLN/MLNMattersArticles/downloads/SE0908.pdf. Published January 2013. Accessed August 17, 2014.
6. Centers for Medicare and Medicaid Services. Revisions and re-issuance of audiology policies-JA6447. http://www.cms.gov/Outreach-and-Education/Medicare-Learning-Network-MLN/MLNMattersArticles/downloads/MM6447.pdf. Published 2010. Accessed August 13, 2014.
7. Centers for Medicare and Medicaid Services. Medicare benefit policy manual, chapter 15 (p. 101). http://www.cms.gov/Regulations-and-Guidance/Guidance/Manuals/Downloads/bp102c15.pdf. Published 2014. Accessed August 21, 2014.
8. Centers for Medicare and Medicaid Services. MLN Matters Number: SE0908. http://www.cms.gov/MLNMattersArticles/downloads/SE0908.pdf. Published 2011. Accessed November 3, 2011.
9. Social Security Act. Payment for physicians' services. Sec. 1848. [42 U.S.C. 1395w–4]. http://www.ssa.gov/OP_Home/ssact/title18/1848.htm. Published 2003. Accessed July 6, 2014.
10. *United States Federal Register.* NPI final rule. http://www.cms.hhs.gov/NationalProvIdentStand/Downloads/NPIfinalrule.pdf. Published 2004. Accessed January 3, 2012.

CHAPTER 18

Office Facial Plastic Surgery

Amit D. Bhrany

Introduction

This chapter describes coding for noncosmetic facial plastic surgery procedures performed in the office setting. Procedures covered in the chapter are those that may be performed under local anesthesia in the office, whereas facial plastic procedures typically performed under sedation or general anesthesia are covered in Chapter 27, "Operative Facial Plastic Surgery." The chapter concludes with some general comments regarding the finances and logistics of cosmetic procedures.

Key Points

- Modifier 25 should be placed on the evaluation and management (E/M) code for an office visit if a procedure is performed as a result of decisions made during the office evaluation.
- The skin biopsy codes (11100, 11101) have a 0-day postoperative global period, per Centers for Medicare and Medicaid Services (CMS) guidelines. Excision of skin lesion codes (114xx, 116xx) and their relevant wound repair codes (intermediate, complex) have a 10-day global period. Repairs involving adjacent tissue transfers have a 90-day global period. Codes with a 10 day global period include suture removal or examination of

the wound once postoperatively, even if that visit occurs outside the 10-day period.
- Multiple excisions of lesions should be billed with separate codes for each lesion.
- Multiple wound repairs of the same type and anatomic locations should be summed, with one code billed for the total length of repair.
- Modifier 58 should be applied to a procedure code if done as a second stage within the global period of a related procedure.
- For most facial plastic surgery diagnoses, *International Classification of Diseases, Tenth Revision, Clinical Modification* (ICD-10-CM) codes are generically converted one-to-one from the *International Classification of Diseases, Ninth Revision, Clinical Modification* (ICD-9-CM) code; however, ICD-10-CM codes often have more specific descriptions of each code and additional language, including laterality of disease.

Key Procedure Codes

Local anesthesia is included in all of these procedural codes.

Skin Lesions

Skin lesions can be biopsied, excised, destroyed, or shaved, and different codes exist for each. If a + is listed before a code, it is an add-on code that is only used in addition to the associated primary code. Excision of skin lesion coding is based on the location of the lesion and the size of the resected diameter. Simple closure is included in all excision codes. If intermediate or complex repair is required, this can be reported separately (see section below, "Wound Repair"). Each lesion is coded separately.

Biopsy

11100 Biopsy of skin, subcutaneous tissue and/or mucous membrane (including simple closure), unless otherwise listed; single lesion
wRVU 0.81; Global 0

> **+11101** each separate/additional lesion (List separately in addition to code for primary procedure)
> *wRVU 0.41; Global ZZZ*

Excision of Benign Skin Lesions

11420 Excision, benign lesion including margins, except skin tag (unless listed elsewhere), scalp, neck, hands, feet, genitalia; excised diameter 0.5 cm or less
wRVU 1.03; Global 10

> **11421** excised diameter 0.6 cm to 1.0 cm
> *wRVU 1.47; Global 10*

> **11422** excised diameter 1.1 cm to 2.0 cm
> *wRVU 1.68; Global 10*

> **11423** excised diameter 2.1 cm to 3.0 cm
> *wRVU 2.06; Global 10*

> **11424** excised diameter 3.1 cm to 4.0 cm
> *wRVU 2.48; Global 10*

> **11426** excised diameter over 4.0 cm
> *wRVU 4.09; Global 10*

11440 Excision, other benign lesion including margins, except skin tag (unless listed elsewhere), face, ears, eyelids, nose, lips, mucous membrane; excised diameter 0.5 cm or less
wRVU 1.05; Global 10

> **11441** excised diameter 0.6 cm to 1.0 cm
> *wRVU 1.53; Global 10*

> **11442** excised diameter 1.1 cm to 2.0 cm
> *wRVU 1.77; Global 10*

> **11443** excised diameter 2.1 cm to 3.0 cm
> *wRVU 2.34; Global 10*

> **11444** excised diameter 3.1 cm to 4.0 cm
> *wRVU 3.19; Global 10*

> **11446** excised diameter over 4.0 cm
> *wRVU 4.80; Global 10*

Excision of Malignant Skin Lesions

11620 Excision, malignant lesion including margins, scalp, neck, hands, feet, genitalia; excised diameter 0.5 cm or less
wRVU 1.64; Global 10

> **11621** excised diameter 0.6 cm to 1.0 cm
> *wRVU 2.08; Global 10*

> **11622** excised diameter 1.1 cm to 2.0 cm
> *wRVU 2.41; Global 10*

> **11623** excised diameter 2.1 cm to 3.0 cm
> *wRVU 3.11; Global 10*

> **11624** excised diameter 3.1 cm to 4.0 cm
> *wRVU 3.62; Global 10*

> **11626** excised diameter over 4.0 cm
> *wRVU 4.61; Global 10*

11640 Excision, malignant lesion including margins, face, ears, eyelids, nose, lips; excised diameter 0.5 cm or less
wRVU 1.67; Global 10

> **11641** excised diameter 0.6 cm to 1.0 cm
> *wRVU 2.17; Global 10*

> **11642** excised diameter 1.1 cm to 2.0 cm
> *wRVU 2.62; Global 10*

> **11643** excised diameter 2.1 cm to 3.0 cm
> *wRVU 3.42; Global 10*

> **11644** excised diameter 3.1 cm to 4.0 cm
> *wRVU 4.34; Global 10*

> **11646** excised diameter over 4.0 cm
> *wRVU 6.26; Global 10*

Wound Repair

Wounds can be repaired with direct closure, local flaps, or tissue grafts. Closure can be accomplished using sutures, staples, tissue adhesives, or a combination of these. One cannot bill for closure if only adhesive strips are used. The wound repair codes are chosen based on anatomical site, size of the repair (sum of lengths of repairs for each group of anatomic sites), and classification of the repair. Thus, if more than one closure is performed on the same subsite, in the same classification, they should be added together and reported for the cumulative length. If more than one classification of repair is performed in the same subsite, then the more complex repair should be billed as the primary procedure and the less complex as a secondary procedure, using modifier 59.

Simple Repair

12001 Simple repair of superficial wounds of scalp, neck, axillae, external genitalia, trunk and/or extremities (including hands and feet); 2.5 cm or less
wRVU 0.84; Global 0

12002 2.6 cm to 7.5 cm
wRVU 1.14; Global 0

12004 7.6 cm to 12.5 cm
wRVU 1.44; Global 0

12005 12.6 cm to 20.0 cm
wRVU 1.97; Global 0

12006 20.1 cm to 30.0 cm
wRVU 2.39; Global 0

12007 over 30.0 cm
wRVU 2.90; Global 0

12011 Simple repair of superficial wounds of face, ears, eyelids, nose, lips and/or mucous membranes; 2.5 cm or less
wRVU 1.07; Global 0

12013 2.6 cm to 5.0 cm
wRVU 1.22; Global 0

12014 5.1 cm to 7.5 cm
wRVU 1.57; Global 0

12015 7.6 cm to 12.5 cm
wRVU 1.98; Global 0

12016 12.6 cm to 20.0 cm
wRVU 2.68; Global 0

12017 20.1 cm to 30.0 cm
wRVU 3.18; Global 0

12018 over 30.0 cm
wRVU 3.61; Global 0

Intermediate Repair

12031 Repair, intermediate, wounds of scalp, axillae, trunk and/or extremities (excluding hands and feet); 2.5 cm or less
wRVU 2.00; Global 10

12032 2.6 cm to 7.5 cm
wRVU 2.52; Global 10

12034 7.6 cm to 12.5 cm
wRVU 2.97; Global 10

12035 12.6 cm to 20.0 cm
wRVU 3.50; Global 10

12036 20.1 cm to 30.0 cm
wRVU 4.23; Global 10

12037 over 30.0 cm
wRVU 5.00; Global 10

12041 Repair, intermediate, wounds of neck, hands, feet and/or external genitalia; 2.5 cm or less
wRVU 2.10; Global 10

12042 2.6 cm to 7.5 cm
wRVU 2.79; Global 10

12044 7.6 cm to 12.5 cm
wRVU 3.19; Global 10

12045 12.6 cm to 20.0 cm
wRVU 3.75; Global 10

12046 20.1 cm to 30.0 cm
wRVU 4.30; Global 10

12047 over 30.0 cm
wRVU 4.95; Global 10

12051   Repair, intermediate, wounds of face, ears, eyelids, nose, lips and/or mucous membranes; 2.5 cm or less
wRVU 2.33; Global 10

> **12052**   2.6 cm to 5.0 cm
> *wRVU 2.87; Global 10*
>
> **12053**   5.0 cm to 7.5 cm
> *wRVU 3.17; Global 10*
>
> **12054**   7.6 cm to 12.5 cm
> *wRVU 3.50; Global 10*
>
> **12055**   12.6 cm to 20.0 cm
> *wRVU 4.50; Global 10*
>
> **12056**   20.1 cm to 30.0 cm
> *wRVU 5.30; Global 10*
>
> **12057**   over 30.0 cm
> *wRVU 6.00; Global 10*

Complex Repair

All complex repair codes are for wounds 1.1 cm or longer. In the past 13150 described a complex repair of a wound less than 1.0 cm. This code has since been deleted. As a result, for wounds 1.0 cm or less, a simple or intermediate repair code should be reported.

13120   Repair, complex, scalp, arms, and/or legs; 1.1 cm to 2.5 cm
wRVU 3.23; Global 10

> **13121**   2.6 cm to 7.5 cm
> *wRVU 4.00; Global 10*
>
> **+13122**   each additional 5 cm or less (List separately in addition to code for primary procedure)
> *wRVU 1.44; Global ZZZ*

13131   Repair, complex, forehead, cheeks, chin, mouth, neck, axillae, genitalia, hands and/or feet; 1.1 cm to 2.5 cm
wRVU 3.73; Global 10

> **13132**   2.6 cm to 7.5 cm
> *wRVU 4.78; Global 10*
>
> **+13133**   each additional 5 cm or less (List separately in addition to code for primary procedure)
> *wRVU 2.19; Global ZZZ*

13151   Repair, complex, eyelids, nose, ears, and/or lips; 1.1 cm to 2.5 cm
wRVU 4.34; Global 10

> **13152**   2.6 cm to 7.5 cm
> *wRVU 5.34; Global 10*
>
> **+13153**   each additional 5 cm or less (List separately in addition to code for primary procedure)
> *wRVU 2.38; Global ZZZ*

Adjacent Tissue Transfer

These codes are used for excision (including lesion) and/or repair by adjacent tissue transfer or rearrangement. One cannot use these codes and then bill separately for the lesion excision. When done to repair lacerations, one must use additional incisions to use these codes, as simply undermining alone does not constitute a tissue transfer. If a full-thickness repair of a lip or eyelid is performed, separate codes exist for these in the appropriate anatomic subsection. The coding is based on anatomic site as well as on the size of the repair. The size is determined by adding the primary defect to the secondary defect (that which is created from flap design).

14020   Adjacent tissue transfer or rearrangement, scalp, arms, and/or legs; defect 10 sq cm or less
wRVU 7.22; Global 90

> **14021**   defect 10.1 sq cm to 30.0 sq cm
> *wRVU 9.72; Global 90*

14040   Adjacent tissue transfer or rearrangement forehead, cheeks, chin, mouth, neck, axillae, genitalia, hands and/or feet; defect 10 sq cm or less
wRVU 8.60; Global 90

> **14041**   defect 10.1 sq cm to 30.0 sq cm
> *wRVU 10.83; Global 90*

14060   Adjacent tissue transfer or rearrangement eyelids, nose, ears and/or lips; defect 10 sq cm or less
wRVU 9.23; Global 90

14061 defect 10.1 sq cm to 30.0 sq cm
wRVU 11.48; Global 90

14301 Adjacent tissue transfer or rearrangement, any area; defect 30.1 sq cm to 60.0 sq cm
wRVU 12.65; Global 90

> **+14302** each additional 30.0 sq cm, or part thereof (List separately in addition to code for primary procedure)
> *wRVU 3.73; Global ZZZ*

Surgical Preparation

Surgical preparation codes are used for excision of an open wound in preparation for closure. The preparation describes the initial services related to preparing a clean and viable wound surface for placement of an autograft, flap, or skin substitute graft or for negative pressure therapy. The intent of this code is to create a cavity that can then be closed by primary intention. This code is not to be used when the wound is left to heal by secondary intention, though the closure can be delayed. In some cases, closure can be accomplished using adjacent tissue transfer or complex repair. Additionally, the code is not to be used for wound debridement as preparing the wound is included in all surgical *Current Procedural Terminology* (CPT) codes.

15004 Surgical preparation or creation of recipient site by excision of open wounds, burneschar, or scar (including subcutaneous tissues), or incisional release of scar contracture, face, scalp, eyelids, mouth, neck, ears, orbits, genitalia, hands, feet and/or multiple digits; first 100 sq cm or 1% of body area of infants and children
wRVU 4.58; Global 0

> **+15005** each additional 100 sq cm, or part thereof, or each additional 1% of body area of infants and children (List separately in addition to code for primary procedure)
> *wRVU 1.60; Global ZZZ*

Grafts/Flaps/Other Office Skin Procedures

15240 Full thickness graft, free, including direct closure of donor site, forehead, cheeks, chin, mouth, neck, axillae, genitalia, hands, and/or feet; 20 sq cm or less
wRVU 10.41; Global 90

15260 Full thickness graft, free, including direct closure of donor site, nose, ears, eyelids, and/or lips; 20 sq cm or less
wRVU 11.64; Global 90

15576 Formation of direct or tubed pedicle, with or without transfer; eyelids, nose, ears, lips, or intraoral
wRVU 9.37; Global 90

15630 Delay of flap or sectioning of flap (division and inset); at eyelids, nose, ears, or lips
wRVU 4.08; Global 90

15780 Dermabrasion; total face (eg, for acne scarring, fine wrinkling, rhytids, general keratosis)
wRVU 8.73; Global 90

15781 Dermabrasion; segmental, face
wRVU 5.02; Global 90

Nasal Fracture Treatment

21310 Closed treatment of nasal bone fracture without manipulation
wRVU 0.58; Global 0

21315 Closed treatment of nasal bone fracture; without stabilization
wRVU 1.83; Global 10

> **21320** with stabilization
> *wRVU 1.88; Global 10*

21337 Closed treatment of nasal septal fracture, with or without stabilization
wRVU 3.39; Global 90

Eyelid and Brow Procedures

15822 Blepharoplasty, upper eyelid;
wRVU 4.62; Global 90

15823   with excessive skin weighting down lid
wRVU 6.81; Global 90

21282   Lateral canthopexy
wRVU 4.27; Global 90

67900   Repair of brow ptosis (supraciliary, mid-forehead, or coronal approach)
wRVU 6.82; Global 90

67912   Correction of lagophthalmos with implantation of upper eyelid lid load (eg, gold weight)
wRVU 6.36; Global 90

67917   Repair of ectropion; extensive (eg, tarsal strip operations)
wRVU 5.93; Global 90

67950   Canthoplasty (reconstruction of canthus)
wRVU 5.99; Global 90

67999   Unlisted procedure, eyelids
wRVU 0; Global YYY

Key Modifiers

25   Significant, Separately Identifiable Evaluation and Management Service by the Same Physician or Other Qualified Health Care Professional on the Same Day of the Procedure or Other Service
This can be appended to an E/M code, such as office visit, when doing a significant, separately identifiable E/M service on the same day as a minor procedure (one with a 0- or 10-day global period).

51   Multiple Procedures
Use when multiple procedures, other than E/M services, are performed at the same session, by the same individual. Append modifier 51 to the secondary procedure or service code(s).

58   Staged or Related Procedure or Service by the Same Physician or Other Qualified Health Care Professional During the Postoperative Period
This modifier is appended to a procedure code(s) when that procedure is done within the global

period of a previous related code, such as in the second stage of a paramedian forehead flap (15731) reconstruction when the pedicle is divided (15630-58).

59   Distinct Procedural Service
This is appended to a procedure code to indicate the procedure is a distinct, separate service to allow for codes to be reported that typically would not be allowed to be reported together for the same session (eg, 13132 and 14040 for a complex forehead repair and an adjacent tissue transfer of the cheek, respectively, for repairs of 2 separate wounds). Refer to Chapter 11, "Demystifying Modifiers," for more information.

79   Unrelated Procedure or Service by the Same Physician or Other Qualified Health Care Professional During the Postoperative Period
This is appended to a procedure code when that procedure is done during the global period of a different, unrelated procedure.

Key ICD-9-CM/ICD-10-CM Codes

For most facial plastic surgery diagnoses, ICD-10-CM codes are generically converted one-to-one —that is, 173.31 Basal cell carcinoma of unspecified parts of the face (ie, cheek) becomes C44.310. But ICD-10-CM codes often have more specific descriptions of each code and additional language, including laterality of disease. For instance, 173.31 would also be an adequate description for a basal cell carcinoma of the nose and/or cheek using ICD-9-CM. With ICD-10-CM, C44.311 is a more specific diagnosis to the nose with a change in the sixth character of the code. For the ears and eyes, the sixth character denotes laterality of the cancer with "1" being unspecified and "2" and "9" corresponding to right and left, respectively. Therefore, a basal cell carcinoma of the left eyelid (173.11 in ICD9) would be coded as C44.119, and a basal carcinoma of the right eyelid would be coded as C44.112. Below, when laterality should be specified this space is left with a "-".

For trauma and open wound codes, laterality clarification is also described with the sixth character of the code, with a "1" or "2" denoting right and left, respectively. If the side is unspecified, "9" is placed as the sixth character.

For example, a laceration of the right eyelid (870.0 in ICD-9-CM) would be coded as S01.111, and a laceration of the left eyelid (870.0 in ICD-9-CM) would be coded as S01.112. Furthermore, a seventh character "A", "D", or "S" is required for all injury codes (except fractures that use A, B, D, G, K, and S) in ICD-10-CM, indicating initial encounter, subsequent encounter, or sequela, respectively. Below is a list of some of the commonly used ICD-9-CM/ICD-10-CM diagnosis codes in office facial plastic surgery:

239.2/D49.2   Neoplasm of unspecified behavior of bone, soft tissue, and skin

173.01/C44.01   Basal cell carcinoma of skin of lip
(excludes vermilion 140.0/C00.0 -140.1/C00.01)

173.02/C44.02   Squamous cell carcinoma of skin of lip
(excludes vermilion 140.0/C00.0 -140.1/C00.01)

173.11/C44.11-   Basal cell carcinoma of skin of eyelid, including canthus

173.12/C44.12-   Squamous cell carcinoma of skin of unspecified eyelid, including canthus

173.21/C44.21-   Basal cell carcinoma of skin of ear and external auditory canal

173.22/C44.22-   Squamous cell carcinoma of skin of ear and external auditory canal

173.31/C44.310   Basal cell carcinoma of skin of unspecified parts of face

(for ICD-10-CM, C44.311 is used to specify basal cell carcinoma of skin of nose)

173.32/C44.320   Squamous cell carcinoma of skin of unspecified parts of face

(for ICD-10-CM, C44.321 is used to specify squamous cell carcinoma of skin of nose)

173.41/C44.41   Basal cell carcinoma of scalp and skin of neck

173.42/C44.42   Squamous cell carcinoma of skin of scalp and neck

172.0/C43.0   Malignant melanoma of lip
(excludes vermilion 140.0/C00.0 -140.1/C00.01)

172.1/C43.1-   Malignant melanoma of eyelid, including canthus

172.2/C43.2-   Malignant melanoma of ear and external auditory canal

172.3/C43.30   Malignant melanoma of unspecified part of the face
(for ICD-10-CM, C43.31 is used to specify melanoma of nose)

172.4/C43.4   Malignant melanoma of scalp and neck

870.0/S01.119A   Laceration without foreign body of unspecified eyelid and periocular area, initial encounter

870.1/S01.119A   Laceration without foreign body of unspecified eyelid and periocular area, initial encounter

872.01/S01.309A   Unspecified open wound of unspecified ear, initial encounter

873.0/S01.00XA   Unspecified open wound of scalp, initial encounter

873.20/S01.20XA   Unspecified open wound of nose, initial encounter

873.40/S09.93XA   Unspecified injury of face, initial encounter

874.8/S11.80XA   Unspecified open wound of other specified part of neck, initial encounter
Note that the above open wound codes require the seventh character change to D for subsequent encounters and S for sequela. Refer to this volume, Chapter 3, "Transition to ICD-10-CM," for more information about the seventh character requirements for injury codes.

802.0/S02.2XXA   Fracture of nasal bones, initial encounter for closed fracture

802.1/S02.2XXB   Fracture of nasal bones, initial encounter for open fracture
Note that the above fracture codes require the seventh character change to D, G, or K for subsequent encounters and S for sequela. Refer to this volume, Chapter 3," Transition to ICD-10-CM,"

for more information about the seventh character requirements for injury codes.

470/J34.2   Deviated nasal septum

374.10/H02.10-   Unspecified ectropion of eyelid

374.21/H02.23-   Paralytic lagophthalmos of eyelid

374.30/H02.40-   Unspecified ptosis of eyelid

374.87/H02.83-   Dermatochalasis of eyelid
The required sixth character for many of the eye ICD-10-CM codes are specific for right and left eyes as well as upper and lower eyelids. Refer to an ICD-10-CM source for more specific codes.

Definition of Procedure Codes

1. Biopsy of lesions (11100, 11101)
   a. *Definitions*—Biopsy codes are used when the procedure is performed to obtain integumentary tissue for diagnosis.
   b. *Key points*—Tissue is sent for histologic review, and biopsy is commonly performed by shaving or punching without removing the entire lesion. If the entire lesion is removed, an excision code (11420–11646) should be used instead. ICD-9-CM/ICD-10-CM diagnosis code 239.2/D49.2 (Neoplasm of uncertain nature, bone, soft tissue, and skin) is commonly associated with biopsy procedure codes. Report 11100 once for the first lesion biopsied and report the add-on code, 11101, for each addition lesion biopsied at the same session.

2. Excision of lesions (11420–11646)
   a. *Definitions*—Excision is defined as full-thickness (through the dermis) removal of a lesion, including margins and includes simple (nonlayered) closure when performed. When multiple lesions are excised at one setting, separately report each lesion excised using modifier 51 (unless a more appropriate modifier is available or required by the payer).

   b. *Key points*—Code selection is determined by measuring the greatest clinical diameter of the apparent lesion plus that margin required for adequate excision based on the physician's judgment. The measurement of the lesion plus margin is made prior to excision, and modifications to the excision for wound repair only (eg, lengthening the excision as an ellipse to facilitate wound closure) should not be added to diameter of lesion excised. If the added length of incision is a part of the margin required for adequate removal, it should be included within the diameter of excision. To code for an excision of a malignant lesion, it is best to have a tissue diagnosis either from a prior biopsy or excision. If a preexcision diagnosis is not available, wait to code the excision after pathology confirms a malignant diagnosis. If excision is being performed for wider margin clearance of a previous diagnosed malignant lesion, a malignant excision CPT code can be used even if no additional malignancy is identified histologically, because removal is being performed for definitive excision of the preexisting malignant lesion.

   Excision codes include simple (nonlayered) closures. When intermediate or complex repairs are required, these repair codes should be reported separately in addition to the excision code. If an adjacent tissue transfer is required for repair of an excision defect, only the adjacent tissue transfer repair code is reported for that specific lesion excision and repair. If multiple separate excisions are performed at one setting with one excision requiring an adjacent tissue transfer repair and the other excisions requiring only an intermediate or complex repair, the excisions and repairs not requiring adjacent tissue transfer are also reported separately for each lesion with 59 modifiers.

3. Wound repair (12001–13153)
   a. *Definitions*—The repair of wounds may be classified as simple, intermediate, or complex.

The wound repair codes require use of sutures, staples, or tissue adhesives (eg, Dermabond), either singly or in combination with each other, or in combination with adhesive strips. Report an E/M code, instead of a wound repair code, if only adhesive strips (eg, Steri-Strips) are used.

Simple repair is used when the wound requires simple 1-layer closure. This includes local anesthesia and chemical or electrocauterization of wounds not closed.

Intermediate repair includes the repair of wounds that require layered closure of one or more of the deeper layers of subcutaneous tissue and superficial (nonmuscle) fascia, in addition to the skin (epidermal and dermal) closure. Single-layer closure of heavily contaminated wounds that have required extensive cleaning or removal of particulate matter also constitutes intermediate repair.

Complex repair includes the repair of wounds requiring more than layered closure. Complex repair may include scar revision with excision of scar creating a defect, removal of standing cutaneous deformities for wound closure, debridement (eg, traumatic lacerations or avulsions), extensive undermining to obtain tension free closure or placement of stents or retention sutures. Extensive excision of an open wound in preparation for closure (15004) should be reported separately. Complex repair must be at least 1.1 cm in length; if the wound is smaller, the appropriate intermediate or simple closure code should be used. Intermediate and complex repair can be reported in addition to coding for an excision of a lesion if this is necessary to close the wound.

b. *Key points*—The repaired wound(s) should be measured and recorded in centimeters, whether linear, curved, angular or stellate. When multiple wounds of the same classification (simple, intermediate, complex) and anatomic group are repaired, sum the lengths of all repairs in order to report the appropriate wound repair code.

For example, if a 1.3 cm complex repair of the forehead is being performed at the same setting as a 2.4 cm cheek repair, these 2 repairs should be summed to 3.7 cm and coded with 13132 (Repair, complex, forehead, cheeks, chin, mouth, neck, axillae, genitalia, hands and/or feet; 2.6–7.5 cm).

Repairs from different groupings of anatomic sites (eg, forehead and nose) should not be summed and codes should be reported separately. Using the example above, if the 1.3 cm complex repair of the forehead was being performed at the same setting of a 2.4 cm complex nasal repair instead, the 2 separate anatomic sites should be coded since they are not grouped together: CPT 13131 for the forehead repair (Repair, complex, forehead, cheeks, chin, mouth, neck, axillae, genitalia, hands and/or feet; 1.1–2.5 cm) and 13151 used for the nasal repair (Repair, complex, eyelids, nose, ears, and/or lips; 1.1–2.5 cm).

Also, lengths of different repair classifications (simple, intermediate, complex) should not be summed but should be reported separately. When more than one classification of wounds is repaired, list the more complicated as the primary procedure and the less complicated as the secondary procedure, using modifier 59.

4. Adjacent tissue transfer (14020–14302)
   a. *Definitions*—An adjacent tissue transfer is defined as a method of repair that requires additional incisions and tissue rearrangement with closure of a primary and secondary defect (eg, a local flap).
   b. *Key points*—The primary defect may be due to a traumatic wound, laceration, or a surgically created wound resulting from excision of a lesion or scar. These wound repairs typically require the formation of local flaps, for example, advancement (eg, unipedicle, bipedicle, V-Y), pure rotational, rotational-advancement (eg, cervicofacial), and transposition (eg, bilobed, Z-plasty, rhombic, nasolabial) flaps.

   Once the most appropriate type of tissue transfer (eg, local flap) is designed, the adjacent skin and subcutaneous tissue are incised and elevated resulting in a secondary defect, then mobilized into the primary defect. Closure of the primary defect creates a secondary defect from which the flap was harvested. The areas of both primary and secondary defects must be documented in the procedure note. The surrounding tissue is undermined to allow for adequate mobilization of the skin flaps, and the secondary defect is closed. The length and width of the primary and secondary defects are measured to determine the respective areas. Then these are summed, in square centimeters (sq cm), to determine the appropriate adjacent tissue transfer code. Report one code per primary defect repaired; this may involve one or more secondary defects to repair the primary defect. If the secondary defect cannot be closed primarily, it may require a separately reportable skin graft code (15120, 15240, 15260) when obtained through a separate incision. The excision of a benign lesion (11420–11446) or a malignant lesion (11620–11646) is not separately reportable with adjacent tissue transfer codes for the same site.

If an adjacent tissue transfer is performed repairing a single primary defect that encompasses different anatomically grouped sites (eg, nose and cheek), only one adjacent tissue transfer code is used, measuring the entire primary and secondary defect area. The code selected is based on the larger anatomical site repaired, or if the total transfer is greater than 30 sq cm but no more than 60.0 sq cm, 14301 (Adjacent tissue transfer or rearrangement, any area; defect 30.1 sq cm to 60.0 sq cm) is reported.

If multiple adjacent tissue transfers are performed for separate primary defects of different anatomical grouping with each requiring separate incisions and flaps, each adjacent tissue transfer is coded and reported separately. For example, if a 16 sq cm transfer is performed on the cheek

and an 8 square centimeter adjacent tissue transfer is performed on the nose, 14041 (Adjacent tissue transfer or rearrangement forehead, cheeks, chin, mouth, neck, axillae, genitalia, hands and/or feet; defect 10.1 to 30.0 sq cm) would be reported for the cheek repair and 14060 (Adjacent tissue transfer or rearrangement, eyelids, nose, ears and/or lips; defect 10 sq cm or less) for the nose repair.

If multiple adjacent tissue transfers are performed within one anatomical grouping, but each at a separate site requiring separate incisions, each adjacent tissue transfer is not summed to report one code. The adjacent tissue transfers are coded separately using modifier 59 for the smaller repair(s), or other appropriate modifier per CPT and/or payer guidelines.

For example, if a 16 sq cm transfer is performed on the cheek and an 8 sq cm adjacent tissue transfer is performed on the forehead, 14041 (Adjacent tissue transfer or rearrangement forehead, cheeks, chin, mouth, neck, axillae, genitalia, hands and/or feet; defect 10.1 to 30.0 sq cm) would be reported for the cheek repair and 14040 with a 59 modifier (Adjacent tissue transfer or rearrangement, forehead, cheeks, chin, mouth, neck, axillae, genitalia, hands and/or feet; defect 10 sq cm or less) for the forehead repair. This distinction holds even when one of the separate adjacent tissue transfers is greater than 30 sq cm, requiring a 14301 code, with codes for both repairs being reported separately, again the smaller repair code being reported with a 59 modifier, or other appropriate modifier per payer requirements.

5. Surgical wound preparation (15004)
   a. *Definitions*—15004 is used to code for surgical wound preparation with the intent of primary reconstruction/closure. It describes services related to preparing a clean and viable wound surface for placement of an autograft, flap, or skin substitute graft, or for negative pressure wound therapy.

b. *Key points*—In some cases, closure may be possible using adjacent tissue transfer (14020–14302) or complex repair (13120–13153). Appreciable nonviable tissue is removed to optimize healing and reconstruction. An example includes the removal of a nonhealing wound of the neck after radiation therapy prior to placement of a flap or skin graft. CPT 15004 is not reportable for removal of nonviable tissue/debris in a chronic wound (eg, venous or diabetic) when the wound is left to heal by secondary intention.

6. Full-thickness skin grafts (15240, 15260)
    a. *Definitions*—A full-thickness skin graft is defined by harvest of a graft that includes the entire dermis.
    b. *Key points*—The graft may be thinned of some of its dermal layers, but differs from a split-thickness graft where only a part of the dermis is harvested, typically using a dermatome. Full-thickness grafts are usually harvested free hand with a knife. Primary repair of the donor site is included within the code, unless a local flap or additional graft is required for closure of the donor site and obtained through a separate incision.

7. Delay or sectioning of flap (15630)
    a. *Definitions*—Delay of flap refers to a staged division of a flap to enhance vascular supply. Delay involves incising or partially dividing the flap and then laying it back at its donor site to enhance circulation prior to transfer to the recipient site. Sectioning of flap refers to division of a previously inset pedicled flap (eg, paramedian forehead flap, 15731; tubed pedicled flap, 15576) and inset at the recipient site.
    b. *Key points*—The code used refers to the recipient site at which the flap is inset (15630 for flaps used for nasal repair). If additional repair is required at the donor site, a separately reportable wound repair or skin graft may be applied if obtained through a separate incision. Once inset, if

the flap requires secondary revision (eg, debulking or scar revision) at a later date, typically complex repair (13131–13153) or adjacent tissue transfer codes (14040–14302) are used. If 2 flaps are divided for a nasal reconstruction (eg, a paramedian forehead flap for skin coverage and a pedicled internal lining flap for mucosal reconstruction, the 15630 code should be reported twice with modifier 59 applied to the second code (or other appropriate modifier per CPT and/or payer guidelines).

8. Dermabrasion (15780, 15781)
    a. *Definitions*—Dermabrasion is controlled removal (abrading) of the superficial layers of the skin including the epidermis and papillary dermis. It is performed for scar improvement or skin rejuvenation. Dermabrasion can be performed with a rotary diamond fraise, wheel, or wire brush, but sterilized sandpaper is effective as well.
    b. *Key points*—Some payers consider dermabrasion a cosmetic procedure, and preauthorization prior to performing is recommended. With the advent of lasers, dermabrasion has become less popular but remains a simple, effective tool for the facial plastic surgeon.

9. Nasal/septal fractures (21310, 21315, 21320, 21337)
    a. *Definitions*—CPT 21320 describes closed reduction of a displaced nasal bone fracture, stabilized either with packing, internal or external splints. If no stabilization but manipulation method is used, 21315 should be used. If no manipulation but stabilization is used, then report 21310. CPT 21337 describes closed reduction of a nasal septal fracture, with or without stabilization using sutures, packing, or splints.
    b. *Key points*—If closed reduction of the nasal injury involves repair of a nasal septal fracture and nasal bone fracture, report the appropriate 21310–21320 code and 21337. Even though CPT implies both codes may be reported, many payers bundle the nasal

bone fracture repair code with the nasal septal repair code.

10. Upper blepharoplasty (15822, 15823)
    a. *Definitions*—A functional upper blepharoplasty is performed for the removal of excess, redundant skin from the upper eyelid when it is obscuring the superior portion of the visual field.
    b. *Key points*—For an upper blepharoplasty to be considered medically necessary and not cosmetic by most payers, visual field obstruction must be documented. Photographs demonstrating excess upper eyelid skin resting on or above eyelashes or upper eyelid dermatitis are useful. Visual field testing with eyelids taped up and untapped demonstrating a 20% improvement with taping the eyelid skin will typically satisfy payer requirements for medical necessity. CPT 15822 is not performed as often because it does not include removal of excessive skin.

11. Lateral canthopexy (21282)
    a. *Definitions*—A lateral canthopexy is performed to suspend and support the lateral canthus to the lateral orbital rim of the zygoma. A suture is placed through the lateral canthal tendon attaching it to the medial aspect of the lateral orbital rim. It is often performed in patients with facial paralysis with existing lower lid retraction. It is also performed in patients with excess lower lid laxity when undergoing lower eyelid reconstruction to help prevent postoperative lower eyelid retraction and/or ectropion.
    b. *Key points*—Although the terms are frequently used interchangeably, a lateral canthopexy differs from a lateral canthoplasty (67950). A lateral canthopexy refers to supporting the lateral canthal tendon to the lateral orbital rim alone. If there is a recreation of the lateral canthal angle during the procedure, the lateral canthoplasty (67950) code should be used. The lateral canthopexy code is also included in 67917 (repair of ectropion) and cannot be

billed separately when an extensive ectropion repair (eg, tarsal strip procedure) is performed.

12. Canthoplasty (reconstruction of canthus) (67950)
    a. *Definitions*—A canthoplasty is performed to reconstruct the medial or lateral canthus.
    b. *Key points*—As described above, lateral canthopexy and lateral canthoplasty are terms that are often used interchangeably by surgeons. But if a lateral canthotomy and inferior cantholysis have been performed with recreation of the lateral canthal angle, canthoplasty is the correct term, and 67950 should be used as opposed to a canthopexy (21282). The canthoplasty code is also included in 67917 (repair of ectropion) and cannot be billed separately when an extensive ectropion repair (eg, tarsal strip procedure) is performed on the same side.

13. Repair of brow ptosis (supraciliary, mid-forehead or coronal approach) (67900)
    a. *Definitions*—An incision is made in the forehead (direct or supraciliary, mid-forehead, or coronal) to elevate the eyebrow.
    b. *Key points*—Functional brow ptosis repair is performed to elevate the eyebrow and upper eyelid skin when brow ptosis is contributing to superior visual field impairment. This procedure is commonly performed in patients with facial paralysis. If an endoscopic approach is used for repair of brow ptosis, the appropriate code is 67999 (Unlisted procedure, eyelids).

14. Correction of lagophthalmos, with implantation of upper eyelid lid load (eg, gold weight) (67912)
    a. *Definitions*—Lagophthalmos is defined as the inability to complete eyelid closure. It often occurs as a result of facial paralysis weakness to the orbicularis oculi muscle. Upper lid loading with a gold or platinum weight allows for complete eye closure upon effort.
    b. *Key points*—The weight is placed through a tarsal crease incision and secured in a sub-

orbicularis oculi muscle pocket, either fixed to the tarsus or in a supratarsal position.

15. Repair of ectropion; extensive (eg, tarsal strip operation) (67917)
    a. *Definitions*—An ectropion occurs when the lid margin is everted away from the globe. There are a variety of methods of repair, and a tarsal strip procedure is commonly employed.
    b. *Key points*—The tarsal strip procedure starts with a lateral canthotomy followed by an inferior cantholysis. The lid margin, anterior lamella, and conjunctiva of the eyelid are removed. A strip of tarsus is maintained and amount chosen for removal based on how much the eyelid needs to be tightened. The tarsal strip is then fixed to the inside of the lateral orbital rim and the lateral canthal angle reconstructed. This code includes a canthopexy (21282) and canthoplasty (67950) on the ipsilateral side.

Controversial Areas

Cosmetic Procedures

Several facial cosmetic procedures are office-based, performed with either local or no anesthesia. These are not covered by third-party payers, and examples include

- Injectable facial rejuvenation
  - Botulinum toxin
  - Facial fillers
- Facial skin procedures
- Laser hair removal
- Skin pigmentation/tattoo laser removal
- Vascular lesion laser removal
- Laser skin resurfacing/tightening
- Chemical peels

1. General considerations
   a. In many ways, the logistics and finances for cosmetic procedures are more straightforward than coding and billing for insurance-based procedures. The patient directly pays for care at a price that is predetermined by the practitioner. The goal is to provide affordable, competitive pricing that permits the practice to deliver the desired patient experience while optimizing financial solvency. The goal of office-based cosmetic procedures is to not only make the patient look better, but feel better. These procedures offer a temporary escape from reality for the patient, and affordable pricing is essential to achieving maximum gratification and repeat business. But aesthetic medicine is not a commodity and having significantly discounted prices to become instantly more competitive risks turning an aesthetic practice's services into nothing more than that. An aesthetic physician must find a reason to bring value to their product if charging a greater price—this typically translates to either more convenience or a better overall experience. Thus, assigned fees for procedures will vary individually for practices and be dependent on practice expense and the surrounding market.

2. Fee structuring
   a. *Injectable therapies*—For injectable therapies (botulinum toxin and facial fillers), costs are typically based per unit of botulinum toxin injected and per syringe of facial filler used. Prices will generally be similar across practices within a region, with most charging approximately double the cost of the product per unit or syringe. Manufacturer discounts are often passed through to the patient, and many practices will discount prices for higher volume of botulinum toxin or facial filler provided.
   b. *Facial skin procedures*—Laser treatment pricing is determined by the amount of surface area treated and/or number of pulses used. The cost associated with buying and maintaining the specific laser affects price per use. Hair and vascular laser treatments tend to be less expensive, whereas superficial skin resurfacing/tightening procedures tend to be more costly. Because many laser treatments require

more than one treatment for full efficacy, they are often priced in packages of multiple treatments with a discount provided if a full package is bought from the outset.

3. Payment
   a. *Form of Payment*—Cash, checks, and credit cards are accepted for office-based cosmetic procedures. Credit card payment is the most common because of the convenience and ability for the patient to finance payment. Credit card transactions also provide a sense of security for the practice and its patients, but they are associated with transaction fees (eg, 2%–3%) charged to the provider. Another potential downside with credit card transactions is that unhappy or debt-ridden patients may dispute charges

to avoid payment, which at the minimum results in a loss of time for the practice. The easiest way to avoid disputes is to have a contract for services, but in an aesthetic practice, defining return procedures with patients is a nuanced conversation.
   b. *Payment Plans*—Payment for office-based procedures is collected at the time of procedure after it is completed. This is in contrast to cosmetic surgical procedures that are paid for in advance. Payment plans are not typically used for office-based cosmetic procedures due to their lower relative cost and since payment plans come at a price to the practice. Payment plans, if offered, are reserved for higher-priced surgical procedures with practices typically establishing a minimum amount that can be financed.

CHAPTER 19

Office Head and Neck Surgery

Marc A. Cohen and Abtin Tabaee

Introduction

Effective practice management in head and neck surgical oncology necessitates a thorough understanding of coding and billing in the various pre- and postoperative situations. Common to the care of head and neck patients is a high level of medical decision-making complexity and a multidisciplinary treatment paradigm. The head and neck surgeon is typically involved throughout the entire course of the medical care including pretreatment evaluation, performance of the surgical aspects of treatment, postoperative care, and finally, long-term follow-up for disease surveillance. The nuances of coding and billing in the office care of a patient with a head and neck neoplasm are reviewed in this chapter. This includes fine needle aspiration (FNA) with or without ultrasound (US), biopsy or resection of lesions of the oral cavity and oropharynx, tracheostomy care management, salivary gland procedures, and other procedures performed under local anesthesia in the office. Practice management strategies are also explored.

Key Points

- Appropriate use of modifiers is integral to appropriate coding and billing, including patients receiving office evaluation (modifier 24) and procedures (modifier 79) in the postoperative global period.

- If a FNA is performed in multiple areas, report 10021 or 10022 for each site taken, and append modifier 59.
- There are distinct codes for biopsy of oral cavity and oropharyngeal lesions (40808, 41100, 41105, 41108, 42100, 42800) as compared to excision of these lesions. All codes are differentiated based on anatomic location. There are distinct codes for excision without closure (40810, 41110, 42104), simple repair (40812, 41112, 41113, 42106), and complex repair (40814).
- When performing sialoendoscopy, the unlisted salivary gland code (42699) should be used, and the provider should anticipate the need for appropriate documentation and dialogue with the insurance carrier.
- The tracheotomy tube change code (31502) can only be used if performed before establishment of a fistula tract (approximately prior to 1 week). Tracheostomy tube changes after establishment of the tract cannot be billed as a procedure but can be incorporated into the evaluation and management (E/M) visit.
- Office staff should be trained to maximize system efficiency: this includes obtaining outside radiology, pathology, and notes with in-house review of all information.
- The surveillance follow-up schedule after treatment for head and neck cancer should be determined by appropriate clinical factors.

- Local anesthesia is included in all office surgical *Current Procedural Terminology* (CPT) codes and is not separately reported by the otolaryngologist.
- Appropriate infrastructure with respect to facilities, staffing, instrumentation, skill set, and emergency protocols should be in place prior to performing in-office procedures.

Key Procedure Codes

The following procedures are commonly performed in the office setting in a head and neck surgical oncology practice. Office-based endoscopy procedures as well as management of laryngeal and skin lesions are reviewed in other chapters.

Office-Based Biopsy Without Imaging

Note: A nasal biopsy is for one done with the use of a headlight. If an endoscope is needed for a biopsy, then the endoscopic biopsy code 31237 should be used instead.

10021 Fine needle aspiration; without imaging guidance
wRVU 1.27; Global XXX

21550 Biopsy, soft tissue of neck or thorax
wRVU 2.11; Global 10

30100 Biopsy, intranasal
wRVU 0.94; Global 0

38500 Biopsy or excision of lymph node(s); open, superficial
wRVU 3.79; Global 10

  38505 by needle, superficial (eg, cervical, inguinal, axillary)
  wRVU 1.14; Global 0

40808 Biopsy, vestibule of mouth
wRVU 1.01; Global 10

41100 Biopsy of tongue; anterior two-thirds
wRVU 1.42, Global 10

41105 posterior one-third
wRVU 1.47; Global 10

41108 Biopsy of floor of mouth
wRVU 1.1; Global 10

42100 Biopsy of palate, uvula
wRVU 1.36; Global 10

42400 Biopsy of salivary gland; needle
wRVU 0.78; Global 0

  42405 incisional
  wRVU 3.34; Global 10

42800 Biopsy; oropharynx
wRVU 1.44; Global 10

60100 Biopsy thyroid, percutaneous core needle
wRVU 1.56; Global 0

Endoscopy

31231 Nasal endoscopy, diagnostic, unilateral or bilateral
wRVU 1.10; Global 0

31237 Nasal/sinus endoscopy, surgical; with biopsy, polypectomy or debridement (separate procedure)
wRVU 2.60; Global 0

31575 Laryngoscopy, flexible fiberoptic; diagnostic
wRVU 1.10; Global 0

  31576 with biopsy
  wRVU 1.97; Global 0

92511 Nasopharyngoscopy with endoscope (separate procedure)
wRVU 0.61; Global 0

Office-Based Imaging

76536 Ultrasound, soft tissues of head and neck (eg, thyroid, parathyroid, parotid), real time with image documentation
wRVU 0.56; Global XXX

Office-Based Biopsy With Imaging

10022 Fine needle aspiration; with imaging guidance
wRVU 1.27; Global XXX

76942 Ultrasonic guidance for needle placement (eg, biopsy, aspiration, injection, localization device), imaging supervision and interpretation
wRVU 0.67; Global XXX

Office-Based Excision of Oral Cavity and Oropharyngeal Lesions

40810 Excision of lesion of mucosa and submucosa, vestibule of mouth; without repair
wRVU 1.36; Global 10

    40812 with simple repair
    wRVU 2.37; Global 10

    40814 with complex repair
    wRVU 3.52; Global 90

40820 Destruction of lesion or scar of vestibule of mouth by physical methods (eg, laser, thermal, cryo, chemical)
wRVU 1.34; Global 10

42808 Excision or destruction of lesion of pharynx, any method
wRVU 2.35; Global 10

41110 Excision of lesion of tongue without closure
wRVU 1.42; Global 10

41112 Excision of lesion of tongue with closure; anterior two-thirds
wRVU 2.83; Global 90

    41113 posterior one-third
    wRVU 3.29; Global 90

41116 Excision, lesion of floor of mouth
wRVU 2.52; Global 90

42104 Excision, lesion of palate, uvula; without closure
wRVU 1.69; Global 10

    42106 with simple primary closure
    wRVU 2.15; Global 10

42160 Destruction of lesion, palate or uvula (thermal, cryo or chemical)
wRVU 1.85; Global 10

Office-Based Excision of Cervical Lesions

21555 Excision, tumor, soft tissue of neck or anterior thorax, subcutaneous; less than 3 cm
wRVU 3.96; Global 90

    #21552 3 cm or greater
    wRVU 6.49; Global 90

60300 Aspiration and/or injection, thyroid cyst
wRVU 0.97; Global 0

Office-Based Salivary Gland Procedures

Note. There is no code for salivary endoscopy. Thus, the unlisted code 42699 should be used for this procedure.

42330 Sialolithotomy; submandibular (submaxillary), sublingual or parotid, uncomplicated, intraoral
wRVU 2.26; Global 10

    42335 submandibular (submaxillary), complicated, intraoral
    wRVU 3.41; Global 90

42500 Plastic repair of salivary duct, sialodochoplasty; primary or simple
wRVU 4.42; Global 90

    42505 secondary or complicated
    wRVU 6.32; Global 90

42650 Dilation salivary duct
wRVU 0.77; Global 0

42699 Unlisted procedure, salivary glands or ducts
wRVU 0.00; Global Y Y Y

Office-Based Tracheotomy Management

17250 Chemical cauterization of granulation tissue (proud flesh, sinus or fistula)
wRVU 0.5; Global 0

31502 Tracheotomy tube change prior to establishment of fistula tract
wRVU 0.65; Global 0

31820 Surgical closure tracheostomy or fistula; without plastic repair
wRVU 4.64; Global 90

31825 with plastic repair
wRVU 7.07; Global 90

31830 Revision of tracheostomy scar
wRVU 4.62; Global 90

Drainage Procedures

10140 Incision and drainage of hematoma, seroma or fluid collection
wRVU 1.58; Global 10

10160 Puncture aspiration of abscess, hematoma, bulla, or cyst
wRVU 1.25; Global 10

10180 Incision and drainage, complex, postoperative wound infection
wRVU 2.3; Global 10

Other Codes

99441 Telephone evaluation and management service by a physician or other qualified health care professional who may report evaluation and management services provided to an established patient, parent, or guardian not originating from a related E/M service provided within the previous 7 days nor leading to an E/M service or procedure within the next 24 hours or soonest available appointment; 5-10 minutes of medical discussion
wRVU 0.25; Global XXX

99442 11-20 minutes of medical discussion
wRVU 0.50; Global XXX

99443 21-30 minutes of medical discussion
wRVU 0.75; Global XXX

99367 **Medical team conference** with interdisciplinary team of health care professionals, patient and/or family not present, 30 minutes or more; participation by physician
wRVU 1.10; Global XXX

Key Modifiers

24 Unrelated Evaluation and Management Service by the Same Physician or Other Qualified Health Care Professional During a Postoperative Period
Most major head and neck oncology surgeries are associated with a 90-day global period. Routine office visits during this period cannot be billed separately. However, office evaluations for non-routine, different diagnosis conditions may be billed and should be appended with the 24 modifier. This includes conditions that are completely unrelated to the underlying neoplasm or surgery (eg, sinusitis in a postop thyroidectomy patient). However, billing for an office visit for a nonroutine issue related to the underlying condition is payer specific. This includes management of complications related to the surgery. Medicare, for example, encompasses all services related to the patient's procedure within the global period, unless there is a return to the operating room, in which case a modifier 78 is used for the second surgical procedure. Otherwise, all office care following the initial surgical procedure is encompassed within the global period.

25 Significant, Separately Identifiable Evaluation and Management Service by the Same Physician or Other Qualified Health Care Professional on the Same Day of the Procedure or Other Service

This modifier is commonly used in head and neck oncology patients when an office procedure is performed at the same setting of a related or unrelated office evaluation. In these situations, the practitioner is justifiably seeking payment for both the E/M and procedure components of the visit. However, the 25 modifier must be substantiated with appropriate medical justification and distinct diagnosis codes.

26 Professional Component
This modifier can appended to 76942 when a professional performs an ultrasound guided biopsy but is billing only for the radiology supervision and interpretation, as the hospital owns the equipment.

51 Multiple Procedures
Modifier 51 may be appended to the lower-valued CPT code when multiple surgical procedures are performed by the same practitioner at the same visit. Within a head and neck surgical practice, this may include performance of an endoscopy and biopsy on different anatomic structures during the same visit. For example, a flexible fiberoptic laryngoscopy (31575) is performed at the same visit as a fine needle aspiration without imaging (10021-51).

59 Distinct Procedural Service
The 59 modifier is appended to a procedure code to identify it as distinct from a different procedure performed by the same practitioner at the same visit. In the office management of a surgical oncology patient, this may be used if multiple, independent procedures with a similar CPT descriptor are performed including multiple biopsies or drainage procedures in distinctly different anatomic areas.

79 Unrelated Procedure or Service by the Same Physician or Other Qualified Health Care Professional During the Postoperative Period
This modifier is used when a procedure is performed during the global period that is unrelated to routine postoperative care and is being submitted for payment. This may include management of an unrelated condition or a complication. For example, this may include performance of nasal endoscopy (31231) for a sinusitis episode in a patient who is in the 90-day global period following a head and neck oncologic procedure.

Key ICD-9-CM/ICD-10-CM

140.5/C00.5   Malignant neoplasm; of lip, unspecified, inner aspect

140.9/C00.2   of external lip, unspecified

141.0/C01   of base of tongue

141.4/C02.3   of anterior two-thirds of tongue, part unspecified

142.0/C07   of parotid gland

142.1/C08.0   of submandibular gland

142.2.0/C08.1   of sublingual gland

143.0/C03.0   of upper gum

143.1/C03.1   of lower gum

144.9/C04.0   of floor of mouth, unspecified

145.0/C06.0   of cheek mucosa

145.2/C05.0   of hard palate

145.3/C05.1   of soft palate

145.6/C06.2   of retromolar area

145.8/C06.89   of overlapping sites of other parts of mouth

145.9/C06.9   of mouth, unspecified

146.0/C09.9   of tonsil, unspecified

146.1/C09.0   of tonsillar fossa

146.2/C09.1   of tonsillar pillar (anterior) (posterior)

146.3/C10.0   of vallecula

146.4/C10.1   of anterior aspect of epiglottis

146.5/C10.8   of overlapping sites of oropharynx

146.7/C10.3   of posterior wall of oropharynx

146.8/C10.4   of branchial cleft

146.8/C10.8   of overlapping sites of oropharynx

147.0/C11.0   of superior wall of nasopharynx

147.1/C11.1   of posterior wall of nasopharynx

147.2/C11.2   of lateral wall of nasopharynx

147.3/C11.3   of anterior wall of nasopharynx

147.8/C11.8   of overlapping sites of nasopharynx

148.0/C13.0   of postcricoid region

148.1/C12   of pyriform sinus

148.2/C13.1   of aryepiglottic fold, hypopharyngeal aspect

148.3/C13.1   of posterior wall of hypopharyngeal

148.8/C13.8   of overlapping sites of hypopharynx

150.0/C15.3   of upper third of esophagus

160.0/C30.0   of nasal cavity

160.2/C31.0   of maxillary sinus

160.3/C31.1   of ethmoidal sinus

160.4/C31.2   of frontal sinus

160.5/C31.3   of sphenoid sinus

160.8/C31.8   of overlapping sites of accessory sinuses

161.0/C32.0   of glottis

161.1/C32.1   of supraglottis

161.2/C32.2   of subglottis

161.3/C32.3   of laryngeal cartilage

161.8/C32.8   of overlapping sites of larynx

170.0/C41.0   of bones of skull and face

170.1/C41.1   of mandible

171.0/C49.0   of connective and soft tissue of head, face, and neck

173.0/C44.00   Unspecified malignant neoplasm of skin of lip

173.02/C44.02   Squamous cell carcinoma of skin; of lip

173.22/C44.22-   of ear and external auditory canal

173.22C44.22-   of ear and external auditory canal

173.42/C44.42   of scalp and neck

193/C73   Malignant neoplasm of thyroid gland

196.0/C77.0   Secondary and unspecified malignant neoplasm of lymph nodes of head, face, and neck

210.2/D11.9   Benign neoplasm; of major salivary gland, unspecified

210.4/D10.30   of unspecified part of mouth

210.4D10.39   of other parts of mouth

212.0/D14.0   of middle ear, nasal cavity and accessory sinuses

225.1/D33.3   of cranial nerves

225.2/D32.0   of cerebral meninges

225.2/D32.9   of meninges, unspecified

226/D34   of thyroid gland

227.3/D35.2   of pituitary gland

227.3/D35.3   of craniopharyngeal duct

235.0/D37.030   Neoplasm of uncertain behavior; of the parotid salivary glands

235.0/D37.031   of the sublingual salivary glands

235.0/D37.032   of uncertain behavior of the submandibular salivary glands

235.0/D37.039   of uncertain behavior of the major salivary glands, unspecified

235.1/D37.01   of uncertain behavior of lip

235.1/D37.02   of uncertain behavior of tongue

235.1/D37.04   of uncertain behavior of the minor salivary glands

235.1/D37.05   of uncertain behavior of pharynx

235.6/D38.0   of uncertain behavior of larynx

238.2/D48.5   of uncertain behavior of skin

239.0/D49.0   of uncertain behavior of digestive system

239.1/D49.1   of uncertain behavior of respiratory system

239.7/D49.7   of uncertain behavior of endocrine glands and other parts of nervous system

241.0/E04.1   Nontoxic single thyroid nodule

241.1/E04.2   Nontoxic multinodular goiter

242.00/E05.00   Thyrotoxicosis with diffuse goiter without thyrotoxic crisis or storm

242.20/E05.20   Thyrotoxicosis with toxic multinodular goiter without thyrotoxic crisis or storm

237.4/D44.0   Neoplasm of uncertain behavior; of thyroid gland

237.4/D44.2   of parathyroid gland

237.4/D44.9   of unspecified endocrine gland

527.2/K11.20   Sialoadenitis, unspecified

527.3/K11.3   Abscess of salivary gland

527.5/K11.5   Sialolithiasis

527.6/K11.6   Mucocele of salivary gland

528.3/K12.2   Cellulitis and abscess of mouth

528.6/K13.21   Leukoplakia of oral mucosa, including tongue

528.79/K13.29   Other disturbances of oral epithelium, including tongue

528.9/K13.70   Unspecified lesions of oral mucosa

528.9/K13.79   Other lesions of oral mucosa

682.0/K12.2   Cellulitis and abscess of mouth

682.0/L03.211   Cellulitis of face

682.0/L03.212   Acute lymphangitis of face

682.1/L03.221   Cellulitis of neck

682.1/L03.222   Acute lymphangitis of neck

701.5/L92.9   Granulomatous disorder of the skin and subcutaneous tissue, unspecified

784.2/R22.0   Localized swelling, mass and lump, head

784.2/R22.1   Localized swelling, mass and lump, neck

784.8/R04.1   Hemorrhage from throat

785.6/R59.9   Enlarged lymph nodes, unspecified

909.3/T88.9XXS   Complication of surgical and medical care, unspecified, sequela

998.11   Hemorrhage complicating a procedure

998.12   Hematoma complicating a procedure

998.13/T88.8XXA   Other specified complications of surgical and medical care, not elsewhere classified, initial encounter

998.51, 998.59/T81.4XXA   Infection following a procedure, initial encounter

998.6/T81.83XA   Persistent postoperative fistula, initial encounter

998.83/T81.89XA   Other complications of procedures, not elsewhere classified, initial encounter

V10.02/Z85.818   Personal history of malignant neoplasm; of other sites of lip, oral cavity, and pharynx

V10.2/Z85.819   of unspecified site of lip, oral cavity, and pharynx

V10.21/Z85.21   Personal history of malignant neoplasm of larynx

V67.9/Z08   Encounter for follow-up examination after completed treatment for malignant neoplasm

V67.2/Z09   Encounter for follow up examination after completed treatment for conditions other than malignant neoplasm

Definition of Procedure Codes

1. Needle and Lymph Node Biopsy (10021, 10022, 38500, 38505)
   a. *Definition*—Needle biopsy is a percutaneous procedure that uses a fine needle (generally a 22 or 25 gauge) and a syringe to obtain a sample of cells from a solid mass or from cyst fluid. If the lesion cannot be palpated or the clinician wishes to sample a certain area of the lesion that cannot be discerned by palpation alone, the procedure is performed with imaging, usually in the head and neck oncologist practice, under ultrasound guidance. Needle biopsy procedures can be done with or without local anesthesia.

   Open biopsy of lymph nodes in the office involves making a small incision overlying a superficial lymph node. The tissue is then dissected to the lymph node of interest. A piece or the entirety of the node is removed and the wound is closed in layers. This may be done with local anesthesia alone depending on the location of the lesion.
   b. *Key points*—FNA without image guidance (10021) is typically performed when a thyroid nodule, lymph node, salivary lesion, or other head and neck mass is palpable. FNA with image guidance is used for smaller and nonpalpable lesions. CPT 10021 is used when the imaging modality is used only for guidance in identifying the lesion and placement of the needle. CPT 76942 encompasses the above procedures as well as formal interpretation of the findings. These codes are distinct from core biopsy (60100). When 10021 or 10022 are performed with another identifiable surgical procedure, the highest value code is listed first, and the remainder of the codes are listed with a 51 modifier. If multiple biopsies are performed, modifier 59 is used. There is no stated minimum or maximum number of passes on biopsy of the same lesion, all of which would be considered one code. Report 76942 without a global modifier when the physician owns the equipment and performs the radiological supervision and interpretation. Append modifier 26 (professional component) to 76942 if the physician performs only the radiological supervision and interpretation because another entity (eg, hospital outpatient department) owns the equipment.

   In the office, an open lymph node biopsy should be performed only if adequate instrumentation and nursing support exists. In addition, biopsy of a deep cervical node (38510) would not be performed in the office setting. CPT 38500 is the appropriate code for biopsy of superficial node. There is no code distinction between incisional or excisional biopsy. This single open lymph node biopsy code includes multiple lymph nodes excised or multiple biopsies performed.

2. Oral Cavity/Pharynx Biopsy (40808, 41100, 41105, 41108, 42100, 42800)
   a. *Definition*—These codes refer to biopsy procedures performed in the oral cavity and oropharynx. A portion of the lesion is removed for diagnostic purposes. These codes are defined by anatomic location. Of note, the vestibule is defined as mucosal and submucosal tissue of the lips and cheeks. It excludes cutaneous lip and dento-alveolar structures as there are separate codes for these procedures.
   b. *Key points*—The procedure codes encompass all aspects of the biopsy procedure including local anesthesia, the biopsy itself, hemostasis, and closure (if performed). The codes are the same regardless of the instrument used for the procedure or the place of service it is performed (office vs operating room). Appropriate excision codes should be used if the lesion is fully excised, even for diagnostic procedures (eg, excisional biopsy). The 59 modifier should be used if multiple biopsies are performed from a single anatomic subsite on separate lesions. Multiple biopsies on the same lesion are reported with one CPT code.

3. Excision of Lesions of the Oral Cavity and Oropharynx (40810, 40812, 40814, 40820, 41110, 41112, 41113, 41116, 42104, 42106, 42160, 42808)
   a. *Definition*—These codes encompass excision of lesions from the different subsites of the oral cavity and oropharynx, regardless of the place of service (office vs operating room). Excision of the entirety of a lesion, in contrast to biopsy, is required to use these codes. These codes are based on the location of the lesion and, in some cases, whether repair was performed. For excision of lesions with no repair, the codes are as follows: 40810 for oral vestibule, 41110 for lesion of the tongue, and 42104 for lesion of the palate. If a simple repair is performed (ie, use of a sutured closure), the codes are 40812 for oral vestibule, 41112 for oral tongue, 41113 for base of tongue, and 42106 for palate. If repair is complex (eg, requires the use of rearrangement of tissue, advancement of tissue flaps, or use of complex suturing techniques), a complex code is used: 40814 for vestibular lesions. When excising a floor of mouth lesion, there is only one code that entails excision and closure: 41116.

   The codes for destruction of lesion or scar by laser, thermal technique such as electrocautery, cryotherapy, or chemical is also dependent on anatomic subsite. CPT 40820 is for oral vestibule, 42160 for the palate or uvula, 42808 for the pharynx (meaning any area of the nasopharynx, oropharynx, or laryngopharynx not specified). These codes include any closure performed as well.
   b. *Key points*—The ability to excise oral cavity and oropharynx lesions is critical to office management of otolaryngology patients. Excision of lesions of the oral cavity or oropharynx can be done in a variety of methods (cautery, scalpel, etc). Distinct codes are used to specify the anatomic locations. Both benign and malignant lesions are included with these excisional codes. Local anesthesia is included in these codes. Use of 42808, destruction of pharynx lesion, denotes any area of the nasopharynx, oro-

pharynx, or laryngopharynx not specified in another code.

4. Office-Based Salivary Gland Procedures (42330, 42335, 42500, 42505, 42650, 42699)
   a. *Definition*—In-office salivary gland procedures include removal of submandibular gland stones. In uncomplicated sialolithotomy of submandibular, parotid, or sublingual glands, a stone is removed after an incision is made overlying the gland or duct. Tissue is dissected, and the stone is removed (42330). When a submandibular gland stone is large and a significant amount of complex dissection is required for sialolithotomy, 42335 is used. When the salivary duct requires sialodochoplasty, or repair and marsupialization of the outflow tract, this can be done over a plastic or silicone tube. Complex sialodochoplasty, 42505, is distinguished from simple repair (42500) in the need for local flaps or delayed reconstruction. When there is a focal narrowing of salivary duct, sequential dilation of this region with larger probes can be performed (42650). For completeness sake, 42699, or unlisted salivary gland code, may be an appropriate code for sialoendoscopy (see section entitled "Controversial Areas"). Sialoendoscopy, although more commonly performed in the operating room, is a minimally invasive technique that enables a camera to be cannulated in a salivary gland duct in order to treat sialoliths or strictures.
   b. *Key points*—Distinction between simple and complex sialolithotomy depends on size of stone and the amount of soft tissue that needs to be dissected. Multiple salivary codes are sometimes applicable to the same patient such as a sialodochoplasty (42500) and sialolithotomy (42335). When this occurs a 51 modifier is appropriate to add onto the lower-value code. Appropriate documentation and close coordination with insurance carriers are required for sialoendoscopy, as the coding remains an unlisted salivary gland code for diagnostic procedures.

5. Tracheotomy Care (17250, 31502, 31820, 31825, 31830)
   a. *Definition*—CPT 17250 is a general code used to designate cauterization of granulation tissue, regardless of anatomic location or disease. CPT 31502 refers to changing of the tracheotomy tube prior to establishment of a fistula tract. CPT does not define the time frame for this code to be appropriate, and it is based on clinical judgment. For most patients, this will be relevant only a single time, typically within 7 days of the procedure. Primary surgical closure of a tracheotomy wound is distinguished by whether the repair was simple (31820), such as sutures, or performed with a plastics technique (31825), such as a complex repair or adjacent tissue transfer (included in the code). A single code exists for revision of a tracheotomy scar (31830) regardless of the complexity of the technique used for closure.
   b. *Key points*—Common to the care of patients with head and neck tumors is airway management, including planned and emergent tracheotomy procedures. Office follow-up for these patients encompasses management of the tracheotomy tube and tracheotomy wound itself. Nursing care is also necessary including patient education and supply coordination. Elements of this care can be billed as distinct procedures, and other elements are not billable beyond the office visit component. Most tracheotomy procedures have a 0-day global period (eg, 31600), but postoperative patients are often under a 90-day global period if the tracheotomy procedure was performed as, and included as, part of a head and neck oncologic surgery. The tracheotomy-related procedures that can be billed include management of granulation tissue (17250), tracheotomy tube change prior to the establishment of a fistula tract (31502), and various wound closure procedures. If performed within a global period of a separate head and neck oncologic procedure, 31502 is appended with a 79 modifier. Tracheotomy tube changes that are performed

after establishment of a fistula tract do not have a separate CPT code and are included the office visit E/M component. In terms of wound closure, there is no separate procedure code for decannulation and wound care associated with secondary closure. CPT 31820 and 31825 refer to a surgical closure of the tracheotomy wound, often including scar excision, tissue mobilization, and closure. If a revision procedure is performed, 31830 is used.

6. Drainage Procedures (10140, 10160, 10180)
   a. *Definition*—10140 is a general code to describe incision and drainage of hematoma, seroma, or a fluid collection regardless of location in the body. Other codes are used for drainage procedures when the collection is an abscess, including in the postoperative setting (10180). Other incision and drainage codes are used for primary abscess events (eg, not as a complication of surgery) and are based on anatomic location. The various incision and drainage codes encompass all aspects of the procedure including incision, dissection, drainage, and packing, and is used regardless of the setting (office vs OR). CPT 10160 is used to describe drainage of any type of fluid from any anatomic location when performed with a needle. Different CPT codes are used when the needle procedure is performed with guidance (76942 ultrasound, 77012 CT, 77021 MRI).
   b. *Key points*—There are a number of distinct CPT codes for drainage procedures in the head and neck region. Choosing the correct code is based on the anatomic location of the collection, the nature of the collection, method of drainage, and whether the collection is de novo or postoperative.
   There are several distinct incision and drainage CPT codes for head and neck abscesses, including for primary infection (not listed here). Choosing the correct code is generally straightforward and is based on anatomic location of the abscess. In situations where multiple, distinct, and separate abscesses are managed, the CPT codes

are appended by the 59 modifier to denote the separate procedures. CPT 10180 is used in the setting of a postoperative abscess, regardless of anatomic location. If this procedure is performed within the global period of the initial head and neck surgery, a 78 modifier is appended to the drainage code when performed in the operating room. Medicare's global surgical package includes care of the patient for all services related to the procedure, and that includes problems or complications treated in the office setting, unless a return to the operating room occurs (then use modifier 78). Therefore, office drainage procedures are encompassed in the global period and should not be billed.

Practice Management in Head and Neck Surgery

Office Setup

Imperative to management of a head and neck oncology practice is scheduling efficiency. As office visits for head and neck cancer patients involve complex evaluation and counseling sessions, success in practice requires ancillary staff training to maximize system efficiency. Prior to the patient visit, the office staff should have a package of materials for each new patient. This should include radiology reports and images, outside pathology report with slide review in hospital, and outside notes including operative reports if pertinent. Ideally, nursing staff or physician office assistants should be educated on material required prior to the office visit for each specific diagnosis. The specifics vary depending on clinician preference. Utilization of institutional electronic medical record (EMR) greatly assists in this process with internal referrals.

Telephone Encounters and Tumor Board Conferences

There are codes for time spent on the telephone in medical discussion with patients, 99441 (5-10 minutes), 99442 (11-20 minutes of medical discus-

sion) and 99443 (21-30 minutes of medical discussion). These codes can be used provided that the patient was not seen within the previous 7 days and the patient is not seen within 24 hours following the call. Medicare considers telephone care to be part of the E/M service and does not provide reimbursement for these codes; however, some plans are beginning to pay clinicians for calls and electronic communication (https://www.acponline.org/running_practice/technology/comm_electronic.pdf). If a medical team has a conference regarding patient management (multidisciplinary tumor conference), there are codes that can be applied provided the team's discussion about that single patient is at least 30 minutes in duration. Use of 99367 requires the conference be composed of at least 3 health care professionals from different specialties. Only one individual from each specialty can report this code, and participants need to have performed in-person evaluation of the patient within the previous 60 days.

Billing an E/M Code Based on Time

As reviewed in detail in Chapter 9, "The Office Visit," there are situations that the physician may appropriately bill for an office visit based on counseling time. This is common in head and neck surgery where the counseling of patients regarding the disease and treatment may require an extensive discussion. Key elements of billing based on time include the following:

- Greater than 50% of the billing provider's time spent face to face with the patient and/or family must be spent on counseling and/or coordination of care, and this must be appropriately documented in the medical record.
- Elements of counseling that can be included in the time calculation include reviewing with the patient any test results, the nature of the patient's condition, treatment considerations, informed consent, patient/family education, and instructions (including postoperative instructions).
- Elements of the visit that may be included in the total time calculation

but *not* the counseling time calculation (>50%) include obtaining the history, reviewing the past records/test results internally, logistical aspects of treatment (coordinating appointments), and telephone calls. Also excluded are elements of the care that are coordinated outside of the examination room, including, but not limited to, the time provided by the nurse, midlevel provider, or resident.

Billing for Surveillance Visits

A common aspect of head and neck surgical oncology care is the need for long-term surveillance. For many lesions, this may include elements of office evaluation, endoscopy, and imaging. In patients who present for a routine visit without any concerning findings or symptoms on office examination and endoscopy, the practitioner might only bill for either the E/M or the endoscopy procedure, but not both, since the 25 modifier may not always be justifiable in this situation. Exceptions to this may include a patient who has an unrelated issue at the same visit as a surveillance follow-up (eg, sinusitis and a history of larynx cancer), or a patient with a new symptom or concerning examination finding (eg, dysphagia and a history of larynx cancer), or a patient with whom you are evaluating multiple issues (eg, dysphonia and a history of larynx cancer). In these scenarios, adequate documentation must be provided, and distinct diagnosis codes should be reported (eg, Z08 for surveillance and Z85.21 for personal history cancer of the larynx and other diagnosis codes for conditions evaluated). Medical justification and standard of care principles apply and should conform to appropriate practice for frequency of surveillance visits. International Classification of Diseases (ICD) guidelines state that if a patient does not currently have cancer or is not being actively treated for cancer, the surveillance code and history of cancer code should be used.

Infrastructure for Office Procedures

Performing in-office procedures for head and neck oncology patients requires the appropri-

ate infrastructure. Surgeon skill set and learning curve principles apply for performance of the procedure in an awake patient, use of local anesthesia, and complication management. In addition, experience will dictate which interventions are reasonable to perform in an office setting. If the clinician is unsure about the suitability to perform a procedure, it should be completed in the operating room. Clinicians need to select patients appropriately and must always disclose the possibility preemptively that the intervention will need to be performed in the operating room if not tolerated in the office. Protocols are required for unanticipated events requiring medical intervention (cardiovascular or pulmonary events, loss of airway, vasovagal events, etc). The head and neck oncology patient population in particular is at risk for respiratory and cardiac issues, and emergency airway instrumentation should be available. Staff should undergo regular training as to the appropriate measures to take during an emergency. In addition to technical skill and protocols to manage complications, the presence of nurses or technicians trained in assisting with procedures is critical. Infrastructure should include staff charged with ensuring appropriate instrumentation is ordered, on hand, and maintained, so available when needed. Finally, the presence of appropriate instrumentation, including thermocautery with a Bovie or bipolar as well as surgical tools appropriate for intervention should be confirmed prior to consideration of a procedure.

Controversial Areas

Coding for sialoendoscopy, which is most frequently performed in the operating room, has the potential for controversy. Some practitioners are of the mindset that use of sialoendoscopy is just a tool to extract a stone as would be performed if merely a ductal cut down were performed. In that setting, the standard sialolithiasis codes are appropriate (42330, 42335, 42500, 42505, 42650). However, surgeons who practice sialoendoscopy note that use of this technology to perform extraction of a proximal stone requires significantly greater resource and skill. Sialoendoscopy often does not require a cut down, and removal of a proximal stone can often obviate the need for removal of the gland. In contrast to an in-office intervention, sialoendoscopy requires general anesthesia and can often take a significant amount of time. In this setting, many commercial payers have been reimbursing the utilization of the unlisted code (42699) with appropriate documentation and dialogue with the insurance carriers. It is not appropriate to use this code with the other sialolithiasis codes. It seems likely that a unique sialoendoscopy code will be developed in the future as this intervention becomes increasingly popular.

CHAPTER 20

Office Pediatric Otolaryngology

John P. Dahl and Sanjay R. Parikh

Introduction

This chapter outlines procedural codes performed in clinic for pediatric patients. As with adult patients, billing for procedural codes in children includes facility and equipment charges when the services are provided in the physician office (place of service 11). Physician services provided in a hospital outpatient department (HOPD) or provider-based clinic (eg, place of service 22) are paid by Medicare and other payers at a lower rate because the facility is submitting a separate charge.

The majority of procedures performed on adults in the clinic or physician office are both safe and acceptable to perform on pediatric patients. In order to appropriately bill for clinic-based procedures, informed consent should be obtained from a parent or legal guardian including appropriate documentation in the procedure note describing the procedure and the name/relation to the patient of the person providing consent. The details of each procedure should also be recorded, including the indications, a description of the technique and equipment, anesthesia, key findings, complications, and disposition. If the 63 modifier (see below) is being used, you must document the weight of the patient at the time of the procedure in either the clinic or procedure note.

Key Points

- The majority of clinic based otolaryngologic procedures can safely be performed on pediatric patients. Childhood compliance may limit one's ability to provide in-office procedural services without anesthesia.
- Centers for Medicare and Medicaid Services' (CMS) postoperative global periods are the same for pediatric patients as adult patients because the global period is assigned to a *Current Procedural Terminology* (CPT) code regardless of patient age.

Key Procedure Codes

Neck

10021 Fine needle aspiration; without imaging guidance
wRVU 1.27; Global XXX

    10022 with imaging guidance
wRVU 1.27; Global XXX

76942 Ultrasonic guidance for needle placement (eg, biopsy, aspiration, injection, localization device), imaging supervision and interpretation
wRVU 0.67; Global XXX

10060 Incision and drainage of abscess (eg, carbuncle, suppurative hidradenitis, cutaneous or subcutaneous abscess, cyst, furuncle, or paronychia); simple or single
wRVU 1.22; Global 10

207

Skin

Skin lesions and wound repair have codes based on diameter. The codes for smaller lesions/repair are listed below, as these are more typically performed in the office. For larger diameters, please see Chapter 18, "Office Facial Plastic Surgery," and Chapter 27, "Operative Facial Plastic Surgery."

10120   Incision and removal of foreign body, subcutaneous tissue; simple
wRVU 1.22; Global 10

10160   Puncture aspiration of abscess, hematoma, bulla, or cyst
wRVU 1.25; Global 10

11200   Removal of skin tags, multiple fibrocutaneous tags, any area; up to and including 15 lesions
wRVU 0.82; Global 10

11420   Excision, benign lesion including margins, except skin tag (unless listed elsewhere), scalp, neck, hands, feet, genitalia; excised diameter 0.5 cm or less
wRVU 1.03; Global 10

> **11421**   excised diameter 0.6 to 1.0 cm
> *wRVU 1.47; Global 10*

11440   Excision, other benign lesion including margins, except skin tag (unless listed elsewhere), face, ears, eyelids, nose, lips, mucous membranes; excised diameter 0.5 cm or less
wRVU 1.05; Global 10

> **11441**   excised diameter 0.6 to 1.0 cm
> *wRVU 1.53; Global 10*

11900   Injection, intralesional; up to and including 7 lesions
wRVU 0.52; Global 0

12011   Simple repair of superficial wounds of scalp, neck, axillae, external genitalia, trunk and/or extremities (including hands and feet); 2.5 cm or less
wRVU 1.07; Global 0

17106   Destruction of cutaneous vascular proliferative lesions (eg, laser technique); less than 10 sq cm
wRVU 3.69; Global 90

17250   Chemical cauterization of granulation tissue (proud flesh, sinus or fistula)
wRVU 0.50; Global 0

Nose

21315   Closed treatment of nasal bone fracture; without stabilization
wRVU 1.83; Global 10

> **21320**   with stabilization
> *wRVU 1.88; Global 10*

30100   Biopsy, intranasal
wRVU 0.94; Global 0

30110   Excision, nasal polyp(s), simple
wRVU 1.68; Global 10

30300   Removal foreign body, intranasal; office type procedure
wRVU 1.09; Global 10

30901   Control nasal hemorrhage, anterior, simple (limited cautery and/or packing) any method
wRVU 1.10; Global 0

30999   Unlisted procedure, nose
wRVU 0; Global YYY

31231   Nasal endoscopy, diagnostic, unilateral or bilateral (separate procedure)
wRVU 1.10; Global 0

31237   Nasal/sinus endoscopy, surgical; with biopsy, polypectomy or debridement (separate procedure)
wRVU 2.60; Global 0

64505   Injection, anesthetic agent; sphenopalatine ganglion
wRVU 1.36; Global 0

92511   Nasopharyngoscopy with endoscope (separate procedure)
wRVU 0.61; Global 0

Larynx/Trachea

31502   Tracheotomy tube change prior to establishment of fistula tract
wRVU 0.65; Global 0

31575 Laryngoscopy, flexible fiberoptic; diagnostic
wRVU 1.10; Global 0

31579 Laryngoscopy, flexible or rigid fiberoptic, with stroboscopy
wRVU 2.26; Global 0

31615 Tracheobronchoscopy through established tracheostomy incision
wRVU 2.09; Global 0

31820 Surgical closure tracheostomy or fistula; without plastic repair
wRVU 4.64; Global 90

Mouth

40490 Biopsy of lip
wRVU 1.22; Global 0

41010 Incision of lingual frenum (frenotomy)
wRVU 1.11; Global 10

41100 Biopsy of tongue; anterior two-thirds
wRVU 1.42; Global 10

41110 Excision of lesion of tongue without closure
wRVU 1.56; Global 10

41112 Excision of lesion of tongue with closure; anterior two-thirds
wRVU 2.83; Global 90

41115 Excision of lingual frenum (frenectomy)
wRVU 1.79; Global 10

41520 Frenoplasty (surgical revision of frenum, eg, with Z-plasty)
wRVU 2.83; Global 90

42000 Drainage of abscess of palate, uvula
wRVU 1.28; Global 10

42700 Incision and drainage abscess; peritonsillar
wRVU 1.67; Global 10

Neck

60300 Aspiration and/or injection, thyroid cyst
wRVU 0.97; Global 0

64611 Chemodenervation of parotid and submandibular salivary glands, bilateral
wRVU 1.03; Global 10

Ear

69000 Drainage external ear, abscess or hematoma; simple
wRVU 1.50; Global 10

69145 Excision soft tissue lesion, external auditory canal
wRVU 2.70; Global 90

69200 Removal foreign body from external auditory canal; without general anesthesia
wRVU 0.77; Global 0

69210 Removal impacted cerumen requiring instrumentation, unilateral
wRVU 0.61; Global 0

69220 Debridement, mastoidectomy cavity, simple (eg, routine cleaning)
wRVU 0.83; Global 0

69420 Myringotomy including aspiration and/ or eustachian tube inflation
wRVU 1.38; Global 10

69433 Tympanostomy (requiring insertion of ventilation tube), local or topical anesthesia
wRVU 1.57; Global 10

69610 Tympanic membrane repair, with or without site preparation of perforation for closure, with or without patch
wRVU 4.47; Global 10

92504 Binocular microscopy (separate diagnostic procedure)
wRVU 0.18, Global XXX

Key Modifiers

22   Increased Procedural Services
Service provided is greater than usually required for the procedure.

24 Unrelated Evaluation and Management Service by the Same Physician or Other Qualified Health Care Professional During a Postoperative Period

This is used when a patient is seen during a global period for a visit unrelated to the surgical procedure.

25 Significant, Separately Identifiable Evaluation and Management Service by the Same Physician or Other Qualified Health Care Professional on the Same Day of the Procedure or Other Service

This is used when a procedure is done at the same setting as an office visit that can stand alone as separate from the procedure.

50 Bilateral Procedure

Used typically when a therapeutic code is used (eg, ear tube placement).

51 Multiple Procedures

Used to get reimbursed when 2 separate, non-bundled procedures are performed on the same patient at the same setting.

63 Procedure Performed on Infants less than 4 kg

Patient weight is less than 4 kg (must document patient weight in procedure note).

Key ICD-9-CM/ICD-10-CM

Note. The diagnosis codes in both *International Classification of Diseases, Ninth Revision, Clinical Modification* (ICD-9-CM) and *International Classification of Diseases, Tenth Revision, Clinical Modification* (ICD-10-CM) are the same for adult and pediatric patients. Following is a list of diagnosis codes relevant to the pediatric population. Please refer to Chapters 12 to 19 and 21 in this section for subspecialty specific codes that can be used for children.

474.00/J35.01   Chronic tonsillitis

474.01/J35.02   Chronic adenoiditis

474.02/J35.03   Chronic tonsillitis and adenoiditis

474.10/J35.3   Hypertrophy of tonsils with hypertrophy of adenoids

474.11/J35.1   Hypertrophy of tonsils

474.12/J35.2   Hypertrophy of adenoids

474.2/J35.8   Other chronic diseases of tonsils and adenoids

475/J36   Peritonsillar abscess

478.0/J34.3   Hypertrophy of nasal turbinates

478.31/J38.01   Paralysis of vocal cords and larynx, unilateral

478.32/J38.01   Paralysis of vocal cords and larynx, unilateral

478.33/J38.02   Paralysis of vocal cords and larynx, bilateral

478.34/J38.02   Paralysis of vocal cords and larynx, bilateral

478.5/J38.3   Other diseases of vocal cords

478.74/J38.6   Stenosis of larynx

519.01/J95.02   Infection of tracheostomy stoma

527.2/K11.20   Sialadenitis, unspecified

527.6/K11.6   Mucocele of salivary gland (*eg, ranula*)

527.7/K11.7   Disturbances of salivary secretions

527.7/R68.2   Dry mouth, unspecified

530.81/K21.9   Gastro-esophageal reflux disease without esophagitis

683/L04.9   Acute lymphadenitis, unspecified

744.01/Q16.0   Congenital absence of (ear) auricle

744.1/Q17.0   Accessory auricle

744.23/Q17.2   Microtia

744.41/Q18.0   Sinus, fistula and cyst of branchial cleft

744.42/Q18.0   Sinus, fistula and cyst of branchial cleft

744.43/Q18.2 Other branchial cleft malformations

744.46/Q18.1 Preauricular sinus and cyst

744.47/Q18.1 Preauricular sinus and cyst

748.0/Q30.0 Choanal atresia

748.3/Q31.1 Congenital subglottic stenosis

748.3/Q31.3 Laryngocele

748.3/Q31.8 Other congenital malformations of larynx

748.3/Q32.1 Other congenital malformations of trachea

748.3/Q32.4 Other congenital malformations of bronchus

749.0/Q35.1-Q35.9 Cleft palate

749.1/Q36.0-Q36.9 Cleft lip

749.2/Q37.0-Q37.9 Cleft palate with cleft lip

750.0/Q38.1 Ankyloglossia

750.15/Q38.2 Macroglossia

754.1/Q68.0 Congenital deformity of sternocleidomastoid muscle

756.0/Q75.0 Craniosynostosis

756.0/Q75.2 Hypertelorism

756.0/Q75.9 Congenital malformation of skull and face bones, unspecified

759.2/Q89.2 Congenital malformations of other endocrine glands

784.2/R22.0 Localized swelling, mass and lump, head

748.2/R22.1 Localized swelling, mass and lump, neck

784.42/R49.0 Dysphonia

784.43/R49.21 Hypernasality

786.0/J98.9 Respiratory disorder, unspecified

786.09/R06.00 Dyspnea, unspecified

786.09/R06.09 Other forms of dyspnea

786.09/R06.3 Periodic breathing

786.09/R06.83 Snoring

786.09/R06.89 Other abnormalities of breathing

786.1/R06.1 Stridor

931/T16.1XXA Foreign body in right ear, initial encounter

931/T16.2XXA Foreign body in left ear, initial encounter

931/T16.9XXA Foreign body in ear, unspecified ear, initial encounter

V55.0/Z43.0 Encounter for attention to tracheostomy

—/Z93.0 Encounter for attention to tracheostomy

—/J95.00 Unspecified tracheostomy complication

—/J95.01 Hemorrhage from tracheostomy stoma

—/J95.02 Infection of tracheostomy stoma

—/J95.03 Malfunction of tracheostomy stoma

—/J95.04 Tracheo-esophageal fistula following tracheostomy

—/J95.09 Other tracheostomy complication

Definition of Procedure Codes

1. Tympanostomy Tube Otorrhea
   a. *Definitions*—This is a common situation encountered by any otolaryngologist who places tympanostomy tubes in children.
   b. *Key points*—There is not a current CPT code for suctioning or clearing such otorrhea from the external auditory canal. For these situations the CPT code for binocular microscopy (92504) may be used if documented and appropriately used.

2. Flexible Airway Endoscopy (31575, 31231, 92511, 31615)
   a. *Definitions*—The indications for flexible endoscopy are the same for children as

they are for adults. Such evaluations are a key component of the diagnostic services offered by otolaryngologists. When clinically indicated, diagnostic nasal endoscopy (31231), nasopharyngoscopy (92511), flexible fiberoptic laryngoscopy (31575), or tracheobronchoscopy via a tracheotomy (31615) should be performed and appropriately billed.

   b. *Key points*—When these procedures are accompanied by a significant, separately identifiable Evaluation and Management (E/M) service by the same physician on the same day of the procedure, the 25 modifier should be appended to the E/M code. If however, the patient presents to the clinic for sole purpose of undergoing the endoscopy, the E/M code should not be billed.

3. In-Office Ear Tube Removal
   a. *Definition*—There is no current CPT code for removing a pressure equalization tube in clinic. The only current code for pressure equalization tube removal (69424) is for removal under general anesthesia. However, it is both safe and efficient to remove pressure equalization tubes in children during clinic visits.
   b. *Key points*—The CPT code for removal of external auditory canal foreign body (69200) cannot be used in such situations. The binocular microscopy code (92504) can be used in such cases when documented. If impacted cerumen is encountered and its removal is necessary, then impacted cerumen removal (69210) can be reported for because there is not a code for in-office ear tube removal. The documentation for the procedure must support the impacted cerumen removal code.

4. Binocular Microscopy (92504)
   a. *Definitions*—Many otolaryngologists feel that binocular microscopy is a component of the standard physical examination and should not be coded as a separate procedure. If binocular microscopy is the otolaryngologist's standard method for ear examination, then it should not be

separately coded. However, if binocular microscopy is necessary after otoscopic exam, then it may be separately reported with 92504.
   b. *Key points*—In such cases, a procedure note that details the indications (medical necessity) should be included in the visit documentation. The documentation should state that the microscope was used because the otoscopic exam performed was inadequate to evaluate the underlying pathology. Appending modifier 25 to the E/M code is payer dependent. CMS does not recognize 92504 as a code where the postoperative global period concept applies; therefore, modifier 25 is not required.

5. Cauterization of Tracheostoma Granulation Tissue (17250)
   a. *Definitions*—Pediatric patients who have undergone tracheotomy require a great deal of clinical follow-up. The majority of such care can be provided in the outpatient setting.
   b. *Key points*—There are at least 2 ICD-9-CM codes that can be used for the E/M during an office visit that requires attention to a pediatric tracheotomy: attention to tracheotomy (V55.0) and respiratory abnormality (786.0). ICD-10-CM has more specificity, and thus there are multiple codes for patients with tracheostomy, including J95.00-J95.09 Tracheostomy complications (see individual codes for specific complication); Z43.0 Encounter for attention to tracheostomy; and Z93.0 Tracheostomy status. In addition, CPT codes for tracheobronchoscopy via a tracheotomy (31615) and chemical cauterization of granulation tissue (17250) can both be used when clinically indicated. However, there is no current CPT code for outpatient tracheotomy tube change in an established fistula tract; CPT 31502 is reported for the tracheotomy tube change prior to the establishment of the fistula tract. The E/M code will be appended with modifier 25, while the second procedure code is appended with modifier 51 (eg, 31615 and 17250-51) as long as both proce-

dures are clinically indicated and a significant separately identifiable E/M service is also rendered. In the case of tracheotomy patients, a separate E/M service can be performed and linked to the reason for the tracheotomy or an additional otolaryngologic condition for which the patient is being evaluated.

6. Lingual Frenulectomy (41010, 41115, 41520)
   a. *Definitions*—This procedure can be safely performed in clinic in neonates. Older children tend to have a thicker lingual frenulum that must be taken into consideration when determining whether to do this procedure in the clinic versus the operating room.
   b. *Key points*—There are three separate CPT codes for lingual frenulectomy: incision of lingual frenulum (41010), excision of lingual frenulum (41115), and frenuloplasty (surgical revision of frenulum, eg, with Z-plasty, 41520). The vast majority of clinic-performed frenulectomies would be considered incision of lingual frenulum (41010) as the surgeon is simply lysing the frenulum with a scissor.

Controversial Areas

Multiple Procedures on Same Day of Service

Billing diagnostic nasal endoscopy (31231) and flexible fiberoptic laryngoscopy (31575) during the same visit is controversial. At a minimum, separate, unrelated indications must be present and documented. Two separate procedure notes must be generated. Furthermore, 2 separate scopes must be used—a rigid scope for the nasal endoscopy and a flexible scope for the fiberoptic laryngoscopy. However, even with this, reimbursement

from commercial carriers for both procedures is unlikely. Finally, repetitive double billing may incur an audit. On the other hand, flexible fiberoptic laryngoscopy (31575) and tracheobronchoscopy via a tracheotomy (31615) can be billed in the same visit with a 51 modifier because different anatomic areas are examined with 2 different scopes.

Evaluation of adenoid hypertrophy is best coded as a nasopharyngoscopy (92511). However, if the adenoid tissue is evaluated during a nasal endoscopy for nasal symptoms, or during a laryngeal evaluation, then a diagnostic nasal endoscopy (31231) or flexible fiberoptic laryngoscopy (31575) may be reported instead of 92511 depending on the indication for the procedure. The procedure documentation should include the specific indication as well as an accurate description of the extent of the endoscopic examination.

Postoperative Global Period

The postoperative global period as established by Centers for Medicare and Medicaid Services (CMS) is the same for both pediatric and adult patients and is CPT code dependent; it is 90 days for adenotonsillectomy, 10 days for pressure equalization tube placement, and 0 days for most endoscopic sinus procedures, microdirect laryngoscopy, and bronchoscopy. As with adults, when you are seeing a patient for a postoperative visit during the global period, you cannot bill for the E/M related to that procedure. However, if a patient is seen for a new complaint related to a separately identifiable diagnosis, the clinic visit E/M code can be appended with modifier 24 while an unrelated procedure code is appended with modifier 79. If you see a patient in clinic who requires hospital admission, you may code for either the outpatient consult or the admission but not both on the same day.

CHAPTER 21

Office Sleep Medicine

Anit T. Patel

Introduction

The practice of sleep medicine has significantly evolved over the past 20 years. This chapter will describe coding and billing for sleep medicine in both the sleep lab and office settings. Coding and billing for sleep surgery is detailed in a separate chapter. This chapter will discuss some of the nuances in managing and billing for sleep studies including the initial polysomnogram (PSG), continuous positive airway pressure (CPAP) titration study, split studies, multiple sleep latency test (MSLT), maintenance of wakefulness test (MWT), and home-based sleep studies. Also reviewed will be office-based procedures for sleep medicine including palatal- and tongue-based procedures along with fitting patients for mandibular repositioning devices. Insurance company authorization and approval for these various sleep medicine procedures are not always straightforward and a conversation with your local insurance representatives is highly recommended to determine payer medical necessity for coverage and reimbursement.

Key Points

- Most insurance companies in geographic areas with high penetration of managed care will require an in-facility PSG to be preauthorized. If the patient's symptoms are consistent with obstructive sleep apnea, they may only approve an at-home PSG.
- Most insurance companies do not cover oral appliance devices unless they are created and provided by a dentist or oral surgeon. An otolaryngology practice may fit patients with these devices, but usually the patient has to pay out of pocket.
- At-home sleep testing is safe and convenient but can underestimate the degree of obstructive sleep apnea (OSA). If the at-home test is negative and there is a high pretest probability of OSA, an in-facility PSG should be performed.
- The coding page of the American Academy of Sleep Medicine (AASM) website (www.aasmnet.org/coding.aspx) includes a guide to searching the Medicare Physician Fee Schedule to find payment for services. The fee schedule search feature allows you to search for national payment or local payment specific to your region.
- All codes for sleep testing (95800–95811, 95782, 95783) include recording of data, scoring of data, interpretation of data, and the official report. Most insurance companies require reporting the sleep test code as a global code. However, other payers may request that you bill the code on two lines with the modifier 26 (professional component) on one line

and with the modifier TC (technical component) on the second line. The date of service and/or place of service might also differ for each component of service provided. For example, Medicare requires the place of service to be "home" for certain sleep tests while the place of service for the interpretation is the physician office or hospital outpatient department (depending on the location of the physician's office). Guidance from your local insurance representatives can help.

Key Procedure Codes

Codes that start with a letter are Healthcare Common Procedure Coding System (HCPCS) Level II codes and not *Current Procedural Terminology* (CPT) codes.

In-Lab Testing

95805 Multiple sleep latency or maintenance of wakefulness testing, recording, analysis and interpretation of physiological measurements of sleep during multiple trials to assess sleepiness
wRVU 1.20; Global XXX

95807 Sleep study, simultaneous recording of ventilation, respiratory effort, ECG or heart rate, and oxygen saturation, attended by a technologist
wRVU 1.28; Global XXX

95810 Polysomnography; age 6 years or older, sleep staging with 4 or more additional parameters of sleep, attended by a technologist
wRVU 2.50; Global XXX

95811 6 years or older, sleep staging with 4 or more additional parameters of sleep, with initiation of continuous positive

airway pressure therapy or bilevel ventilation, attended by a technologist
wRVU 2.60; Global XXX

#95782 younger than 6 years, sleep staging with 4 or more additional parameters of sleep, attended by a technologist
wRVU 2.60; Global XXX

#95783 younger than 6 years, sleep staging with 4 or more additional parameters of sleep, with initiation of continuous positive airway pressure therapy or bi-level ventilation, attended by a technologist
wRVU 2.83; Global XXX

Home Testing

#95800 Sleep study, unattended, simultaneous recording; heart rate, oxygen saturation, respiratory analysis (eg, by airflow or peripheral arterial tone), and sleep time
wRVU 1.05; Global XXX

#95801 minimum of heart rate, oxygen saturation, and respiratory analysis (eg, by airflow or peripheral arterial tone)
wRVU 1.00; Global XXX

95806 Sleep study, unattended, simultaneous recording of, heart rate, oxygen saturation, respiratory airflow, and respiratory effort (eg, thoracoabdominal movement)
wRVU 1.25; Global XXX

G0398 Home sleep study test (HST) with type II portable monitor, unattended; minimum of 7 channels: EEG, EOG, EMG, ECG/ heart rate, airflow, respiratory effort and oxygen saturation
wRVU 0.00; Global XXX

G0399 Home sleep test (HST) with type III portable monitor, unattended; minimum of 4 channels: 2 respiratory movement/

airflow, 1 ECG/heart rate and 1 oxygen saturation
wRVU 0.00; Global XXX

G0400 Home sleep test (HST) with type IV portable monitor, unattended with minimum of 3 channels
wRVU 0.00; Global XXX

Device Codes

21085 Impression and custom preparation oral surgical splint
wRVU 8.99; Global 10

E0485 Oral device/appliance used to reduce upper airway collapsibility, adjustable or non-adjustable, prefabricated, includes fitting and adjustment

E0486 Oral device/appliance used to reduce upper airway collapsibility, adjustable or non-adjustable, custom fabricated, includes fitting and adjustment

Office Procedures

41530 Submucosal ablation of the tongue base, radiofrequency, 1 or more sites, per session
wRVU 4.51; Global 10

42140 Uvulectomy, excision of uvula
wRVU 1.70; Global 90

42299 Unlisted procedure, palate, uvula
wRVU 0.00; Global YYY

S2080 Laser-assisted uvulopalatoplasty (LAUP)
wRVU 0.00; Global XXX

Key Modifiers

26 Professional Component
Used when billing only the professional component of the sleep test (eg, the interpretation of the

test) or when subdividing the professional and technical components out as indicated by the individual payer.

TC Technical Component
Used for billing the technical component of the sleep test (ie, the test itself).

52 Reduced Services
Used for reduced services such as less than 4 nap opportunities for MSLT or MWT; less than 6 hours of sleep testing for codes 95800–95811, less than 7 hours of sleep testing for children under the ages of 6 (95782, 95783).

Key ICD-9-CM/ICD-10-CM Codes

For sleep medicine–related disorders, most *International Classification of Diseases, Ninth Revision, Clinical Modification* (ICD-9-CM) to *International Classification of Diseases, Tenth Revision, Clinical Modification* (ICD-10-CM) codes are converted one-to-one, such as 327.23 obstructive sleep apnea (adult) (pediatric) becomes G47.33. Sleep-related breathing disorders, central disorders of hypersomnolence, circadian rhythm sleep-wake disorders, parasomnias, and movement disorders generally convert one-to-one. However, alcohol- and substance-induced sleep disorders do not convert one-to-one. For example, the ICD-9-CM code for drug-induced sleep disorders, 292.85, can convert to more than 27 codes in ICD-10-CM depending on the type of the substance.

278.03/E66.2   Morbid (severe) obesity with alveolar hypoventilation

307.41/F51.02   Adjustment insomnia

307.41/F51.09   Other insomnia not due to a substance or known physiological condition

307.42/F51.01   Primary insomnia

307.42/F51.03   Paradoxical insomnia

307.42/F51.09   Other insomnia not due to a substance or known physiological condition

307.44/F51.11   Primary hypersomnia

307.44/F51.12   Insufficient sleep syndrome

307.44/F51.19   Other hypersomnia not due to a substance or known physiological condition

307.46/F51.3   Sleepwalking (somnambulism)

307.46/F51.4   Sleep arousal disorder

307.47/F51.58   Other sleep disorders not due to a substance or known physiological condition

327.11/G47.11   Idiopathic hypersomnia with long sleep time

327.12/G47.12   Idiopathic hypersomnia without long sleep time

327.13/G47.13   Recurrent hypersomnia

327.14/G47.14   Hypersomnia due to medical condition

327.21/G47.31   Primary central sleep apnea

327.22/G47.32   High altitude periodic breathing

327.23/G47.33   Obstructive sleep apnea (adult) (pediatric)

327.24/G47.34   Idiopathic sleep related nonobstructive alveolar hypoventilation

327.26/G47.36   Sleep related hypoventilation in conditions classified elsewhere

327.27/G47.37   Central sleep apnea in conditions classified elsewhere

327.29/G47.39   Other sleep apnea

327.31/G47.21   Circadian rhythm sleep disorder, delayed sleep phase type

327.32/G47.22   Circadian rhythm sleep disorder, advanced sleep phase type

327.33/G47.23   Circadian rhythm sleep disorder, irregular sleep wake type

327.34/G47.24   Circadian rhythm sleep disorder, free running type

327.35/G47.25   Circadian rhythm sleep disorder, jet lag type

327.36/G47.26   Circadian rhythm sleep disorder, shift work type

327.42/G47.52   REM sleep behavior disorder

327.43/G47.53   Recurrent isolated sleep paralysis

327.51/G47.61   Periodic limb movement disorder

327.52/G47.62   Sleep related leg cramps

327.53/G47.63   Sleep related bruxism

327.59/G47.69   Other sleep related movement disorders

333.94/G25.81   Restless legs syndrome

347.00/G47.419   Narcolepsy without cataplexy

347.01/G47.411   Narcolepsy with cataplexy

770.81/P28.3   Primary sleep apnea of newborn

780.51/G47.30   Sleep apnea, unspecified

780.52/G47.00   Insomnia, unspecified

780.53/G47.30   Sleep apnea, unspecified

780.54/G47.10   Hypersomnia, unspecified

780.55/G47.20   Circadian rhythm sleep disorder, unspecified type

780.57/G47.30   Sleep apnea, unspecified

780.58/F51.8   Other sleep disorders not due to a substance or known physiological condition

780.59/G47.8   Other sleep disorders

786.04/R06.3   Periodic breathing

786.09/R06.00   Dyspnea, unspecified

786.09/R06.09   Other forms of dyspnea

786.09/R06.3   Periodic breathing

786.09/R06.83   Snoring

786.09/R06.89   Other abnormalities of breathing

788.36/N39.44   Nocturnal enuresis

Definition of Codes

1. Polysomnography In-Lab Testing (95807, 95810, 95811, 95782, 95783)
   a. *Definition*—A sleep test that involves the continuous, simultaneous recording of physiologic parameters for a minimum of 6 hours in a sleep laboratory and is monitored by a technician who is in close enough proximity to the patient so that he or she can physically respond to emergencies or technical issues. The parameters measured include electroencephalogram (EEG), electrooculogram (EOG), electromyography (EMG) and at least 4 additional parameters. The additional parameters are usually electrocardiogram (EKG), nasal or oral airflow, respiratory effort, oxygen saturation or anterior tibialis EMG.
   b. *Indications*—The AASM practice parameters state that PSG is routinely indicated for the diagnosis of sleep-related breathing disorders; for CPAP titration in patients with sleep-related breathing disorders; for the assessment of treatment results in some cases; with a multiple sleep latency test in the evaluation of suspected narcolepsy; in evaluating sleep-related behaviors that are violent or otherwise potentially injurious to the patient or others; and in certain atypical or unusual parasomnias. Polysomnography may be indicated in patients with neuromuscular disorders and sleep-related symptoms; to assist in the diagnosis of paroxysmal arousals or other sleep disruptions thought to be seizure related; in a presumed parasomnia or sleep-related seizure disorder that does not respond to conventional therapy; or when there is a strong clinical suspicion of periodic limb movement sleep disorder.
   c. *Key points*—Polysomnography is not routinely indicated to diagnose chronic lung disease; in cases of typical, uncomplicated, and noninjurious parasomnias when the diagnosis is clearly delineated; for patients with seizures who have no specific complaints consistent with a sleep disorder; to diagnose or treat restless legs syndrome; for the diagnosis of circadian rhythm sleep disorders; or to establish a diagnosis of depression.
   d. Diagnostic testing in patients older then 6 (95807, 95810). CPT 95807 is a sleep study attended by a technologist with simultaneous recording of ventilation, respiratory effort, ECG or heart rate, and oxygen saturation. Sleep staging does not occur in 95807. CPT 95810 requires sleep staging with at least 4 additional parameters of sleep.
   e. CPAP, bilevel positive airway pressure (BiPAP) or split study in the sleep lab (95811). Polysomnogram performed in patients age 6 years or older with initiation of positive airway pressure (PAP).
   f. Pediatric sleep study in the sleep lab (95782). In 2013, this code was added to CPT. Therefore, the previous code for polysomnogram (95810) is now specifically for patients 6 years or older.
   g. Pediatric CPAP, BiPAP, or split study in the sleep lab (95783). This was a new code in 2013; therefore, the existing code for CPAP titration study (95811) is now specifically for patients 6 years or older.

2. Multiple Sleep Latency Test (MSLT) or Maintenance of Wakefulness Test (MWT) (95805)
   a. *Definition*—Multiple sleep latency or maintenance of wakefulness test, recording, analysis, and interpretation of physiological measurements of sleep during multiple trials to assess sleepiness.
   b. *Indications*—The MSLT and MWT tests are the primary objective tests for assessing sleepiness (MSLT) and alertness (MWT). This can help determine whether a patient is too sleepy to drive or not alert enough to perform certain functions. The transportation industry has used the MWT to evaluate treatment response or to assess a patient's ability to remain awake for safety purposes. The MSLT also helps diagnose narcolepsy vs idiopathic hypersomnia.
   c. *Key points*—Usually, the MSLT is performed the morning after a polysomnogram and done in the facility. Therefore,

preauthorizations from the insurance company should be obtained for both 95810 and 95805.

3. Home sleep testing (HST) (95800, 95801, 95806, G0398–G0400)
   a. *Definitions*—CPT 95800 should be used for an unattended sleep study that includes simultaneous recording of heart rate, oxygen saturation, respiratory analysis (eg, by airflow or peripheral arterial tone), and sleep time. CPT 95801 is the most basic of the home sleep testing codes. It includes everything in CPT 95800 except for sleep time. So if sleep time is not part of the HST, then use CPT 95801. CPT 95806 is the most comprehensive of the home sleep study codes. It includes everything in CPT 95800 and in addition includes respiratory effort (eg, thoracoabdominal movement). The respiratory effort helps to differentiate obstructive from central sleep apnea. If your HST module includes respiratory effort, use CPT 95806. All three of these CPT codes include both the professional and technical components. Medicare utilizes G-codes for at home sleep testing. These codes should be billed to Medicare patients instead of the standard CPT codes above.
   b. *Indications*—Home sleep testing is indicated for patients who have a high pretest probability of obstructive sleep apnea. If the HST is negative, the patient should have an attended polysomnogram to definitively rule out OSA. The American Academy of Sleep Medicine states that HST is not appropriate for diagnosis of OSA in patients with comorbid diseases that may reduce the accuracy of the HST. These conditions include but are not limited to pulmonary disease, neuromuscular disease, or congestive heart failure. Also, HST is not appropriate if other sleep disorders are suspected such as central sleep apnea, periodic limb movement disorder, insomnia, circadian rhythm disorder, or narcolepsy. Please see the flowchart in Figure 21–1 for the recommended pathway of patients considered for HST.

4. Oral appliances for obstructive sleep apnea
   a. *Definitions*—Custom-made or custom-fit oral appliances may improve the upper airway by increasing the diameter of the upper airway or by reducing the collapsibility of the upper airway. This should improve obstructive sleep apnea.
      i. Mandibular repositioning devices attach to the upper and lower teeth and hold the mandible in a forward position during sleep. This opens up the airway by forward movement of the suprahyoid and genioglossus muscles and helps minimize obstructive episodes.
      ii. Tongue-retaining devices fit around the tongue and keep the tongue forward by means of suction. This prevents gravitational effects of the tongue and helps minimize obstructive episodes. These devices are generally indicated for patients who wear dentures or have contraindications for a mandibular repositioning device (eg, patients who have significant TMJ).
   b. *Indications*—The AASM states that oral appliances, although not as efficacious as CPAP, are indicated in patients
      i. With mild to moderate OSA who prefer oral appliances to CPAP
      ii. Who do not respond to CPAP
      iii. Who are not appropriate candidates for CPAP
      iv. Who fail CPAP or behavioral measures such as weight loss or sleep position change
      To ensure adequate treatment with an oral appliance, the patient should undergo an attended or at-home PSG with the oral appliance in. This should be performed after final adjustments to the appliance have been made.
   c. HCPCS E0485—Oral device/appliance used to reduce upper airway collapsibility for sleep apnea, adjustable or nonadjustable, prefabricated, includes fitting and adjustment. The key here is a prefabricated device and not a custom-made appliance.
   d. HCPCS E0486 Impression and custom preparation of an oral appliance for sleep

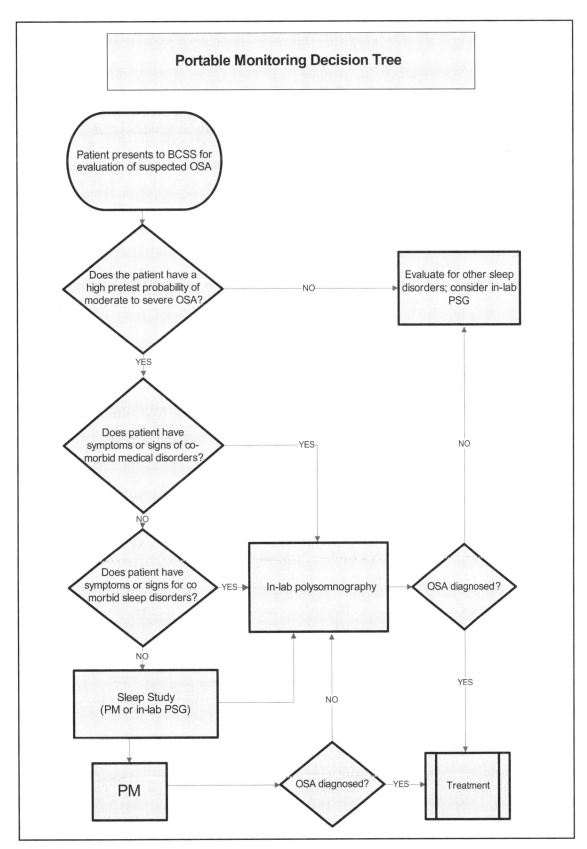

Figure 21–1. Recommended pathway of patients considered for home sleep test (also known as portable monitoring). (BCSS = Board Certified Sleep Specialist, PM = portable monitoring). From Collop et al. (2007). Clinical Guidelines for the Use of Unattended Portable Monitors in the Diagnosis of Obstructive Sleep Apnea in Adult Patients. *Journal of Clinical Sleep Medicine*, Vol. 3, No. 7, p. 741.

apnea which is individually and uniquely made for a specific patient. It is a mandibular advancement device for OSA. Effective July 1, 2012, the coding guideline is revised to state: It involves taking an impression of the patient's teeth and making a positive model to produce the final product. Custom fabrication requires more than trimming, bending, or making other modifications to a substantially prefabricated item. A custom-fabricated oral appliance may include a prefabricated component (eg, the mechanism).

e. CPT 21085—Impression and custom preparation of oral prosthesis for treatment of OSA. This code is a CPT code. It is the equivalent of the HCPCS code E0486. Medicare only covers custom appliances under E0486. Check with your local private insurance representatives whether they utilize the HCPCS or CPT code.

5. Office-based procedures for snoring and obstructive sleep apnea
   a. CPT 41530—Submucosal ablation of the tongue base, radiofrequency. Includes somnoplasty of the tongue base which utilizes controlled radiofrequency current to reduce tissue volume. Many insurers do not cover this code; therefore, preauthorization for this procedure should be attempted. If it is a noncovered benefit, then the patient will have to decide if he or she wants to pay for the entire procedure out of pocket.
   b. CPT 42299—Unlisted procedure, palate, uvula. This includes various procedures such as injection snoreplasty, somnoplasty of soft palate, and cautery-assisted palatal stiffening operation (CASPO). The Pillar procedure, which utilizes small implants into the soft palate to reduce snoring and sleep apnea, is also included under this code. Most insurance companies do not cover these procedures and will usually have a standard statement that these are not medically necessary services because there is insufficient clinical data to support

its efficacy. If these procedures are being performed for snoring, not sleep apnea, then the patient should be billed directly as a noncovered service.

c. HCPCS S2080—Laser-assisted uvulopalatoplasty (LAUP). This is the HCPCS II code for the procedure and the CPT code mostly closely related to this procedure is the unlisted code, 42299. There is considerable debate about whether this procedure gives any benefit for OSA patients. The AASM concluded in 2001 that LAUP should not be recommended for treatment of OSA. It should be noted that most insurers do not cover this code. If the procedure is being done for snoring, this should be billed as an out-of-pocket expense to the patient.

Controversial Areas

PAP-Nap

This refers to the acclimation of CPAP therapy in the lab in patients who have trouble tolerating the mask. Although there is no specific code for PAP-Nap, the AASM has identified 95807-52 as the code that most approximates the services being performed. The test is done in the laboratory but usually does not take the full 6 hours that code 95807 describes. Therefore, the modifier 52 (reduced services) is appended to 95807. Medicare has historically reimbursed PAP-Nap services when billed as 95807-52. Sleep centers interested in billing other payers for this service should contact them to determine if this is a covered service.

Split Night Study

This refers to patients who have the diagnostic portion of the PSG and the CPAP titration done during the same night. There is no separate CPT code for split night studies. However, CPT 95811 encompasses everything that was done on that night and is the correct code to use. It is inappropriate to bill both the polysomnogram (95810) and the CPAP titration study (95811) as this would require 6 hours of study time for each code adding up to 12 hours of study time.

Oral Appliances

Payment for oral appliances for obstructive sleep apnea is not always straightforward. Although most medical insurance policies recognize the benefit of oral appliances for mild and moderate OSA, each individual plan varies; therefore, preauthorization should be obtained prior to fabrication of the appliance. It should be noted that as of January 3, 2011, Medicare will only authorize a licensed dentist to bill for E0486. The dentist must first become a Medicare Durable Medical Equipment (DME) supplier in order to bill for oral appliances. Also, effective November 1, 2012, only those appliances and laboratories that have been reviewed and approved through Medicare may be reimbursed.

The American Academy of Otolaryngology-Head and Neck Surgery position statement (http://www.entnet.org/?q=node/216) supports both an otolaryngologist and qualified dentist to fit an oral appliance for OSA:

> Oral appliances are a treatment of the upper airway. An oral appliance device for the medical treatment of Obstructive Sleep Apnea may be fit, adjusted, and medically assessed by an Otolaryngologist or a qualified Dentist with training in Sleep Medicine. An Otolaryngologist is an MD or DO physician who has satisfactorily completed an accredited training program in Otolaryngology-Head and Neck surgery. A qualified Dentist, as defined by The American Academy of Dental Sleep Medicine (AADSM) is a Dentist who maintains certification from the American Board of Dental Sleep Medicine, or one who is the director of an AADSM-accredited dental facility and has completed 30 hours of continuing education (ADA CERP recognized or AGD PACE approved) within the past three years, of which a minimum of 20 credits must be in dental sleep medicine and the rest must be sleep medicine related.

In practical terms, many private payers may not reimburse for oral appliances, and if they do, usually they typically require a dentist to do this. Payment for an oral appliance from an otolaryngology practice will be usually be an out-of-pocket expense for the patient.

Home Sleep Testing

As insurance companies attempt to reduce costs of sleep services, many are requiring a preauthorization process to be completed for any type of sleep test. If the patient has symptoms consistent with obstructive sleep apnea, an elevated BMI and a high score on the Epworth sleepiness scale, they will likely deny an in-facility study and only approve a HST. In some cases, the HST may only be performed by a designated provider that the insurance company has contracted with. Many private payers have designated providers for HST and those networks are closed to any new provider who may be interested in doing HST.

Some outside companies provide the physician with the HST machine and will bill the technical component and allow the physician to bill the professional component. However, Medicare does not allow this and includes the following language regarding DME local coverage determination: "No aspect of an HST, including but not limited to delivery and/or pickup of the device, may be performed by a DME supplier." Some private payers may allow this, but it is important to check with your local insurance representatives.

Physicians Dispensing CPAP as a DME Supplier

Stark laws prohibit physicians from selling PAP devices to Medicare patients because of the risk of overutilization of these devices. If the sleep center is owned by physicians, then they can sell PAP devices to commercial patients (given there are no state laws to the contrary) but not to Medicare patients. If the sleep center is not owned by physicians, then they can sell PAP devices to both Medicare and commercial patients.

CHAPTER 22

In-Office Imaging

Gavin Setzen, Mary Lally, and Michelle M. Mesley-Netoskie

Introduction

In-office imaging such as computed tomography (CT) and ultrasound are valuable diagnostic imaging tools utilized by otolaryngologists to visualize the anatomy and disease processes affecting the maxillofacial and head and neck regions to guide patient management and treatment. The diagnostic quality of the images and the accuracy of the interpretation are critical components to obtaining an appropriate diagnosis for patient management.

Key Points

- Radiology codes are 70010–79999.
- The Centers for Medicare and Medicaid Services (CMS) under the Medicare Improvements for Patients and Providers Act (MIPPA) Law 2008, require in-office imaging accreditation for the following advanced diagnostic imaging modalities: CT, magnetic resonance imaging (MRI), nuclear medicine, and positron emission tomography (PET) imaging for physicians or entities that bill under the Physician Fee Schedule for the technical component (this may not be required by all payers, however).
- An order for the test is required from a clinician before the test is performed.
- For imaging performed using intravenous contrast material, one

may be able to bill for contrast using Healthcare Common Procedure Coding System (HCPCS) codes Q9966 or Q9967 if the provider has incurred the expense for the contrast material.

- Medicare rule on self-referral for advanced imaging (section 6003 of the PPACA, Patient Protection and Affordable Care Act) requires the referring physician to provide written disclosure notice to the patient at the time of the referral. The notice must include a list of 5 other suppliers that provide the same service and are located within a 25-mile radius of the referring physician's office. The notice must include the supplier's name, address, and telephone number.
- Always link the *Current Procedural Terminology* (CPT) code with an appropriate *International Classification of Diseases, Ninth Revision, Clinical Modification* (ICD-9-CM) / *International Classification of Diseases, Tenth Revision, Clinical Modification* (ICD-10-CM) code and document medical necessity for the service ordered.
- CMS requires direct physician supervision for imaging performed with intravenous contrast administration.
- A separate written radiological supervision and interpretation report is required for all radiological services. Notation of the interpretation in the evaluation and management (E/M) note

225

alone is not sufficient for reporting a
radiology code.

- Billing options for otolaryngologists
include
  - Global billing, billing without a
  modifier, includes both the technical
  and professional components
  - Technical component alone, billing
  with modifier TC, with outsourcing
  the interpretation or the professional
  component
  - Participate with a radiologist for
  professional component (digital file
  transfer and image storage options),
  billing with modifier 26

Key Procedure Codes

Plain Films

This is divided into the part of the head and neck
imaged, as well as whether a complete series was
done (3 or more views) or a limited series.

70140 Radiologic examination, facial bones; less
than 3 views
wRVU 0.19; Global XXX

    70150 complete, minimum of 3 views
wRVU 0.26; Global XXX

70160 Radiologic examination, nasal bones,
complete, minimum of 3 views
wRVU 0.17; Global XXX

70210 Radiologic examination, sinuses,
paranasal, less than 3 views
wRVU 0.17; Global XXX

70220 Radiologic examination, sinuses,
paranasal, complete, minimum of 3 views
wRVU 0.25; Global XXX

70360 Radiologic examination; neck, soft tissue
wRVU 0.17; Global XXX

Computed Tomography (CT)

CT coding is based on the area imaged as well
as whether contrast was administered. There are
separate codes for examinations performed with
and without contrast. There is a separate code if
the CT is performed for stereotactic localization.

70450 Computed tomography, head or brain;
without contrast material
wRVU 0.85; Global XXX

    70460 with contrast material(s)
wRVU 1.13; Global XXX

    70470 without contrast material,
followed by contrast material(s)
and further sections
wRVU 1.27; Global XXX

70480 Computed tomography, orbit, sella, or
posterior fossa or outer, middle, or inner
ear; without contrast material
wRVU 1.28; Global XXX

    70481 with contrast material
wRVU 1.38; Global XXX

    70482 without contrast material,
followed by contrast material(s)
and further sections
wRVU 1.45; Global XXX

70486 Computed tomography, maxillofacial
area; without contrast material
wRVU 0.85; Global XXX

    70487 with contrast material(s)
wRVU 1.13; Global XXX

    70488 without contrast material,
followed by contrast material(s)
and further sections
wRVU 1.27; Global XXX

70490 Computed tomography, soft tissue neck;
without contrast material
wRVU 1.28; Global XXX

    70491 with contrast material(s)
wRVU 1.38; Global XXX

    70492 without contrast material
followed by contrast material(s)
and further sections
wRVU 1.45; Global XXX

77011 Computed tomography guidance for
stereotactic localization
wRVU 1.21; Global XXX

Ultrasound

The ultrasound codes for the head and neck include a separate code for diagnostic ultrasound and a second code for needle placement for biopsy:

76536 Ultrasound, soft tissues of head and neck (eg, thyroid, parathyroid, parotid), real time with image documentation
wRVU 0.56; Global XXX

76942 Ultrasonic guidance for needle placement (eg, biopsy, aspiration, injection, localization device), imaging supervision and interpretation
wRVU 0.67; Global XXX

Example of Ultrasound Diagnosis and Procedure Codes for a Thyroid Nodule

For identification or characterization of a thyroid nodule, use the CPT code for ultrasound of soft tissues of head and neck: 76536.

For percutaneous core needle biopsy of the thyroid, use CPT code 60100.

For image-guided, fine needle aspirations, use CPT code 10022.

For ultrasound guidance of a thyroid biopsy or cyst aspiration, use ultrasonic guidance of needle placement CPT code 76942 (report 76942 in addition to the code of the underlying procedure, eg, 60100, 10022).

For diagnostic thyroid ultrasound and an ultrasound-guided fine needle aspiration procedure performed on the same patient, consider using the following CPT codes:

- Diagnostic ultrasound: 76536
- Ultrasound guidance used for needle guidance: 76942
- Underlying procedure code (FNA): 10022

Payment Policies for Ultrasound Services

Medicare Part B will reimburse physicians for medically necessary diagnostic ultrasound services, provided the services are within the scope of the physician's license. Some Medicare carriers require the physician who performs and/or interprets specific types of ultrasound examinations to demonstrate relevant, documented training through recent residency training or postgraduate Continuing Medical Education (CME) and experience. Contact your Medicare Part B carrier for details related to your particular practice environment.

Private insurance payment rules about which specialties may perform and receive reimbursement for ultrasound services vary by payer and plan. Some payers will reimburse providers of any specialty for ultrasound services, and others may restrict imaging procedures to specific specialties or providers possessing specific certifications or accreditations. Some insurers require physicians to submit applications requesting ultrasound exams and procedures be added to their list of services performed in their practice. It is important to contact your private payers before submitting claims to determine their requirements and request that they add ultrasound to your list of services.

Site of Ultrasound Service: Code Selection

In an office setting (place of service 11), a physician who owns the equipment and personally performs the ultrasound examination for guidance or performs the examination through an employed or contracted sonographer may report the global service code and report the CPT code without any modifier.

If the site of service is the hospital (eg, POS 22), modifier 26, indicating only the professional service was provided, must be added by the physician to the CPT code for the ultrasound service. Typically payers will not reimburse physicians for the global service or technical component in the hospital outpatient setting.

If billing for a biopsy or injection procedure on the same day as an office visit, append modifier 25 to the office visit code if a significant, separately identifiable E/M service was performed. However, modifier 25 is not to be used routinely. The E/M service must be "above and beyond the usual preoperative and postoperative care associated with the procedure that was performed." It is very important to document in the patient's record all components of the E/M service.

Regardless of the type of ultrasound equipment that is used, all ultrasound examinations must

- Meet the requirements of medical necessity as set forth by the payer.
- Meet the requirements of completeness for the code that is chosen.
- Be documented in the patient's record as a separate note.

It is the physician's responsibility to select the codes that accurately describe the service performed and the corresponding reason for the study. Under the Medicare program, the physician should select the diagnosis or ICD-9-CM/ICD-10-CM code based upon test results, with 2 exceptions. If the test does not yield a diagnosis or was normal, the physician should use the preservice signs, symptoms, and conditions that prompted the study. If the test is a screening examination ordered in the absence of any signs or symptoms of illness or injury, the physician should select "screening" as the primary reason for the service. If there are test results, they should be recorded as additional diagnoses.

Key Modifiers

TC   Technical component
This is for all nonphysician work, and includes administrative, personnel, and capital (equipment and facility) costs and related malpractice expenses.

26   Professional Component
This is used to reimburse for the physician work interpreting a diagnostic test or performing a procedure, and includes indirect practice and malpractice expense related to that work.

Key ICD-9-CM/ICD-10-CM Codes

Listed below are some common ICD-9-CM codes for ordering radiological examinations. Due to the significant expansion of codes in ICD-10-CM

related to malignant and benign categories of classification, please refer to the ICD-10-CM code set for the most accurate specificity for the patient's condition.

171.0/C49.0   Malignant neoplasm of connective and soft tissue of head, face and neck

193/C73   Malignant neoplasm of thyroid gland

194.1/C75.0   Malignant neoplasm of parathyroid gland

195.0/C76.0   Malignant neoplasm of head, face and neck

226/D34   Benign neoplasm of thyroid gland

227.1/D35.1   Benign neoplasm of parathyroid gland

386.00/H81.09   Meniere's disease, unspecified ear

386.11/H81.13   Benign paroxysmal vertigo, bilateral

388.30/H93.19   Tinnitus, unspecified ear

461.0/J01.00   Acute maxillary sinusitis, unspecified

461.9/J01.90   Acute sinusitis, unspecified

470/J34.2   Deviated nasal septum

471.0/J33.0   Polyp of nasal cavity

473.0/J32.0   Chronic maxillary sinusitis

473.9/J32.9   Chronic sinusitis, unspecified

780.2/R55   Syncope and collapse

784.0/G44.1   Vascular headache, not elsewhere classified

784.0/R51   Headache

784.2/R22.0   Localized swelling, mass and lump, head

784.2/R22.1   Localized swelling, mass and lump, neck

784.7/R04.0   Epistaxis

785.6/R59.9   Enlarged lymph nodes, unspecified

Controversial Areas

Most commercial carriers require precertification or preapproval of advanced imaging. Medicare requires only that the test be medically necessary. As with any diagnostic test, the clinician should clearly document in the patient's chart the reason and the medical necessity for ordering the test.

1. Commercial payers may impose a higher copay or deductible if the patient has the advanced imaging service in the ordering physician's office. Payers typically have preferred sites—free-standing imaging centers that accept a lower copay or none at all.
2. CPT 77011 is not a diagnostic CT code; this code is used in surgical preplanning. A stereotactic CT localization scan is frequently obtained prior to sinus surgery. The data set is then loaded into the navigational workstation in the operating room for use during the surgical procedure. In most cases, the preoperative CT is a technical-only service that does not require separate interpretation by an otolaryngologist or radiologist and is then only reported using CPT 77011. If a diagnostic scan is performed and interpreted, the appropriate diagnostic CT code (eg, CPT 70486) should be used. It is not appropriate to report both CPT 70486 and CPT 77011 for the same CT stereotactic localization imaging session. Furthermore, 3-dimensional (3D) rendering (CPT 76376 or CPT 76377) should not be reported in conjunction with CPT 77011 (or CPT 70486 if used), as the procedure inherently generates a 3D data set.
3. Plain-film sinus x-rays and sinography (an x-ray examination of a body cavity, sinus, using contrast medium, often because of infection) are rarely indicated and not routinely performed for evaluation of nasal and sinus pathology. CPT 70220 is used for 3 or more views, and CPT 70210 is used for less than 3 views.
4. 3D Rendering of CT images is not frequently used in the point-of-care setting. Both CPT codes 76376 and 76377 require concurrent supervision of the image postprocessing 3D manipulation of the volumetric data set and image rendering. These two codes differ in the need for and use of an independent workstation for postprocessing (CPT 76377). The 3D rendering codes should not be used for 2-dimensional (2D) reformatting. Also, 3D rendering is built into the imaging software of many devices and generally only takes a few minutes to do. CPT 76377 can be considered in a patient with complex facial fractures, for example, especially where treatment will be based on preoperative planning for a complex surgical repair.

CT Accreditation and Intersocietal Accreditation Commission (IAC)

The Intersocietal Accreditation Commission (IAC), through its IAC CT division, offers an accreditation program that evaluates the quality of the critical elements of a CT facility. The peer-review process provides a mechanism for facilities performing CT procedures—in private office settings, outpatient imaging centers, and/or hospitals—to be evaluated and recognizes those facilities that demonstrate that they provide quality services. All aspects related to patient care, including medical and technical staff training and experience, medical safety policies, equipment quality assurance, radiation safety, quality imaging, and reporting are evaluated. The IAC grants 3-year accreditation to those facilities that are found to be in substantial compliance with the IAC CT standards through a comprehensive application process including detailed case study and report review.

The IAC is the sole organization to offer an accreditation pathway for facilities that perform CT imaging using volume cone beam CT (CBCT) scanners. In addition, many practices utilizing conventional CT scanners seek accreditation for maxillofacial and temporal bone imaging, as well as soft tissue neck (and other organs systems) through the IAC CT program. The requirements for IAC CT accreditation are consistent, regardless of the type of scanner that the facility uses for imaging.

Medicare Improvements for Patients and Providers Act (MIPPA)

Specific to Medicare reimbursement, the MIPPA was approved by Congress and enacted into law in 2008. The MIPPA law requires imaging accreditation for all nonhospital suppliers that bill for the technical component for advanced diagnostic imaging (ADI) services defined by the Centers for Medicare and Medicaid Services (CMS) as nuclear medicine/PET, MRI, and CT. CMS currently recognizes 4 imaging accreditation organizations: the Intersocietal Accreditation Commission (IAC; http://www.intersocietal.org/ct); the American College of Radiology (ACR; http://www.acr.org/ quality-safety/accreditation); RadSite (http:// www.radsitequality.com/); and the Joint Commission (http://www.jointcommission.org/).

The IAC communicates the status of applicant facilities to CMS through a data share process; therefore, it is important that those physicians or entities that bill under the Physician Fee Schedule for the technical component indicate their national provider identifier (NPI) and Medicare enrollment number in the IAC Online Accreditation portal to ensure accurate data matching and corresponding reimbursements.

There are several national and state-specific, private insurers that require imaging accreditation as a condition of payment. The IAC monitors and publishes reimbursement policy details as they become available but encourages facilities to check with their practice administrator or regional insurance carriers for the most up-to-date payment policies, to ensure compliance. Link to IAC website with payment policies: http://www. intersocietal.org/iac/reimbursement/policies/ IACCT_PaymentPolicies.pdf.

IAC Accreditation Requirements

IAC Standards and Guidelines: http://www.inter societal.org/ct/

Designed to serve facilities as an educational tool, the IAC accreditation program consists of 2 crucial steps. First, facilities conduct a detailed self-assessment using the *IAC Standards and Guidelines* (http://www.intersocietal.org/ct/) and subsequently answer questions and provide data as specified by the Online Accreditation application. Through the accreditation process, facilities assess many aspects of daily operation and their impact on the quality of health care provided to patients. While completing the accreditation application, facilities often identify and correct potential problems, revise processes, and implement ongoing quality improvement programs.

Submission Requirements

- Staff credentials and training documents including CME/CE
- Policies and procedures (eg, pregnancy, medical emergency, quality improvement)
- Equipment quality control, preventive maintenance (PM) report, and physicist survey
- Accreditation agreement and fees
- Case studies and final interpretation reports

Facilities are granted accreditation upon meeting substantial compliance with the *IAC CT Standards and Guidelines for CT Accreditation* (http://www .intersocietal.org/ct/) following a comprehensive peer review which takes an average of 10 to 12 weeks from application submission. Obtaining diagnostic images and providing accurate final reports are crucial components for patient management and the treatment of disease processes and therefore are the most heavily weighted aspects in the IAC accreditation review.

Facilities that fall short of meeting all of the standards are delayed accreditation until compliance with the *IAC CT Standards and Guidelines for CT Accreditation* is evident. Helpful guidance is provided and facilities are given an opportunity to correct any deficiencies noted during the review. The most common oversights are incomplete final reports, physicist surveys, and nondiagnostic or incomplete case studies. Corrective measures of the noncompliant items for most facilities take place within a relatively short time period, generally within weeks.

The most common noncompliant report items include missing physician signature and signature date, the clinical indication not indicated for the study, exceeding the 4-day report turnaround time, lack of report standardization among the physicians, and discrepancies in the report findings.

The submissions of the physicist reports and surveys are often incomplete, lacking a comprehensive patient dose assessment or verification of the protective shielding in the CT room to keep staff and patients safe from unnecessary radiation exposure.

Image quality deficiencies identified include poor visualization of the anatomy of clinical interest, patient or equipment artifacts, poor positioning technique, low signal-to-noise ratio resulting in grainy images and incomplete case study submission.

Related to noncompliance, it is important to recognize that Medicare reimbursements will not be paid until CMS is notified that the imaging facility has been granted accreditation. The MIPPA law and private insurance mandates do not recognize facilities that have submitted an application and are in a delayed status.

As well, the IAC provides frequent, complimentary informational accreditation webinars to assist in completing the online application and help applicant facilities with the process. Participants receive continuing education (CE) credit for attending the webinar.

Sample documents and resources are located on the IAC website: http://www.intersocietal .org/ct/main/sample_documents.htm

- Submit all documentation that is required in the application.
- Carefully review all the material, prior to submission, for accuracy and completeness.
- The policies and procedures must be facility specific and reflect current practices.
- Use the IAC CT resources as guidance for document submission: http://www .intersocietal.org/ct/seeking/sample_ documents.htm.
- Each of the case studies submitted must include all of the images, including reformats used in the interpretation, and the applicable final report.
- The case studies should be of high quality and representative of best work submitted: http://www.intersocietal.org/ ct/seeking/case_studies.htm.
- Images must be submitted on CD or flash drive with the DICOM viewer installed.
- Complete the current Accreditation Agreement downloaded from http:// www.intersocietal.org/iac/legal/ agreement.htm.
- Submit the appropriate accreditation fee: http://www.intersocietal.org/ct/ seeking/fees.htm.
- Contact the IAC CT staff with any questions about the application process toll free at 800-838-2110.

Key Steps to Follow in CT Accreditation Process to Avoid Delay

- Allow adequate time to prepare the application materials for submission.
- Facility staff should verify that they are adhering to the current version of the *IAC CT Standards and Guidelines for CT Accreditation*. The website http://www. intersocietal.org/ct/ contains the current version, and the links within the Online Accreditation application interact with this version.

Conclusion

This guide offers information about coverage and payment for diagnostic imaging services and related procedures and CT imaging accreditation. The information is meant to help determine appropriate codes and other information for reimbursement. There are no guarantees concerning reimbursement or coverage; it is the individual otolaryngologist's responsibility to confirm and submit appropriate codes, modifiers, and claims for services provided.

SECTION III

Surgical Otolaryngology

CHAPTER 23

Basics of Surgical Coding

Seth M. Brown

Introduction

This chapter sets the stage for the third section of the book, surgical coding. It goes through how to properly dictate an operative report and when modifiers should be appended to *Current Procedural Terminology* (CPT) codes. It describes how to best select the code to describe the work done as well as the principles of bundling and unbundling. Furthermore, it will discuss the definition of the surgical global package as well as a global period. Finally, this chapter will discuss the use of unlisted codes and what should be included in the dictation and communication to the payer.

The Operative Report

The operative note is the surgeon's description of what was done to and for the patient. A good operative note allows the surgeon to review the operative details at any time after surgery. Any practitioner who is taking care of the patient will be aware of what was performed during surgery, as will an attorney reviewing the case, an insurance company, or a professional coder; thus, the language, details, and structure are of the utmost importance.

An operative note should include the basics: the physician, the assistant, the type of anesthesia, blood loss, specimens, the preoperative and postoperative diagnoses, the procedure performed, findings, and complications at a minimum. When multiple diagnoses and procedures are used, it is best to list these individually on separate lines. An operative note should also include the indications for surgery and the discussion that was had with the patient, including the discussion of risks, benefits, and alternatives. This is useful as someone can pick up the operative note and not only understand what was done but also why these procedures were done, which is, along with the diagnoses, commonly called "medical necessity."

The body of the note should include patient positioning, the preparation used, that proper patient time-outs were done, and that images were reviewed and present (when applicable). The rest of the note should include a stepwise approach to the procedure including the key equipment used. A reader should be able to conceptually replicate the steps done by the surgeon by reading the operative note.

In many cases, codes are dependent on the structures opened or resected, and thus it is important to document when tissue is removed or an additional area is approached. This is specifically applicable for sinus and ear surgery where there are several codes that are similar, but dependent on the extent of surgery and whether tissue is removed or not. The mentioning of technology is important for certain surgeries as well, for instance, in laryngeal surgery the use of a microscope for a similar procedure is a different code from when one is not used. It is also important to document in the operative note the use of the endoscope for endoscopic sinus procedures because there are codes for endoscopic and non-endoscopic procedures.

Finally, the operative report should conclude with the incision closure and the condition in which the patient was brought to the recovery room (or intensive care). If the procedure was abnormally complex, or if an unlisted code or modifier 22 will likely be used, it is useful to add an additional paragraph describing the unique aspects of this surgery.

The more readable, detailed, and organized the operative report is, the easier it will be for others who need to read it. It is useful to separate different aspects of the surgery by paragraph and highlight critical aspects of the surgery. For instance, when performing a total endoscopic ethmoidectomy, highlight that the orbit and skull base were identified as well as demonstrate that surgery was performed on both sides of the ground lamella (to highlight that a total ethmoidectomy was performed and not just an anterior dissection). Similarly, if tissue such as a polyp was removed from a maxillary or sphenoid sinus, this should be documented as well.

The more you can allow your operative note to be a stand-alone document, that a reader can interpret everything from why you did the surgery to what you did and how you did it, the stronger your supporting evidence will be in either a chart audit, legal suit, or dispute with an insurance company.

How to Select a Surgical Code

How do you select a code to bill? Often this is easy, as you will be using a standard code to describe a surgery. For instance, if you perform a tympanostomy with insertion of a ventilation tube, you will choose one of two codes—69433 or 69436. The difference between these 2 codes is whether general anesthesia is used or not. Using a coding guide or book, such as the American Medical Association (AMA) CPT codebook will describe the procedure for the physician to select.

69433 Tympanostomy (requiring insertion of ventilating tube), local or topical anesthesia
wRVU 1.57; Global 10

69436 Tympanostomy (requiring insertion of ventilating tube), general anesthesia
wRVU 2.01; Global 10

The CPT codebook will oftentimes tell you if the code is unilateral or bilateral and when bilateral, a 50 modifier is applicable, and thus each ear can be billed separately. For both of these codes, there is a descriptive statement below the code "(For bilateral procedure, report 69433 (69436) with modifier 50)."

In some situations, the codes can be a little more challenging. For instance, when performing a tracheostomy, there are 5 different codes that can be selected (31600, 31601, 31603, 31605, 31610). It is thus imperative that the physician consult with a coding book to make sure the proper code is selected. Under this scenario, the various codes differ based on the age of the patient, whether the tracheostomy is planned or emergent, the location of the opening into the trachea, and whether a fenestration procedure with skin flaps is performed.

Coding becomes even more complex when a new procedure is performed, when new technology is used, or for a procedure that does not seem to fit under a specific code. For instance, epistaxis can be controlled with an endoscopic sphenopalatine ligation. One might be tempted to use the code 30920—Ligation arteries; internal maxillary artery, transantral. However, this is an open code, and one should not use a similar code when one does not exist for the procedure performed. In this situation there is not a code that describes the procedure of an endoscopic sphenopalatine ligation, and thus the only appropriate selection is to use an unlisted code (ie, 31299—Unlisted procedure, accessory sinuses). When looking for a code to describe the procedure done, be sure to read the associated clinical vignette (or the explanation of the code) in the CPT codebook; however, not all codes have clinical vignettes. (Note that many of the vignettes are in the AMA's CodeManager product and not in the codebook itself.) If this does not describe the procedure performed, including the work required, then this code should not be used to bill the procedure.

It goes without saying that when performing surgery, only procedures that are medically necessary should be performed. One should not bill or be reimbursed for performing an unnecessary surgery. Furthermore, in most situations, one cannot bill codes for procedures that were done to access a surgical site (eg, billing a sphenoidotomy [31287, 31288] when performing pituitary surgery [61548, 62165]). A sphenoidotomy code implies the procedure is performed to remove disease or provide drainage; it is not to be used to describe access or the approach to another surgical site. One exception is in open skull base surgery where there are codes that were created for access.

Modifiers Typically Used During Surgery

Often, when billing surgery, modifiers are used to notify the insurance company something about the code being used. There are a number of modifiers typically used during surgery billing. For instance, the 50 modifier is used frequently during sinus surgery, to describe that both sides were operated. Depending on the individual payers, each side can be listed on a separate line on the billing sheet or the code listed only once with the 50 modifier.

Another modifier that can be used during surgery billing is the 22 modifier. This modifier lets the insurance company know that the procedure performed was more complex or difficult than the standard procedure. This can be used if the procedure required more time, the patient had complicating factors making this a more challenging procedure, the risks were increased, or more advanced training was needed for this procedure. Often, this will be used by a tertiary referral physician, who is performing a surgery that was too complex for a community-based otolaryngologist. When using the 22 modifier a letter may be needed with the claim explaining why this surgery was outside the norm. This can be included in the operative report as well as in a separate paragraph.

Other modifiers used during surgery billing include modifiers 51 (multiple procedures) and 59 (distinct procedural service), modifier 58 for a staged or planned/anticipated procedure, modifier 62 which tells the insurance company that 2 surgeons (usually of 2 different specialties) worked together to perform the procedure, modi-

fiers 76 and 77 which describe repeat procedures, modifier 78 which describes return to the operating room during a global period, and modifier 79 for an unrelated procedure during the global period.

Please see Chapter 11, "Demystifying Modifiers," for a more in-depth discussion on modifiers and when to use the individual modifiers.

How to Bill Multiple Procedures

Oftentimes during otolaryngologic surgery multiple procedures are performed during the same operative session. For instance, one might perform a septoplasty (30520) along with an uvulopalatopharyngoplasty (42145). One should then use both the septoplasty code along with the code for uvulopalatopharyngoplasty. The correct way to bill this is to list the highest-valued code first followed by the code of next value. This is particularly true in sinus surgery where often multiple separate codes are used. Most payers follow Medicare guidelines and will pay the first code at 100% followed by the next code at 50% and then further reduce the rest of the codes to 25% to 50% depending on how the codes are listed. It is thus important to organize codes in descending fee value and generally not to reduce the billed fee (except for certain modifiers—refer to Chapter 11, "Demystifying Modifiers," for more information). Each payer will reduce the allowed amount based on your contract.

Some payers may require the use of a modifier on multiple or separate procedures to avoid them from getting bundled together. An example of this is the code for concha bullosa which payers, although not Medicare, often bundle with an ethmoidectomy. Modifier 59 may be added to the concha bullosa code depending on the individual payer to avoid a denial on this distinctly separate procedure.

Unbundling

When coding surgery, it is important to look for a code that describes the entire procedure performed. For instance, there are codes for tonsillectomy

(42825, 42826) and adenoidectomy (42830, 42831, 42835, 42836) as well as codes for tonsillectomy with adenoidectomy (42820, 42821). It is *not* appropriate to bill both the tonsillectomy and adenoidectomy codes separately, as this is termed *unbundling* and is not accurate coding. There are many situations, however, in which multiple procedures are performed together and there is not one code to describe the procedure performed, thus each individual code would be separately reported.

The Postoperative Global Period

Most major procedures are associated with a "postoperative global period." This is the period of time following a surgery during which the after care is included in the payment of the procedural code. As a result, when a patient is reevaluated for the condition that he or she had surgery for during this global period (eg, postoperative visits related to the procedure), this visit is included in the payment for the surgical procedure. However, follow-up care for surgical procedures includes only that care which is usually a part of the surgical service. Should the patient suffer a complication or an unrelated condition during the global period and require additional services, this can be separately reported.

Many of the otolaryngology surgery CPT codes carry a 90-day global period, according to Centers for Medicare and Medicaid Services (CMS). This means all the postoperative care whether done in the hospital or office/clinic is included unless there is a return to the operating room that can be separately reported. The majority of commonly used laryngoscopy and sinus endoscopy codes carry a 0-day global period. Therefore, these office visits and procedures such as debridement, nasal endoscopy, and fiberoptic laryngoscopy can be separately billed during the postoperative period.

CMS has been talking about reducing or eliminating global periods. If this happens, postoperative care may be separately reimbursable in the future.

The Global Surgical Package

The global surgical package includes the surgeon's work that is included in the code selected. For instance, when performing surgery it is common to see the patient immediately prior to surgery and then again in the recovery room. These "visits" are not separately billable. They are part of the "global surgical package." In some procedures there may be more extensive time requirements in the immediate preoperative or postoperative periods, and in others this may be only a matter of minutes; however, this variation is built into the nature of each individual code. Evaluation and management (E/M) visits subsequent to the decision for surgery, including the visit on the day before or the day of surgery, are also included. Furthermore, local and topical anesthesia are included in the surgical code.

Billing Unlisted Codes

As mentioned, there are times when a code does not exist for the procedure performed. When this occurs, an unlisted code should be used and not a corresponding "like" or "similar" CPT code. There is essentially an unlisted code for each individual system in the head and neck. The unlisted code selected should thus be the one that is most similar to the method of the procedure performed. For instance, if using an endoscope to perform an advanced sinus procedure, one should use, 31299 —Unlisted procedure, accessory sinuses. The various unlisted codes can be found in the AMA CPT codebook and the individual surgical subsections.

When using an unlisted code, one should select a comparison code to associate with the unlisted code. The surgeon should select the code that best represents the procedure, time, risk, and expertise required to perform the procedure. This is the code that should be preauthorized when contacting the insurance company prior to surgery if the payer will not accept the unlisted code for precertification. The surgeon should then describe in the operative report exactly how the surgery was performed. It is helpful to have an additional paragraph at the end describing how this surgery was different than the comparison procedure code. The surgeon should then submit a paper claim showing the unlisted code along with the operative report and a cover letter describing why an unlisted code was used, the comparison code being used, and the amount of the charge. Check with the payer prior to claim submission as some will accept an electronic claim with a brief explanation in the Remarks box.

The unlisted codes do not have an assigned global period; thus, postoperative care is not typically included in the code. However, if you select a comparison code with a global period and choose a fee that reflects this code, then in essence you are asking for payment for the postoperative care and should not bill for postoperative care. If you feel that more work is required than would typically be included in the fee of the comparison code, then your letter can reflect that you will be billing for postoperative care including office visits, endoscopy, and debridement. If you do not intend to bill these visits, your charges can reflect a standard 90-day global period.

Controversial Areas

The Operative Note

Some physicians dictate the actual procedure and/or diagnosis codes directly in the operative note. The purpose of this is to inform the staff that will be sending this information to the payer the codes the physician feels that they have performed. To do this it requires a physician who is well versed in the individual codes. The staff should review the entire operative note to make sure they agree with the codes selected and that the operative report supports these codes prior to submitting.

However, this can create issues as most physicians have only a cursory understanding of the codes and often select the wrong codes. Secondly, if using a transcription service this can create issues with the transposition of numbers correctly. Also, the operative report is a patient medical record and not a coding tool. There are many better ways to capture surgical charges (eg, apps for the iPhone or iPad, e-mail) than by dictating codes in the operative note. Thus, we do not recommend that the CPT or diagnosis codes be documented in the operative note. More importantly, the code language should be dictated so the appropriate code can be assigned and billed.

Conclusion

Coding for surgery can seem like a daunting task; however, it is too important not to learn and understand how to properly select codes and modifiers as well as to capture all charges for services provided. The surgeon performing the procedure is the only one who knows exactly what was done and the effort and expertise required to perform the surgery. It is essential that the operating surgeon dictates an appropriate operative note and selects the code based on the procedure performed. In addition to risking not getting paid adequately for the procedure performed, falsely or inaccurately selecting codes leaves you open for an audit that can result in financial take-back or in severe cases financial and even criminal penalties.

CHAPTER 24

Operative Rhinology

Jivianne T. Lee

Introduction

This chapter discusses coding and billing for rhinologic procedures performed in the operating room setting. It encompasses both fundamental (eg, turbinate surgery, septoplasty, endoscopic sinus surgery [ESS]) and advanced sinonasal operations (eg, frontal sinus drill-outs, revision sinus surgery). Endoscopic, open, and combined sinus approaches are described. Extended endoscopic transnasal procedures (eg, medial maxillectomy, orbital surgery, cerebrospinal fluid leak repair) are also addressed. However, skull base approaches will be covered in a separate chapter on skull base surgery. Unique aspects of coding for hospital versus ambulatory surgery settings is elucidated, particularly with respect to image guidance. Furthermore, appropriate coding for emerging technologies including balloon sinuplasty and sinus stent implantation is delineated.

As with other otolaryngologic surgeries, *Current Procedural Terminology* (CPT) codes for operative rhinology are designated by the American Medical Association (AMA) and are assigned relative value units (RVUs) by the Centers for Medicare and Medicaid Services (CMS) to describe physician work, practice expense, and professional liability resources associated with each service. Such RVUs are updated on an annual basis and determine physician payment as well as facility (hospital, ambulatory surgery center) vs nonfacility reimbursement. Current RVUs are listed on the CMS website (http://www.cms.gov), and in various AMA publications. Search engines for CPT codes and RVU calculators are also available on the AMA website (https://ocm.amaassn.org/OCM/CPTRelativeValueSearch.do?submitbutton=accept). All rhinologic surgeries should be documented in an operative note describing the indications, risks, benefits, anesthesia, details of the procedure, and any associated complications. There are multiple codes for each sinus, and documentation of the method of opening the sinus, use of an endoscope, and tissue removal is essential. Supplemental documentation may also be necessary when modifiers or unlisted procedure codes are utilized. This may include letters of medical necessity or appeal that describes the procedure being performed.

Key Points

- Endoscopic sinus surgery codes, including debridement, are unilateral and can be billed for each side. If performed bilaterally, modifier 50 should be applied.
- If an endoscope is used during the procedure, corresponding endoscopic CPT codes should be reported as opposed to an open code. If no appropriate endoscopic code exists, an unlisted code may be necessary. Use of the endoscope must be documented in the procedure statement as well as in the body of the operative note.
- Stereotactic computer-assisted navigation (SCAN)/image guidance codes are

241

"add-on" codes that must be billed in conjunction with the primary procedure.

- Balloon sinus dilation codes should be used to describe dilation of sinus ostia via displacement of tissue only. If accompanied by tissue removal, existing endoscopic sinus surgery codes should be reported instead.

- Although introduction of a new CPT code for sinus stent implantation has been proposed, no distinct procedure code has been approved by the AMA at the time of this publication.

Key Procedure Codes

Septoplasty and Turbinate

30520 Septoplasty or submucous resection, with or without cartilage scoring, contouring, or replacement with graft
wRVU 7.01; Global 90

30801 Ablation, soft tissue of inferior turbinates, unilateral or bilateral, any method (eg, electrocautery, radiofrequency ablation, or tissue volume reduction); superficial
wRVU 1.14; Global 10

> **30802** intramural (ie, submucosal)
> *wRVU 2.08; Global 10*

30930 Fracture nasal inferior turbinate(s), therapeutic
wRVU 1.31; Global 10

30130 Excision inferior turbinate, partial or complete, any method
wRVU 3.47; Global 90

30140 Submucous resection inferior turbinate, partial or complete, any method
wRVU 3.57; Global 90

Endoscopic Sinus Surgery

Codes for diagnostic maxillary and sphenoid sinusoscopy (31233, 31235) are rarely used in this day and age. They require puncturing the sinus, typically with a trocar, in order to simply visualize the sinus. Typically, the standard maxillary and sphenoid endoscopic surgery codes should be used for a surgical procedure (31256, 31267, 31287, 31288), and if only for diagnosis, 31231 is generally used. These codes are included below mostly for historical purposes.

31233 Nasal/sinus endoscopy, diagnostic with maxillary sinusoscopy (via inferior meatus or canine fossa puncture)
wRVU 2.18; Global 0

31235 Nasal/sinus endoscopy, diagnostic with sphenoid sinusoscopy (via puncture of sphenoid face or cannulation of ostium)
wRVU 2.64; Global 0

31237 Nasal/sinus endoscopy, surgical; with biopsy, polypectomy, or debridement (separate procedure)
wRVU 2.60; Global 0

> **31238** with control of nasal hemorrhage
> *wRVU 2.74; Global 0*

> **31240** with concha bullosa resection
> *wRVU 2.61; Global 0*

31254 Nasal/sinus endoscopy, surgical; with ethmoidectomy, partial (anterior)
wRVU 4.64; Global 0

> **31255** with ethmoidectomy, total (anterior and posterior)
> *wRVU 6.95; Global 0*

31256 Nasal/sinus endoscopy, surgical with maxillary antrostomy;
wRVU 3.29; Global 0

> **31267** with removal of tissue from maxillary sinus
> *wRVU 5.45; Global 0*

31276 Nasal/sinus endoscopy, surgical with frontal sinus exploration, with or without removal of tissue from frontal sinus
wRVU 8.81; Global 0

31287 Nasal/sinus endoscopy, surgical, with sphenoidotomy;
wRVU 3.91; Global 0

    31288 with removal of tissue from the sphenoid sinus
wRVU 4.57; Global 0

Extended Endoscopic Sinus Surgery

31290 Nasal/sinus endoscopy, surgical, with repair of cerebrospinal fluid leak; ethmoid region
wRVU 18.61; Global 10

    31291 sphenoid region
wRVU 19.56; Global 10

31299 Unlisted procedure, accessory sinuses
wRVU 0.00; Global YYY

Endoscopic Orbital Surgery

31239 Nasal/sinus endoscopy, surgical; with dacryocystorhinostomy
wRVU 9.04; Global 10

31292 Nasal/sinus endoscopy, surgical; with medial or inferior orbital wall decompression
wRVU 15.90; Global 10

    31293 with medial orbital wall and inferior orbital wall decompression
wRVU 17.47; Global 10

    31294 with optic nerve decompression
wRVU 20.31; Global 10

Open Nasal/Sinus Surgery

30117 Excision or destruction (eg, laser), intranasal lesion; internal approach
wRVU 3.26; Global 90

    30118 external approach (lateral rhinotomy)
wRVU 9.92; Global 90

31000 Lavage by cannulation; maxillary sinus (antrum puncture or natural ostium)
wRVU 1.20; Global 10

31030 Sinusotomy, maxillary (antrotomy); radical (Caldwell-Luc) without removal of antrochoanal polyps
wRVU 6.01; Global 90

    31032 radical (Caldwell-Luc) with removal of antrochoanal polyps
wRVU 6.69; Global 90

31040 Pterygomaxillary fossa surgery, any approach
wRVU 9.77; Global 90

31070 Sinusotomy frontal; external, simple (trephine operation)
wRVU 4.40; Global 90

    31075 transorbital, unilateral (for mucocele or osteoma, Lynch type)
wRVU 9.51; Global 90

    31080 obliterative, without osteoplastic flap, brow incision (includes ablation)
wRVU 12.74; Global 90

    31081 obliterative, without osteoplastic flap, coronal incision (includes ablation)
wRVU 14.19; Global 90

    31084 obliterative, with osteoplastic flap, brow incision
wRVU 14.95; Global 90

    31085 obliterative, with osteoplastic flap, coronal incision
wRVU 15.64; Global 90

    31086 nonobliterative, with osteoplastic flap, brow incision
wRVU 14.36; Global 90

    31087 nonobliterative, with osteoplastic flap, coronal incision
wRVU 14.57; Global 90

31205 Ethmoidectomy; extranasal, total
wRVU 10.58; Global 90

31225   Maxillectomy; without orbital
         exenteration
         wRVU 26.70; Global 90

    31230   with orbital exenteration (en bloc)
         wRVU 30.82; Global 90

Balloon Dilation

31295   Nasal/sinus endoscopy, surgical; with
         dilation of maxillary sinus ostium (eg,
         balloon dilation), transnasal or via canine
         fossa
         wRVU 2.70; Global 0

    31296   with dilation of frontal sinus
         ostium (eg, balloon dilation)
         wRVU 3.29; Global 0

    31297   with dilation of sphenoid sinus
         ostium (eg, balloon dilation)
         wRVU 2.64; Global 0

Image Guidance

+61781   Stereotactic computer-assisted
         (navigational) procedure; cranial,
         intradural (List separately in addition
         to code for primary procedure)
         wRVU 3.75; Global ZZZ

    +61782   cranial, extradural (List
         separately in addition to code
         for primary procedure)
         wRVU 3.18; Global ZZZ

Key Modifiers

Modifiers are used to indicate that the procedure performed has been modified by some specific circumstance but has not altered the definition or code of the service. They are composed of 2-digit codes that are appended to 5-digit CPT codes.

22   Increased Procedural Services

Modifier 22 is used to designate an increased service requiring work substantially greater than typically required for the listed procedure. This can potentially encompass anatomical variants, more extensive surgery, and so on, in which no existing code is available to describe the increased work. Additional time alone does not justify use of this modifier. It should also not be utilized if there is already an existing code for the service or to simply indicate that a specialist conducted the procedure. Use of this modifier often requires supplemental documentation (eg, separate statement, special forms) to support the claim and delineate how the service went above and beyond the typical surgery. A Draf III/modified endoscopic Lothrop procedure, for example, could be coded as 31276 with modifier 22 to indicate the increased work involved beyond that typically required of an endoscopic frontal sinusotomy.

50   Bilateral Procedure

Modifier 50 is appended to certain CPT codes to indicate that the service was performed bilaterally. Since all ESS codes describe unilateral procedures, they should be accompanied by modifier 50 if completed bilaterally. Bilateral maxillary antrostomy without removal of tissue, for example, would be coded as 31267 with modifier 50.

51   Multiple Procedures

Modifier 51 is applied when multiple procedures are performed by the same physician during the same operative session. It is typically added to the second and subsequent lower valued operative procedures, when modifier 50 is not being used, to designate progressive discounting (eg, the practice of reducing payment for procedures completed at the same sitting due to presumed savings when multiple services are performed together). Modifier 51 should not be used on add-on codes or services that require modifier 50 since the multiple procedure discount is already included in payment for bilateral procedures. For Medicare, reporting of modifier 51 is not usually necessary as the processing system is automatically programmed to append the modifier to the appropriate CPT codes. If a septoplasty (30520) and submucous resection of the inferior turbinate (30140) are performed at the same sitting by the same surgeon, for example, modifier 51 could be added to 30140.

59 Distinct Procedural Service

Modifier 59 should be reported with a CPT combination to denote distinct procedural services performed at separate sites. This modifier is used to designate a separate procedure not included within the CPT code for the primary service. For example, if septoplasty (30520) is performed in conjunction with inferior turbinate ablation (eg, 30801), modifier 59 can be applied to prevent bundling by certain payers (eg, Medicare).[1]

Key ICD-9-CM/ICD-10-CM Codes

October 1, 2015, was the compliance date for transitioning to the *International Classification of Diseases, Tenth Revision, Clinical Modification* (ICD-10-CM) code sets. Under ICD-10-CM, codes will be longer with more alphanumeric characters (3–7 vs 3–5). These additional descriptors are designed to provide greater specificity and information regarding anatomical location, laterality, associated causes, temporal factors (acute/recurrent/chronic), and so on. Consequently, the coding list is expected to expand from approximately 14,000 *International Classification of Diseases, Ninth Revision, Clinical Modification* (ICD-9-CM) codes to more than 69,000 ICD-10-CM codes. For acute unspecified sinusitis, for example, there was only one code under ICD-9-CM (461.9). However, with ICD-10-CM there will be 3 codes (J01.80 other acute sinusitis, J01.90 acute sinusitis unspecified, J01.91 acute recurrent sinusitis unspecified). The most common ICD-9-CM/ICD-10-CM codes utilized for operative rhinology are listed below.

Acute rhinosinusitis is defined by up to 4 weeks of purulent nasal drainage with nasal obstruction and/or facial pain-pressure-fullness. Recurrent acute rhinosinusitis refers to 4 or more episodes of acute rhinosinusitis in a given year with no signs or symptoms in between episodes.[2] Chronic rhinosinusitis is defined by 12 weeks or more of 2 or more of the following signs and symptoms: mucopurulent drainage, nasal obstruction, facial pain-pressure-fullness, or reduced sense of smell as well as radiographic or endoscopic (purulent mucus, edema, polyps) evidence of sinus inflammation.[2] Pansinusitis refers to inflammation of all the sinuses on one side. ICD-10-CM codes for "other" sinusitis are used when 2 or 3 sinuses on one side are affected.

Nasal Disorders

470/J34.2   Deviated nasal septum

471.0/J33.0   Polyp of nasal cavity

471.9/J33.9   Nasal polyp, unspecified

478.0/J34.3   Hypertrophy of nasal turbinates

478.19/J34.0   Abscess, furuncle and carbuncle of nose

478.19/J34.1   Cyst and mucocele of nose and nasal sinus

478.19/J34.89   Other specified disorders of nose and nasal sinuses

784.7/R04.0   Epistaxis

Acute Sinusitis (Codes are designated by 461.-/JO1.-)

461.0/J01.00   Acute maxillary sinusitis, unspecified

461.0/J01.01   Acute recurrent maxillary sinusitis

461.1/J01.10   Acute frontal sinusitis, unspecified

461.1/J01.11   Acute recurrent frontal sinusitis

461.2/J01.20   Acute ethmoidal sinusitis, unspecified

461.2/J01.21   Acute recurrent ethmoidal sinusitis

461.3/J01.30   Acute sphenoidal sinusitis, unspecified

461.3/J01.31   Acute recurrent sphenoidal sinusitis

461.8/J01.40   Acute pansinusitis, unspecified

461.8/J01.41   Acute recurrent pansinusitis

461.8/J01.80   Other acute sinusitis

461.8/J01.81   Other acute recurrent sinusitis

461.9/J01.90   Acute sinusitis, unspecified

461.9/J01.91   Acute recurrent sinusitis, unspecified

Chronic Sinusitis
(Codes are designated by 473.-/J32.-)

473.0/J32.0   Chronic maxillary sinusitis

473.1/J32.1   Chronic frontal sinusitis

473.2/J32.2   Chronic ethmoidal sinusitis

473.3/J32.3   Chronic sphenoidal sinusitis

473.8/J32.4   Chronic pansinusitis

473.8/J32.8   Other chronic sinusitis

473.9/J32.9   Chronic sinusitis, unspecified

Sinonasal Lesions

160.0/C30.0   Malignant neoplasm of nasal cavity

160.2/C31.0   Malignant neoplasm of maxillary sinus

160.3/C31.1   Malignant neoplasm of ethmoidal sinus

160.4/C31.2   Malignant neoplasm of frontal sinus

160.5/C31.3   Malignant neoplasm of sphenoid sinus

212.0/D14.0   Benign neoplasm of middle ear, nasal cavity, and accessory sinuses

239.1/D49.1   Neoplasm of unspecified behavior of respiratory system

471.0 /J33.0   Polyp of nasal cavity

471.8/J33.8   Other polyp of sinus

471.9/J33.9   Nasal polyp, unspecified

Cerebrospinal Fluid Leak

349.81/G96.0   Cerebrospinal fluid leak

742.0/Q01.9   Encephalocele, unspecified

Orbital Pathology

For the below orbital codes with a "-", the sixth digit represents the location:

- 1—right
- 2—left
- 3—bilateral
- 9—unspecified

375.20/H04.20-   Unspecified epiphora, lacrimal gland

375.30/H04.30-   Unspecified dacryocystitis of lacrimal passage

375.32/H04.32-   Acute dacryocystitis of lacrimal passage

375.42/H04.41-   Chronic dacryocystitis of lacrimal passage

375.33/H04.31-   Phlegmonous dacryocystitis of lacrimal passage

376.21/H05.89   Other disorders of orbit

376.22/H05.89   Other disorders of orbit

Definition of Codes

1. Turbinate Codes (30801, 30802, 30930, 30130, 30140)
   a. *Introduction*—There are numerous turbinate codes to describe whether an ablation, either submucosal or intramural, outfracturing, submucosal dissection, or a partial (or complete) turbinate resection is performed.
   b. *Definition*—CPT 30801 (superficial ablation of inferior turbinates) and 30802 (intramural ablation of inferior turbinates) should be reported for ablation or "reduction"

of inferior turbinates irrespective of the method used (eg, cautery, radiofrequency). These codes are mutually exclusive and should not be reported in conjunction with each other.

c. *Key points*—CPT 30930 may be appended with modifier 51 when reported with 30802 (submucosal ablation inferior turbinate (s)) to indicate that two separate procedures were performed.[1] (However, 30930 may not be billed with 30801 nor should it be billed with modifier 50). That said, many payers will not reimburse the lower valued code (30930) because both procedures were performed on the same anatomical structure (inferior turbinate). Modifier 59 may not be appended to 30930 because the definition of modifier 59 is not met when two procedures are performed on the same structure at the same session.

   i. CPT 30801 can be appended with modifier 59 when used with 30520 (septoplasty) for Medicare claims because procedures on 2 separate anatomical structures (inferior turbinates and septum) were performed. Medicare's CCI edits do not bundle 30802 with 30520 at the time this chapter was written; therefore, modifier 51 may be appended to 30802 in this scenario.

   ii. CPT 30801, 30802, as well as 30930 can refer to either unilateral or bilateral procedures, and therefore the modifier 50 should not be used.[3]

   iii. In contrast, 30130 (partial or complete excision of inferior turbinate) and 30140 (submucous resection of inferior turbinate) refer to unilateral procedures, and require use of modifier 50 if performed bilaterally. CPT 30130 should be used if a portion of the inferior turbinate is resected. CPT 30801, 30802, and 30930 should not be reported with 30130 or 30140.

   iv. As the inferior turbinates are not considered to be inherently part of sinus surgery or septoplasty, 30130 and 30140 can be reported separately from

CPT codes for ESS and septal surgery. In contrast, if the middle turbinate is addressed during endoscopic ethmoidectomy (31254, 31255) or polypectomy (31237), middle turbinate removal should not be reported separately. However, middle turbinectomy is considered distinct from septoplasty or sphenoid, maxillary, and frontal sinus surgery.[1] However, any procedure performed for "access" or "approach" such as middle turbinate lateralization is included in the primary ESS code and not separately reported. There is not a code for middle turbinate removal, only removal of a concha bullosa (31240).

d. *Documentation pearls*—For 30140, it is important to elucidate that the mucosa was incised and preserved, and that underlying soft tissue and/or bone was removed or reduced in the submucosal plane. The diagnosis and indications for performing the turbinate procedure should always be included as well. A sample code combination for septoplasty, bilateral submucous resection of the inferior turbinates, and bilateral outfracturing of the inferior turbinates is shown in the following box.

Sample code combination for septoplasty, bilateral submucous resection of inferior turbinates, and bilateral outfracture of inferior turbinates. Modifier 50 indicates that the procedures were done bilaterally. Modifier 51 designates that multiple procedures were performed during the same operative session. Note that 30930 is not listed in this case because it should not be reported in conjunction with either 30130 or 30140.

Code	Procedure
30520	Septoplasty
30140-51	Submucous resection of inferior turbinate
30140-50	(Bilateral modifier)

---

2. Endoscopic Sinus Surgery Codes (31240–31288)
   a. *Introduction*—There are multiple codes used to describe procedures performed during ESS. These encompass surgical approaches involving the use of an endoscope to open the respective sinuses (ie, endoscopic frontal sinusotomy, sphenoidotomy, maxillary antrostomy and ethmoidectomy) with or without tissue removal.
   b. *Definitions*—ESS codes are unique to each sinus (ie, frontal, sphenoid, ethmoid, maxillary) and refer to unilateral procedures. If performed bilaterally, they should be accompanied by modifier 50.
   c. *Key points*—CPT 31240 (endoscopic resection of concha bullosa) can be reported as a separate procedure if documented appropriately with inclusion of indications, pre-operative diagnosis, computed tomography (CT) findings, and description of concha bullosa excision. Otherwise, middle turbinate surgery performed to improve access to the sinuses should not be coded as a distinct service.
      i. CPT 31267 (endoscopic maxillary antrostomy with removal of tissue from the maxillary sinus) and 31288 (endoscopic sphenoidotomy with removal of tissue from the sphenoid sinus) should only be reported if removal of tissue from the respective sinus is actually performed. Tissue may refer to polyps, cysts, mucocele, fungus ball, and so on, but not mucus, pus, or debris. If no tissue is removed, then 31256 (endoscopic maxillary antrostomy) and 31287 (endoscopic sphenoid sinusotomy) should be used for the maxillary and sphenoid sinuses, respectively.
      ii. CPT 31254 (endoscopic partial/anterior ethmoidectomy), 31255 (endoscopic total ethmoidectomy), and 31276 (endoscopic frontal sinusotomy) may be reported for the ethmoid and frontal sinuses whether or not tissue is removed. CPT 31237 should not be used to separately code for nasal polypectomy as nasal polyp removal is included in the aforementioned codes. A sample code com-

bination for bilateral ESS with tissue removal, septoplasty, and bilateral submucous resection of the inferior turbinates is shown in the following box.
      iii. ESS (31254–31288) and balloon dilation (31295–31297) codes are mutually exclusive for procedures performed on the same sinus and should not be used in conjunction with each other. Existing ESS codes should be reported if balloon dilation is accompanied by removal of bone and/or tissue and additional instrumentation is used to open the sinus ostia.
      iv. At this time, there is no distinct CPT code for revision endoscopic sinus surgery. If particularly difficult, modifier 22 may be considered (see Chapter 11, "Demystifying Modifiers").

Sample code combination for bilateral endoscopic sinus surgery with tissue removal from each of the respective sinuses, septoplasty, and bilateral submucous resection of inferior turbinates:

Code	Procedure
30520	Septoplasty
31276-51	Endoscopic frontal sinusotomy
31276-50	(Bilateral modifier)
30140-51	Submucous resection of inferior turbinate
30140-50	(Bilateral modifier)
31255-51	Endoscopic complete ethmoidectomy
31255-50	(Bilateral modifier)
31267-51	Endoscopic maxillary antrostomy with tissue removal from maxillary sinus
31267-50	(Bilateral modifier)
31288-51	Endoscopic sphenoid sinusotomy with tissue removal from sphenoid sinus
31288-50	(Bilateral modifier)

3. Unlisted Procedure Codes (30999, 31299)
   a. *Introduction*—With continued advances in endoscopic instrumentation and techniques, many procedures traditionally performed with an open approach are now being accomplished endoscopically. Consequently, recent years have witnessed a growing number of endoscopic rhinologic surgeries without available CPT codes to accurately describe the services rendered. For such procedures, use of modifier 22 or an unlisted procedure code (30999, 31299) has been recommended.
   b. *Definitions*—As elucidated in an earlier section, modifier 22 is used to designate an increased service requiring work substantially greater than typically required for the listed procedure (see section on modifiers). CPT 30999 (unlisted procedure, nose) is applied when a nasal procedure is performed that is not currently described by any existing CPT code. Similarly, 31299 (unlisted procedure, accessory sinuses) is used when a sinus procedure is performed that is not accurately described by any existing CPT code.
   c. *Key points*
      i. Do not report more than one unlisted code per operative session.[4] Unlisted codes do not have defined global periods but have been assumed to have the global period consistent with other services in the same group (ie, for endoscopic sinus surgery, 0 days). Ultimately, however, the global period is determined by payer policy and may vary from one carrier to another.
      ii. Procuring compensation for unlisted codes as well as modifier 22 can prove challenging, with extensive documentation and onerous discussions with insurance payers often required to facilitate reimbursement. A claim must typically be submitted along with a detailed operative note describing the work performed and justifying the charge requested. Such paperwork will be subjected to medical review and can lead to significant delays for processing. Template appeal letters for modifier 22 and unlisted codes are available on the American Academy of Otolaryngology-Head and Neck Surgery (AAO-HNS) website.
      iii. To facilitate reimbursement for unlisted codes, be sure to obtain prior authorization for the elective procedure and understand specific carrier requirements. Outline how and why an unlisted code is being used, how the base code was selected, and what factors make the unlisted procedure more or less difficult than the comparison CPT code.[4]

4. Advanced Endoscopic Sinus Surgery Codes
   a. *Introduction*—There are a number of codes that have been developed to describe more advanced endoscopic sinus surgical procedures including cerebrospinal fluid leak repair and orbital surgery. However, there are also several complex endoscopic sinus surgical approaches that currently do not have an existing CPT code.
   b. *Definitions*—CPT 31290 and 31291 should be reported to describe endoscopic CSF leak repair in the ethmoid and sphenoid regions, respectively. With respect to orbital surgery, CPT 31239 should be utilized to code for endoscopic dacryocystorhinostomy. CPT 31292–31293 should be applied when an endoscopic orbital wall decompression is performed and 31294 for optic nerve decompression.
   c. *Key points*
      i. Endoscopic sphenopalatine artery ligation: No available CPT code exists at this time to accurately describe this service. CPT 31238 (Nasal/sinus endoscopy, surgical; with control of nasal hemorrhage) may be reported with use of modifier 22. Alternatively, an unlisted code (30999, 31299) may be applied with the understanding that this will likely have varying degrees of reimbursement depending on payer policy.
      ii. Extended endoscopic maxillary sinus procedures (eg, endoscopic medial

maxillectomy, mega-antrostomy): Currently, there is no CPT code for more advanced endoscopic maxillary procedures. In such situations, 31267 may be used with an option to add modifier 22 or use the unlisted code, 31299 with the understanding that this may have varying degrees of reimbursement depending on payer policy.

iii. Extended endoscopic frontal sinus procedures (frontal sinus drill-out/ endoscopic Lothrop/ Draf III): Such advanced endoscopic frontal sinus procedures also do not have existing CPT codes. Similar to endoscopic medial maxillectomy, the corresponding endoscopic frontal sinusotomy code (31276) may be used with modifier 22 or use the unlisted code, 31299 with the understanding that this will have varying degrees of reimbursement depending on payer policy.

5. Non-endoscopic Nasal/Sinus Surgery Codes (30000–31230)
    a. *Introduction*—Most traditional open approaches already have existing CPT codes that appropriately describe the procedure performed. These codes encompass a broad spectrum of surgeries that involve approaching the nose or sinus through an external incision without the use of an endoscope.
    b. *Definitions*—Similar to the endoscopic surgical codes, CPT codes for open sinus procedures are typically specific to the sinus involved. CPT 31000–31205 describe approaching the various sinuses either transnasal with a headlight or through an extranasal incision. Most of these codes are not used in this day and age, as endoscopic sinus surgery has become the standard of care. There still remain instances when open frontal sinus surgery is done. As there are multiple methods of accessing the frontal sinus via an external approach, distinct codes have been developed for the various procedures performed including trephinations (31070), transorbital Lynch

incisions (31075), and osteoplastic flaps (31084–31087). Open resection of sinus lesions is also covered by this set of codes such as maxillectomy without/with orbital exenteration (31230, 31255), pterygomaxillary fossa surgery (31040), and lateral rhinotomy (30118).
    c. *Key points*—For combined open and endoscopic approaches, the CPT code that best describes the procedure performed should be used. For example, if a nonobliterative osteoplastic flap via a coronal incision is coupled with a transnasal endoscopic frontal sinusotomy, either 31276 or 31087 should be applied, but not both codes. It would be appropriate to append a 22 modifier to the code selected, describing the increased complexity that required the need for an above and below approach.

6. Balloon Procedure Codes (31295–31297)
    a. *Introduction*—The balloon dilation codes were established in 2011 to describe the use of balloon technology in the paranasal sinuses.
    b. *Definitions*—Balloon dilation codes (31295–31297) are sinus specific and describe dilation of the sinus ostium without removal of tissue. They refer to unilateral procedures, and require modifier 50 if performed bilaterally. Tissue may be displaced but not resected. If sinus dilation is accompanied by tissue removal, existing endoscopic sinus surgery codes (31254–31288) should be applied instead.[5,6]
    c. *Key points*
        i. Surgical sinus endoscopy (eg, sinusotomy), diagnostic endoscopy, and fluoroscopy are all included in the balloon procedure codes. Sinus lavage is also considered to be a part of these codes and should not be billed separately just as lavage is included in the traditional ESS codes. The only circumstance in which lavage codes can be reported with balloon procedure codes is if endoscopic dilation is performed on one side, and only an irrigation is conducted on the opposite, contralateral

side.[7] In that scenario, right and left modifiers (and/or modifier 59) would then be applied.[7]

    ii. CPT 31295, 31296, and 31297 describe endoscopic dilation of the maxillary, frontal, and sphenoid sinus ostia, respectively. Only one code can be used per sinus per side. Consequently, 31295 should not be used in conjunction with 31256 (endoscopic maxillary antrostomy) or 31267 (endoscopic maxillary antrostomy with removal of tissue from the maxillary sinus) when performed on the same sinus. Likewise, 31296 should not be reported with 31276 (endoscopic frontal sinusotomy), and 31297 should not be reported with 31287 (endoscopic sphenoidotomy) or 31288 (endoscopic sphenoidotomy with removal of tissue from the sphenoid sinus) when performed on the same sinus.[6,7]

7. SCAN/Image Guidance Codes (61781, 61782)

    a. *Introduction*—The image guidance codes were developed to describe the use of SCAN during sinus surgical procedures.

    b. *Definitions*—The original CPT code used to report image guidance was 61795. However, in January 2011, 61795 was eliminated and replaced by 3 new codes which differentiated among SCAN for cranial intradural (61781), cranial extradural (61782), and spinal (61783) procedures, respectively.[5]

    c. *Key points*—All SCAN codes are "add-on" codes that must be listed separately in addition to the codes reported for the primary procedures (31255–31294). As add-on codes, 61781–61783 are exempt from modifier 51 and not subject to multiple procedure discount formulas. Additionally, both surgeons can fully bill for different SCAN codes without the use of modifier 62 in procedures involving a co-surgeon such as endoscopic skull base surgery performed with a neurosurgeon. However, for this to be billed by both surgeons, each must document their own pre-procedure work as well as intra-procedure use of stereotactic navigation. That said, typically the surgeon who performs the set-up (eg, planning, registration) bills for the service as many payers will not reimburse both surgeons. Use the intradural code (61781) when the pathology being addressed is intradural (eg, pituitary tumor), and use the extradural code (61782) when the pathology being addressed is extradural (eg, sinus disease).

    d. *Documentation*—When SCAN is performed during ESS without intradural navigation, 61782 is the appropriate code to use. Documentation of indications, pre-operative planning, image analysis, registration of data points, instrument calibration, accuracy/target error, and use of interactive navigation for anatomic localization at multiple junctures throughout the procedure must be included in the operative report. Medical necessity (eg, need for navigation around high-risk anatomical areas), pre-planning activities, and any added work involved with use of the navigation system must be documented in the operative report in addition to a description of the stereotactic procedure. An explanation of the clinical circumstances substantiating the need for navigational assistance should be included. Sample documentation of SCAN in an operative note is shown in the following box.

    e. *Indications*—Image-guidance technology should not be reported on a routine basis for all endoscopic sinus surgical cases. Examples of indications in which computer-assisted navigation may be deemed appropriate include the following: revision endoscopic sinus surgery; distorted sinus anatomy secondary to developmental, traumatic, or postoperative sequelae; extensive sinonasal polyposis of sufficient severity to support the need for assisted navigation and precise localization; frontal or sphenoid surgery with documented loss or altered anatomical landmarks, congenital deformities, or severe trauma; pathology in the frontal, posterior, ethmoid, or sphenoid sinuses; disease abutting the carotid artery, optic nerve, orbit, or skull

> **Sample documentation for stereotactic computer-assisted navigation in an operative note.**
>
> Due to extensive scarring and distorted sinonasal anatomy from multiple prior sinus surgeries, computer-assisted surgical navigation was utilized to facilitate intraoperative anatomic localization. Triplanar computed tomography images were reviewed to assist with pre-operative planning. The image guidance headset was placed and reference array secured. Surface registration was performed using a Z-touch wand to an accuracy of 1 mm. Verification was then performed using a straight pointer. Interactive imaging was used to confirm the location of multiple anatomic sites throughout the procedure including the medial orbital wall, the skull base, anterior face of the sphenoid, and frontal sinus ostium.

base; benign and malignant sinonasal neoplasms of sufficient size or in a high-risk location; cerebrospinal fluid rhinorrhea or presence of a skull base defect; transsphenoidal surgery; and skull base surgery.

Controversial Areas

Image Guidance in the Ambulatory Surgical Center (ASC) Setting

When 61795 was still the code for surgical navigation in ESS, CMS allowed physician reimbursement but denied separate facility coverage for SCAN performed at an ASC. This policy carried over to the 3 new codes that replaced 61795 in 2011. Currently, CMS considers 61781-61783 as "packaged" services/equipment already included in the payment for primary procedures when reported in the ASC setting. Consequently, no separate facility reimbursement, by Medicare, for SCAN codes are permitted for sinus surgical procedures performed at ASCs. Other payer policies may vary.

Balloon Procedure Codes

When balloon sinus dilatation was first introduced, controversy emerged regarding appropriate coding for such procedures and whether existing ESS codes or 31299 (unlisted code) should be reported. In 2011, separate balloon sinus dilation (31295-31297) codes were created for use both in the ASC and nonfacility (office) setting. Currently, such codes are reported only if dilation of the sinus ostium occurs with no accompanying tissue resected. If tissue removal is performed, then corresponding traditional ESS codes should be applied.

Advanced Endoscopic Sinus Surgery

Currently, there are no existing CPT codes that accurately describe certain complex endoscopic sinus surgical procedures being performed including the Draf III/modified endoscopic Lothrop, endoscopic medial maxillectomy/mega-antrostomy, sphenopalatine artery ligation, and endoscopic resection of skull base lesions. Although the use of unlisted codes and modifier 22 have been recommended in the interim, creation of new CPT codes that better represent these procedures may be a more viable long-term solution.

Sinus Implantation

In 2011, a steroid-eluting bioabsorbable implant was approved by the US Food and Drug Administration for placement in the ethmoid sinus. A request for a Category I CPT code for this device was subsequently submitted to the AAO-HNS in 2013. However, the AAO-HNS deemed the physician work involved in sinus implantation to already be included in the existing ESS CPT codes when performed in the operating room.[8] Consequently, no distinct Category I CPT code for endoscopic insertion of a drug-eluting sinus implant in the surgical setting has been established by the AMA at this time. There are two Category III codes that were approved, mainly for placement of the implant only (not during an ethmoidectomy) or with debridement. These are explained further in Chapter 12, "Office Rhinology," as this will likely be more applicable in this setting.

References

1. Waguespack R, Koopmann C. CPT for ENT: turbinectomy guidance. http://www.entnet.org/content/cpt-ent-turbinectomy-guidance. Accessed January 20, 2016.
2. Rosenfeld RM, Piccirillo JF, Chandrasekhar S, et al. Clinical practice guideline (Update): Adult sinusitis. *Otolaryngology-Head and Neck Surgery.* 2015;152(2S):S1–S39.
3. CPT for ENT: reporting radiofrequency ablation and out-fracturing of inferior turbinates. http://www.entnet.org//content/cpt-ent-reporting-radiofrequency-ablation-and-out-fracturing-inferior-turbinates. Accessed January 20, 2016.
4. CPT for ENT: utilizing unlisted CPT codes. http://www.entnet.org/content/cpt-ent-utilizing-unlisted-cpt-codes. Accessed January 20, 2016.
5. Batra PS. Coding update for balloon dilatation and image-guided surgery. *American Rhinologic Society Nose News.* 2010;3:4.
6. Setzen M, Sillers M, Stringer S, et al. CPT for ENT: balloon sinus dilation. https://www.entnet.org/content/cpt-ent-balloon-sinus-dilation. Accessed January 20, 2016.
7. CPT for ENT: coding 31000 with balloon dilation procedures. http://www.entnet.org//content/cpt-ent-coding-31000-balloon-dilation-procedures. Accessed January 20, 2016.
8. Denneny J. 3P Update: Academy efforts regarding new technology. *American Academy of Otolaryngology-Head and Neck Surgery Bulletin.* 2013;32:36–37.

CHAPTER 25

Operative Laryngology

Babak Sadoughi and Lucian Sulica

Introduction

This chapter will focus on laryngology procedures performed in the operating room. All procedures must be properly described in the operative note, with specific mention of indications, preoperative and intraoperative findings, techniques, and equipment used, as these factors often have coding implications.

Key Points

- Direct laryngoscopy codes involve the use of a rigid laryngoscope and include suspension, if used. Examination of the tongue base and hypopharynx is included and may not be billed separately.
- Magnified visualization under suspension using an operative microscope or telescope (ie, "suspension microlaryngoscopy") must be documented in order to justify use of relevant *Current Procedural Terminology* (CPT) codes.
- Diagnostic laryngoscopy cannot be billed separately if an operative component (biopsy, ablation, lesion removal, injection, dilation, etc) is being performed via laryngoscopy.
- Unlisted codes should only be used in the absence of an adequate code for the

procedure performed, and are often subject to supplemental documentation requirements.

Key Procedure Codes

31300 Laryngotomy (thyrotomy, laryngofissure); with removal of tumor or laryngocele, cordectomy
wRVU 15.91; Global 90

    31320 diagnostic
wRVU 5.73; Global 90

31367 Laryngectomy; subtotal supraglottic, without radical neck dissection
wRVU 30.57; Global 90

    31368 subtotal supraglottic, with neck dissection
wRVU 34.19; Global 90

31370 Partial laryngectomy (hemilaryngectomy); horizontal
wRVU 27.57; Global 90

    31375 laterovertical
wRVU 26.07; Global 90

    31380 anterovertical
wRVU 25.57; Global 90

    31382 antero-latero-vertical
wRVU 28.57; Global 90

31400 Arytenoidectomy or arytenoidopexy, external approach
wRVU 11.60; Global 90

31420 Epiglottidectomy
wRVU 11.43; Global 90

31525 Laryngoscopy, direct, with or without tracheoscopy; diagnostic, except newborn
wRVU 2.63; Global 0

> **31526** diagnostic with operating microscope or telescope
> *wRVU 2.57; Global 0*

> **31527** with insertion of obturator
> *wRVU 3.27; Global 0*

> **31528** with dilation, initial
> *wRVU 2.37; Global 0*

> **31529** with dilation, subsequent
> *wRVU 2.68; Global 0*

31530 Laryngoscopy, direct, operative, with foreign body removal;
wRVU 3.38; Global 0

> **31531** with operating microscope or telescope
> *wRVU 3.58; Global 0*

31535 Laryngoscopy, direct, operative, with biopsy.
wRVU 3.16; Global 0

> **31536** with operating microscope or telescope
> *wRVU 3.55; Global 0*

31540 Laryngoscopy, direct, operative, with excision of tumor and/or stripping of vocal cords or epiglottis;
wRVU 4.12; Global 0

> **31541** with operating microscope or telescope
> *wRVU 4.52; Global 0*

31545 Laryngoscopy, direct, operative, with operating microscope or telescope, with submucosal removal of non-neoplastic lesion(s) of vocal cord; reconstruction with local tissue flap(s)
wRVU 6.30; Global 0

> **31546** reconstruction with graft(s) (includes obtaining autograft)
> *wRVU 9.73; Global 0*

31560 Laryngoscopy, direct, operative, with arytenoidectomy;
wRVU 5.45; Global 0

> **31561** with operating microscope or telescope
> *wRVU 5.99; Global 0*

31570 Laryngoscopy, direct, with injection into vocal cord(s), therapeutic;
wRVU 3.86; Global 0

> **31571** with operating microscope or telescope
> *wRVU 4.26; Global 0*

31580 Laryngoplasty; for laryngeal web, 2-stage, with keel insertion and removal
wRVU 14.66; Global 90

> **31582** for laryngeal stenosis, with graft or core mold, including tracheotomy
> *wRVU 23.22; Global 90*

> **31584** with open reduction of fracture
> *wRVU 20.47; Global 90*

31587 Laryngoplasty, cricoid split
wRVU 15.27; Global 90

31588 Laryngoplasty, not otherwise specified (eg, for burns, reconstruction after partial laryngectomy)
wRVU 14.99; Global 90

31590 Laryngeal reinnervation by neuromuscular pedicle
wRVU 7.85; Global 90

31595 Section recurrent laryngeal nerve, therapeutic (separate procedure), unilateral
wRVU 8.84; Global 90

31599 Unlisted procedure, larynx
wRVU 0.00; Global YYY

31600 Tracheostomy, planned (separate procedure);
wRVU 7.17; Global 0

31613 Tracheostoma revision; simple, without flap rotation
wRVU 4.71; Global 90

31614 complex, with flap rotation
wRVU 8.63; Global 90

31615 Tracheobronchoscopy through established tracheostomy incision
wRVU 2.09; Global 0

31622 Bronchoscopy, rigid or flexible, including fluoroscopic guidance, when performed; diagnostic, with cell washing, when performed (separate procedure)
wRVU 2.78; Global 0

> **31625** with bronchial or endobronchial biopsy(s), single or multiple sites
> *wRVU 3.36; Global 0*

> **31630** with tracheal/bronchial dilation or closed reduction of fracture
> *wRVU 3.81; Global 0*

> **31631** with placement of tracheal stent(s) (includes tracheal/bronchial dilation as required)
> *wRVU 4.36; Global 0*

> **31635** with removal of foreign body
> *wRVU 3.67; Global 0*

> **31640** with excision of tumor
> *wRVU 4.93; Global 0*

> **31641** with destruction of tumor or relief of stenosis by any method other than excision (eg, laser therapy, cryotherapy)
> *wRVU 5.02; Global 0*

31750 Tracheoplasty; cervical
wRVU 15.39; Global 90

31780 Excision tracheal stenosis and anastomosis; cervical
wRVU 19.84; Global 90

31820 Surgical closure trachostomy or fistula, without plastic repair
wRVU 4.64; Global 90

> **31825** with plastic repair
> *wRVU 7.07; Global 90*

31830 Revision of tracheostomy scar
wRVU 4.62; Global 90

43030 Cricopharyngeal myotomy
wRVU 7.99; Global 90

43130 Diverticulectomy of hypopharynx or esophagus, with or without myotomy; cervical approach
wRVU 12.53; Global 90

43180 Esophagoscopy, rigid, transoral with diverticulectomy of hypopharynx or cervical esophagus (eg, Zenker's diverticulum), with cricopharyngeal myotomy, includes use of telescope or operating microscope and repair, when performed
wRVU 9.03; Global 90

43200 Esophagoscopy, flexible, transoral; diagnostic, including collection of specimen(s) by brushing or washing, when performed (separate procedure)
wRVU 1.52; Global 0

> **43201** with directed submucosal injection(s), any substance
> *wRVU 1.82; Global 0*

> **43202** with biopsy, single or multiple
> *wRVU 1.82; Global 0*

> **43215** with removal of foreign body(s)
> *wRVU 2.54; Global 0*

43450 Dilation of esophagus, by unguided sound or bougie, single or multiple passes
wRVU 1.38; Global 0

> **43499** Unlisted procedure, esophagus
> *wRVU 0.00; Global YYY*

Healthcare Common Procedure Coding System Codes

The Healthcare Common Procedure Coding System (HCPCS) codes do not have relative value units (RVUs) because they are codes for supplies, not physician work.

C1878 Material for vocal cord medialization, synthetic (implantable)

J0585 Injection, onabotulinumtoxinA, 1 unit Botulinum toxin type A (Botox, Dysport, Xeomin) per unit

J0587 Injection, rimabotulinumtoxinB, 100 units Botulinum toxin type B (Myobloc), per 100 units

J3590 Unclassified biologics

Q2026 Radiesse, injectable, 0.1 cc

Q4112 Cymetra, injectable, 1 cc

Key Modifiers

22 Increased Procedural Services
Examples may include bilateral procedures performed where the 50 modifier is not allowed, such as bilateral medialization thyroplasty (31588) for presbylarynx or extensive transoral debridement of diffuse bilateral papilloma (31541).

50 Bilateral Procedure
The vast majority of laryngology procedure terminology does not allow for specification of laterality in coding, with the notable exception of 31545 and 31546, which are the only codes allowing the use of the 50 modifier.

51 Multiple Procedures
Use when more than one procedure is performed at the same operative session. For instance, Suspension microlaryngoscopy with tumor removal (31541) and suspension microlaryngoscopy with steroid injection (31571-51).

52 Reduced Services
A common example for use of the 52 modifier is when performing bronchoscopy (31622) without examination of the airway beyond the trachea. See further details below (Airway endoscopy).

58 Staged or Related Procedure or Service by the Same Physician or Other Qualified Health Care Professional During the Postoperative Period
In staged open laryngotracheal reconstructions, apply modifier 58 to second-stage procedure (sec-

ond look, stent or keel removal) in order to override global period edits if the second procedure is performed within 90 days.

59 Distinct Procedural Service
The phonomicrosurgical excision of a submucosal vocal fold cyst combined with the simple excision of a contralateral vocal fold polyp may be reported using 31545 and 31541-59, respectively, because different procedures were performed on the same structure and the 2 codes are "bundled" according to Medicare's correct coding initiative (CCI) edits; therefore, modifier 59 is more appropriate than modifier 51 on 31541 (the lower valued code).

78 Unplanned Return to the Operating/Procedure Room by the Same Physician or Other Qualified Health Care Professional Following Initial Procedure for a Related Procedure During the Postoperative Period
This modifier typically applies to the management of a related complication in the operating room during the global period of the initial procedure, for instance, drainage of hematoma or removal of extruded implant after medialization laryngoplasty.

79 Unrelated Procedure or Service by the Same Physician or Other Qualified Health Care Professional During the Postoperative Period
Examples could include intercurrent general otolaryngology treatments (cerumen removal, diagnostic nasal endoscopy) performed during the global period of a medialization thyroplasty.

Key ICD-9-CM/ICD-10-CM

Most *International Classification of Diseases, Ninth Revision, Clinical Modification* (ICD-9-CM) codes in laryngology are converted one-to-one, but the new *International Classification of Diseases, Tenth Revision, Clinical Modification* (ICD-10-CM) codes may include multiple descriptions for an old ICD-9-CM code. For instance, aphagia and unspecified dysphagia will have separate ICD-10-CM codes (R13.0 and R13.10, respectively), while both used to fall under the same ICD-9-CM code for unspecified dysphagia (787.20).

Neoplasms

161.0/C32.0   Malignant neoplasm; of glottis

161.1/C32.1   of supraglottis
excludes anterior surface of epiglottis (C10.1); aryepiglottic fold: NOS (C13.1), hypopharyngeal aspect (C13.1), marginal zone (C13.1)

161.2/C32.2   of subglottis

161.3/C32.3   of laryngeal cartilages

161.8/C32.8   of overlapping sites of larynx

161.9/C32.9   of larynx, unspecified

212.1/D14.1   Benign neoplasm of larynx
excludes epiglottis, anterior aspect (D10.5); polyp of vocal cord and larynx (J38.1)

231.0/D02.0   Carcinoma in situ of larynx
excludes aryepiglottic fold: NOS (D00.0), hypopharyngeal aspect (D00.0), marginal zone (D00.0)

235.6/D38.0   Neoplasm of uncertain behavior of larynx

Laryngeal/Tracheal Disorders

478.30/J38.00   Paralysis of vocal cords and larynx; unspecified

478.31/J38.01   unilateral

478.32/J38.01   unilateral

478.33/J38.02   bilateral

478.34/J38.02   bilateral

478.4/J38.1   Polyp of vocal cord and larynx
excludes adenomatous polyps (D14.1)

478.5/J38.3   Other diseases of vocal cords
includes nodules of vocal cords: chorditis (fibrinous) (nodosa)(tuberosa), singer nodes, teacher nodes

478.6/J38.4   Edema of larynx
excludes laryngitis: acute obstructive (croup) (J05.0), edematous (J04.0)

478.70/J38.7   Other disease of larynx
includes abscess, cellulitis, disease NOS, necrosis, pachyderma, perichondritis, ulcer

478.71/J38.7   Other diseases of larynx
includes cellulitis and perichondritis of larynx

478.74/J38.6   Stenosis of larynx
excludes postprocedural subglottic stenosis (J95.5)

478.75/J38.5   Laryngeal spasm

478.79/J38.7   Other diseases of larynx

519.02/J95.03   Malfunction of tracheostomy stoma

519.19/J39.8   Other specified diseases of upper respiratory tract

519.19/J98.09   Other diseases of bronchus, not elsewhere classified

748.2/Q31.0   Web of larynx

748.3/Q31.1   Congenital subglottic stenosis

748.3/Q31.3   Laryngocele

748.3/Q31.8   Other congenital malformations of larynx

748.3/Q32.1   Other congenital malformations of trachea

748.3/Q32.4   Other congenital malformations of bronchus

Vocal Disorders

784.41/R49.1   Aphonia

784.42/R49.0   Dysphonia

784.49/R49.8   Other voice and resonance disorders

Esophagus/Swallowing Disorders

530.5/K22.4   Dyskinesia of esophagus

530.6/K22.5   Diverticulum of esophagus, acquired

787.20/R13.0   Aphagia

787.20/R13.10   Dysphagia, unspecified

787.21/R13.11   Dysphagia, oral phase

787.22/R13.12   Dysphagia, oropharyngeal phase

787.23/R13.13   Dysphagia, pharyngeal phase

787.24/R13.14   Dysphagia, pharyngoesophageal phase

787.29/R13.19   Other dysphagia

Trauma

807.5/S12.8XXA   Fracture of other parts of neck, initial encounter

807.6/S12.8XXA   Fracture of other parts of neck, initial encounter

Definition of Codes

Open (Transcervical) Laryngeal Surgery

1. Laryngotomy/laryngofissure (31300, 31320)
   a. *Definitions*—These codes include an open approach to the thyroid cartilage, division of cartilage, and performance of planned endolaryngeal work as described, followed by cartilage reconstruction and closure using any method (sutures, wires, internal fixation plates).
   b. *Key points*—Do not use laryngeal fracture repair codes in the musculoskeletal system chapter of CPT for the reconstruction portion; do not use concurrent laryngoscopy codes, unless the need for endoscopic examination of an area not visible through the laryngotomy can be justified.

2. Partial laryngectomy (31367, 31368, 31370, 31375, 31380, 31382, 31420)
   a. *Definitions*—These codes pertain exclusively to open conservation surgery of the larynx, and are mutually exclusive of other codes describing removal of vocal fold lesions (eg, 31540/31541 or 31545/31546).

Horizontal partial laryngectomy procedures are listed in 31367-31370 (31370 is best suited for supracricoid partial laryngectomy), and 31375-31382 describes vertical partial laryngectomy procedures.
   b. *Key points*—The usual local reconstruction methods employed, such as cricohyoidopexy, cricohyoidoepiglottopexy, or thyrohyoidopexy are included in each code and should not be billed separately. Similarly, if a transient tracheotomy is performed, it will not be separately billable.

3. Thyroplasty/Laryngoplasty (31400, 31580, 31582, 31584, 31587, 31588, 31750)
   a. *Definitions*—Most laryngeal framework procedures designed to impact voice function (eg, Isshiki type I-IV thyroplasties) will be billed under code 31588. In case of bilateral thyroplasty, use of modifier 50 is not acceptable as the procedure described is performed on an unpaired structure (the larynx); consider use of modifier -22 (increased services). Provide adequate operative report documentation to justify the increased services. See "Controversial Areas" section for additional discussion.
   b. *Key points*—If concurrent medialization thyroplasty (Isshiki type I) and arytenoid adduction/arytenopexy are performed, add a separate 31400 code to 31588. For suture lateralization of arytenoid via external approach (for relief of airway obstruction caused by bilateral vocal fold paralysis), use 31400 alone. Although intraoperative flexible nasolaryngoscopy is often used to assess vocal fold repositioning, the use of 31575 is not appropriate in this instance, since a diagnostic laryngoscopy is not separately reported with the therapeutic laryngoplasty. In staged open laryngotracheal reconstructions, apply modifier 58 to second-stage procedure (second look, stent or keel removal) in order to override global period edits if the second procedure is performed within 90 days. Document anticipated need for follow-up procedure in the initial operative report, and keep in mind that the global period will be reset

to 90 days from the date of the subsequent procedure.

Endoscopic Procedures

1. Airway endoscopy (31525–31531, 31540, 31560, 31561, 31599, 31622, 31630, 31641)
   a. *Definitions*—Tracheoscopy is included in some laryngoscopy code descriptions (31525–31529), and in those instances, bronchoscopy should not be reported separately unless significant bronchial examination (distal to the carina) is performed. When tracheoscopy is not included in the code (31530–31571) and visualization of the tracheal lumen is necessary, for instance to rule out tracheal stenosis, tumor, or foreign body, consider the additional use of a bronchoscopy code (31622) with modifier 52 (reduced services). Clearly describe the indication and technique of tracheoscopy/bronchoscopy in the operative report.
   b. *Key points*—Procedures performed to relieve subglottic stenosis by radial laser incisions followed by balloon dilation are best addressed by use of 31528/31529, although the description does not include laser incisions. In that instance, consider use of modifier 22 or the unlisted larynx procedure code (31599). Always ensure proper documentation of procedure and consider predetermination/ preauthorization of procedure by insurance carrier. If stenosis involves the trachea (ie below the inferior border of the cricoid cartilage), then 31641 is the appropriate code to use.

   Please note that there is no CPT code describing lysis of adhesions, synechiae, or scar tissue from the larynx. Therefore, relief of glottic stenosis, posterior cordotomy, or radial incisions of stenosis using CO_2 laser should be submitted through an unlisted code, 31599, with the usual requirements to ensure recognition at the payer level. If a laser medial arytenoidectomy is performed in conjunction with posterior cordotomy, then 31560/31561 should be used. When scar tissue is actually excised rather than

divided or ablated, use of 31540/31541 may be appropriate.

2. Operative laryngoscopy/phonomicrosurgery (31535, 31536, 31540, 31541, 31545, 31546, 31599)
   a. *Definitions*—Lesions addressed by ablation with laser or radiofrequency (eg, for recurrent respiratory papillomatosis), rather than actual excision resulting in a surgical tissue specimen, should be reported using unlisted procedure code 31599 with usual documentation requirements. Excision codes such as 31540/31541 or 31545/31546 may be reported only if a lesion is in fact excised, regardless of the method use to perform the excision (cold knife, laser, or microdebrider). Biopsies performed under laryngoscopy are coded uniformly with 31535/31536, whether one or multiple specimens are removed, and whether the lesions are unilateral or bilateral. This typically involves sampling a lesion using a cupped forceps. If the biopsy is excisional in nature (complete removal of leukoplakia, for instance), then 31540/31541 may be reported instead.
   b. *Key points*—Operative laryngoscopy codes do not allow the use of modifier 50 for bilateral lesions, with the exception of 31545/31546, typically pertaining to so-called "microflap" procedures. For the latter, be sure to report the technique description in detail, including subepithelial infusion, mucosal flap elevation and preservation, and/or use of mucosal flap or graft (eg, temporalis fascia or buccal mucosal graft) for defect reconstruction. Codes 31545 and 31546 are only to be used when a flap is created for excision of a submucosal lesion of the vocal fold proper, or a flap or graft is used for reconstruction following excision or for preexisting lesion. Modifier 50 may be reported with 31545 or 31546 when performed bilaterally. When a lesion is mucosal in nature, and removed without preservation of an overlying mucosal flap or concurrent reconstruction, the use of codes 31540/31541 is more appropriate than 31545/31546.

Subepithelial infusion/hydrodissection with local anesthetic or saline solution is considered a routine preparatory step of the procedure and cannot be billed separately with 31570/31571. For bilateral benign lesions of different nature, addressed via different techniques, consider use of modifier 59. For instance, the phonomicrosurgical excision of a submucosal vocal fold cyst combined with the simple excision of a contralateral vocal fold polyp may be reported using 31545 and 31541-59, respectively. The use of different techniques in the same setting should be clearly documented, and warranted by the nature of the lesions rather than for billing convenience.

3. Vocal fold injections/injection laryngoplasty (31570, 31571)
   a. *Definitions*—Describe indication for injection (eg, volume augmentation for glottic insufficiency or vocal fold paralysis; steroid injection to prevent or treat reactive inflammatory granuloma formation; botulinum toxin injection for spasmodic dysphonia). These codes are for procedures performed using a direct approach with a rigid scope which requires general anesthesia.
   b. *Key points*—Modifier 50 is not applicable even if bilateral injection is performed. CPT 31570/31571 may be used for steroid injection in conjunction with a lesion removal code (eg, 31540/31541 or 31545) if independently justified (eg, medical necessity is documented) and documented. As indicated earlier, preliminary hydrodissection by subepithelial injection of vasoconstrictors or isotonic saline solution is not separately billable.

Esophagus Procedures/(43030, 43130, 43180, 43200)

1. Cricopharyngeal Myotomy/Zenker Diverticulum Management

   a. *Definitions*—External cricopharyngeal myotomy is included in 43130. If performed alone, for instance for achalasia without the presence of a diverticulum, use 43030. Open management of a diverticulum without resection (diverticulopexy) may be best reported by the adjunction of –modifier 52 (reduced services) to 43130.
   b. *Key points*—Endoscopic management of Zenker diverticulum, whether by laser or stapler myotomy should be reported with the new dedicated 43180 code, released on January 1, 2015. It is unclear how to best report an isolated endoscopic myotomy without the presence of a diverticulum; possible options include appending modifier 52 to 43180, or the use of an unlisted code, 43499. Proper documentation is required in both situations to maximize chances of successful claim processing.

   Trials of cricopharyngeal chemodenervation via rigid esophagoscopy in order, for example, to evaluate a patient's candidacy for definitive myotomy, are appropriately coded using 43201. See below remarks relating to coding for botulinum toxin products.

Controversial Areas

Transoral Laser Microsurgery/ Robotic Surgery

The use of transoral techniques for partial laryngectomy, whether using line-of-sight CO_2 laser or robotic assistance, has not yet been recognized by the current CPT iteration. Thus, most endoscopic procedures involving resections beyond a simple lesion excision, such as transoral supraglottic laryngectomy, should be reported using 31599. Alternatively, some centers have reported successful submission of corresponding codes relating to external partial laryngectomy; however, this practice remains discretionary and does not follow conventional CPT coding guidelines.

Injection Material

C1878 - Material for vocal cord medialization, synthetic implantable

J0585 Botulinum toxin type A (Botox, Dysport, Xeomin), per unit

J0587 Botulinum toxin type B (Myobloc), per 100 units

J3590 Unclassified biologics

Q2026 Radiesse, per 0.1 ml

Q4112 Cymetra, per 1 ml

The cost of the material used for vocal fold augmentation or chemodenervation will typically be covered by the facility when the procedure is performed in the operating room. However, if your practice is providing the injectate, then use the appropriate J code. Insurance carriers have variable and often restrictive policies for reimbursement of synthetic augmentation material, and predetermination/preauthorization is recommended. It is a common mistake to submit C1878 as part of a professional (physician) services claim, when this Healthcare Common Procedure Coding System (HCPCS) Level II code is only designed for facility billing purposes. Billing C1878 by physicians will invariably result in denial of payment because it is not appropriate for the provider to use this code. Use J3590 instead for any commercially available "filler" except Cymetra (micronized cadaveric dermis collagen), which now has a dedicated code (Q4112). Radiesse (calcium hydroxylapatite) is also being increasingly recognized for injection laryngoplasty under its generic Q2026 code by commercial payers—not CMS. For accurate claim submission after chemodenervation with botulinum toxin, remember to use modifier JW for any amount of discarded product.

Medialization Thyroplasty

At this writing, the 3158x series of codes are undergoing re-evaluation by the Relative Value Scale Update Committee (commonly known as the RUC). As part of this process, a specific code for medialization thyroplasty, distinct from 31588, is anticipated. It may go into effect during the course of 2016. Until then, the vast majority of clinicians performing the procedure recommend the use of 31588. If this code is not felt to completely reflect the procedure being performed, the unlisted 31599 code can be used, with the usual anticipation of more stringent documentation requirements and inconsistent reimbursement practices.

CHAPTER 26

Operative Otology

Christopher R. Thompson and Charles A. Syms III

Introduction

This chapter describes coding for operative otologic procedures.

Key Points

- Graft harvesting can only be billed for if a separate incision is required to harvest the graft (eg, tragal cartilage, temporalis fascia when a transcanal procedure is performed).
- Eustachian tube balloon dilation currently should be billed with an unlisted code (69799), as the previous eustachian tube codes were removed in 2015; the description describing the procedure should give an equivalent such as balloon dilatation of the frontal sinus ostia (31296).

Key Procedure Codes

External Ear

69005   Drainage external ear, abscess or hematoma; complicated
wRVU 2.16; Global 10

69020   Drainage external auditory canal, abscess
wRVU 1.53; Global 10

69100   Biopsy external ear
wRVU 0.81; Global 0

69105   Biopsy external auditory canal
wRVU 0.85; Global 0

69110   Excision external ear; partial simple repair
wRVU 3.53; Global 90

69120   complete amputation
wRVU 4.14; Global 90

69140   Excision exostosis(es), external auditory canal
wRVU 8.14; Global 90

69145   Excision soft tissue lesion, external auditory canal
wRVU 2.70; Global 90

69150   Radical excision external auditory canal lesion; without neck dissection
wRVU 13.61; Global 90

69155   with neck dissection
wRVU 23.35; Global 90

69205   Removal foreign body from external auditory canal; with general anesthesia
wRVU 1.21; Global 10

69222   Debridement, mastoidectomy cavity, complex (eg, with anesthesia or more than routine   cleaning)
wRVU 1.45; Global 10

69300   Otoplasty, protruding ear, with or without size reduction
wRVU 6.69; Global YYY

265

69310   Reconstruction of external auditory canal (meatoplasty) (eg, for stenosis due to injury, infection) (separate procedure)
wRVU 10.97; Global 90

69320   Reconstruction external auditory canal for congenital atresia, single stage
wRVU 17.18; Global 90

69399   Unlisted procedure, external ear
wRVU 0.00; Global YYY

69540   Excision aural polyp
wRVU 1.25; Global 10

Middle Ear

Basic

69421   Myringotomy including aspiration and/ or Eustachian tube inflation requiring general anesthesia
wRVU 1.78; Global 10

69424   Ventilating tube removal requiring general anesthesia
wRVU 0.85; Global 0

69436   Tympanostomy (requiring insertion of ventilating tube), general anesthesia
wRVU 2.01; Global 10

69440   Middle ear exploration through postauricular or ear canal incision
wRVU 7.71; Global 90

69450   Tympanolysis, transcanal
wRVU 5.69; Global 90

Mastoidectomy/Tympanoplasty

69501   Transmastoid antrotomy (simple mastoidectomy)
wRVU 9.21; Global 90

69502   Mastoidectomy; complete
wRVU 12.56; Global 90

69505   modified radical
wRVU 13.17; Global 90

69511   radical
wRVU 13.70; Global 90

69530   Petrous apicectomy including radical mastoidectomy
wRVU 20.38; Global 90

69601   Revision mastoidectomy; resulting in complete mastoidectomy
wRVU 13.45; Global 90

69602   resulting in modified radical mastoidectomy
wRVU 13.76; Global 90

69603   resulting in radical mastoidectomy
wRVU 14.20; Global 90

69604   resulting in tympanoplasty
wRVU 14.20; Global 90

69605   with apicectomy
wRVU 18.69; Global 90

69610   Tympanic membrane repair, with or without site preparation of perforation for closure, with or without patch
wRVU 4.47; Global 10

69620   Myringoplasty (surgery confined to drumhead and donor area)
wRVU 6.03; Global 90

69631   Tympanoplasty without mastoidectomy (including canalplasty, atticotomy, and/ or middle ear surgery), initial or revision; without ossicular chain reconstruction
wRVU 10.05; Global 90

69632   with ossicular chain reconstruction (eg, postfenestration)
wRVU 12.96; Global 90

69633   with ossicular chain reconstruction and synthetic prosthesis (eg, partial ossicular replacement prosthesis [PORP], total ossicular replacement prosthesis [TORP])
wRVU 12.31; Global 90

69635   Tympanoplasty with antrotomy or mastoidotomy (including canalplasty, atticotomy, middle ear surgery, and/ or tympanic membrane repair); without ossicular chain reconstruction
wRVU 13.51; Global 90

69636 with ossicular chain reconstruction
wRVU 15.43; Global 90

69637 with ossicular chain reconstruction and synthetic prosthesis (eg, partial ossicular replacement prosthesis [PORP], total ossicular replacement prosthesis [TORP])
wRVU 15.32; Global 90

69641 Tympanoplasty with mastoidectomy (including canalplasty, middle ear surgery, tympanic membrane repair); without ossicular chain reconstruction
wRVU 12.89; Global 90

69642 with ossicular chain reconstruction
wRVU 17.06; Global 90

69643 with intact or reconstructed canal wall, without ossicular chain reconstruction
wRVU 15.59; Global 90

69644 with intact or reconstructed canal wall, with ossicular chain reconstruction
wRVU 17.23; Global 90

69645 radical or complete, without ossicular chain reconstruction
wRVU 16.71; Global 90

69646 radical or complete, with ossicular chain reconstruction
wRVU 18.37; Global 90

Stapes

69650 Stapes mobilization
wRVU 9.80; Global 90

69660 Stapedectomy or stapedotomy with reestablishment of ossicular continuity, with or without use of foreign material;
wRVU 12.03; Global 90

69661 with footplate drill out
wRVU 15.92; Global 90

69662 Revision of stapedectomy or stapedotomy
wRVU 15.60; Global 90

Facial Nerve

64864 Suture of facial nerve; extracranial
wRVU 13.41; Global 90

64865 infratemporal, with or without grafting
wRVU 16.09; Global 90

69720 Decompression facial nerve, intratemporal; lateral to geniculate ganglion
wRVU 14.71; Global 90

69725 including medial to geniculate ganglion
wRVU 27.64; Global 90

69740 Suture facial nerve, intratemporal, with or without graft or decompression; lateral to geniculate ganglion
wRVU 16.27; Global 90

69745 including medial to geniculate ganglion
wRVU 17.02; Global 90

61458 Craniectomy, suboccipital; for exploration or decompression of cranial nerves
wRVU 28.84; Global 90

61460 for section of 1 or more cranial nerves
wRVU 30.24; Global 90

Additional Procedures

69535 Resection temporal bone, external approach
wRVU 37.42; Global 90

69550 Excision aural glomus tumor; transcanal
wRVU 11.15; Global 90

69552 transmastoid
wRVU 19.81; Global 90

69554 extended (extratemporal)
wRVU 35.97; Global 90

69666 Repair oval window fistula
wRVU 9.89; Global 90

69667 Repair round window fistula
wRVU 9.90; Global 90

69670 Mastoid obliteration (separate procedure)
wRVU 11.73; Global 90

69676 Tympanic neurectomy
wRVU 9.69; Global 90

69700 Closure postauricular fistula, mastoid (separate procedure)
wRVU 8.37; Global 90

69799 Unlisted procedure, middle ear
wRVU 0.00; Global YYY

Inner Ear

69801 Labyrinthotomy, with perfusion of vestibuloactive drug(s); transcanal
wRVU 2.06; Global 0

69805 Endolymphatic sac operation; without shunt
wRVU 14.71; Global 90

> **69806** with shunt
> *wRVU 12.63; Global 90*

69820 Fenestration semicircular canal
wRVU 10.52; Global 90

69840 Revision fenestration operation
wRVU 10.44; Global 90

69905 Labyrinthectomy; transcanal
wRVU 11.26; Global 90

> **69910** with mastoidectomy
> *wRVU 13.91; Global 90*

69915 Vestibular nerve section, translabyrinthine approach
wRVU 22.77; Global 90

69949 Unlisted procedure inner ear
wRVU 0.00; Global YYY

+69990 Microsurgical techniques, requiring use of operating microscope (List separately in addition to code for primary procedure)
wRVU 3.46; Global ZZZ

Implants

69710 Implantation or replacement of electromagnetic bone conduction hearing device in temporal bone
wRVU 0.00; Global XXX

69711 Removal or repair of electromagnetic bone conduction hearing device in temporal bone
wRVU 10.62; Global 90

69714 Implantation, osseointegrated implant, temporal bone, with percutaneous attachment to external speech processor/cochlear stimulator; without mastoidectomy
wRVU 14.45; Global 90

> **69715** with mastoidectomy
> *wRVU 18.96; Global 90*

69717 Replacement (including removal of existing device), osseointegrated implant, temporal bone, with percutaneous attachment to external speech processor/cochlear stimulator; without mastoidectomy
wRVU 15.43; Global 90

> **69718** with mastoidectomy
> *wRVU 19.21; Global 90*

69930 Cochlear device implantation, with or without mastoidectomy
wRVU 17.73; Global 90

Acoustic Neuroma and Skull Base

Please see Chapter 30, "Skull Base Surgery," for a full discussion of the correct use of the approach/definitive procedure codes and co-surgeon coding and billing.

61520 Craniectomy for excision of brain tumor, infratentorial or posterior fossa; cerebellopontine angle tumor
wRVU 57.09; Global 90

61526 Craniectomy, bone flap craniotomy, transtemporal (mastoid) for excision of cerebellopontine angle tumor
wRVU 54.08; Global 90

62100 Craniotomy for repair of dural/
cerebrospinal fluid leak, including
surgery for rhinorrhea/otorrhea
wRVU 23.53; Global 90

64999 Unlisted procedure, nervous system
wRVU 0.00; Global YYY

Grafts

15120 Split-thickness autograft, face, scalp,
eyelids, mouth, neck, ears, orbits,
genitalia, hands, feet, and/or multiple
digits; first 100 sq cm or less, or 1% of
body area of infants and children (except
15050)
wRVU 10.15; Global 90

20926 Tissue grafts, other (eg, paratenon, fat,
dermis)
wRVU 5.79; Global 90

21235 Graft; ear cartilage, autogenous, to nose
or ear (includes obtaining graft)
wRVU 7.50; Global 90

Key Modifiers

50 Bilateral Procedure
This indicates a bilateral procedure. An example
of when to use this would be when performing placement of bilateral tympanostomy tubes
(69436-50 or 69436 with 69436-50 depending on
payer preference).

59 Distinct Procedural Service
This indicates a distinct procedure that is not
usually reported separately. This is used when a
normally bundled procedure requires a separate
incision. For example, this would be used if a pressure equalization (PE) tube is placed on the left ear
and a tympomastoidectomy is done on the right
ear under the same general anesthesia. The 69436
code would then be appended with modifier 59. If
the PE tube is done on the same ear as the tympomastoidectomy, this is bundled and should not be
separately reported. Modifiers RT (right) and LT

(left) may also be used for additional description
of laterality.

Key ICD-9-CM/ICD-10-CM Codes

*International Classification of Diseases, Ninth Revision,
Clinical Modification* (ICD-9-CM) to *International
Classification of Diseases, Tenth Revision, Clinical
Modification* (ICD-10-CM) conversion is simple
for operative otology coding. There is a 1:1 trans-
lation for the most part. Conductive hearing loss
has become simpler as it has lost some specificity.
The major diagnosis where multiple new nuances
have been added is in otitis media. Many of these
additional diagnoses apply more appropriately to
the outpatient setting. They are not involved in
the current discussion and can be found in Chapter 16, "Office Otology." The last digit on most of
the codes defines location (left, right, bilateral,
or unspecified, and this would replace the "-").
Another major change to the ear diagnosis codes is
the presence of "acute recurrent" conditions such
as otitis media as well as combination codes for
acute recurrent suppurative/nonsuppurative otitis media with spontaneous rupture of ear drum.

Additionally, there are new ICD-10-CM
guidelines for all middle ear diagnosis codes
which instruct the user to use an additional code
to identify

- exposure to environmental tobacco
  smoke (Z77.22)
- exposure to tobacco smoke in the
  perinatal period (P96.81)
- history of tobacco use (Z87.891)
- occupational exposure to environmental
  tobacco smoke (Z57.31)
- tobacco dependence (F17.-)
- tobacco use (Z72.0)

Linking ICD-10-CM diagnoses to the specific *Current Procedural Terminology* (CPT) codes outlined
in this chapter is currently undergoing testing in
our office at the time this chapter was written, but
our plan is to use the equivalent ICD-10-CM diagnoses, mapped from ICD-9-CM diagnoses that
we know have worked, unless we see a recurrent
problem with denials.

External Ear

173.20/C44.201 Unspecified malignant neoplasm of skin of ear and external auditory canal

216.2/D23.2 Other benign neoplasm of skin of ear and external auditory canal

232.2/D04.20 Carcinoma in situ of skin of ear and external auditory canal

380.10/H60.0 Abscess of external ear

380.14/H60.2 Malignant otitis externa

380.21/H60.4 Cholesteatoma of external ear

380.31/H61.12 Hematoma of pinna

380.4/H61.2 Impacted cerumen

380.50/H61.30 Acquired stenosis of external ear canal, unspecified

380.50/H61.39 Other acquired stenosis of external ear canal

380.52/H61.39 Other acquired stenosis of external ear canal

380.81/H61.81 Exostosis of external canal

Middle Ear

—/H65.0 Acute serous otitis media, recurrent (*right ear H65.04, left ear H65.05, bilateral H65.06, unspecified ear H65.07*)

381.10/H65.2 Chronic serous otitis media

381.20/H65.3 Chronic mucoid otitis media

382.1/H66.1 Chronic tubotympanic suppurative otitis media

382.2/H66.2 Chronic atticoantral suppurative otitis media

385.10/H74.1 Adhesive middle ear disease

385.30/H71.9 Unspecified cholesteatoma

385.31/H71.0 Cholesteatoma of attic

385.32/H71.1 Cholesteatoma of tympanum

385.32/H74.4 Polyp of middle ear

Tympanic Membrane

384.20/H72.9 Unspecified perforation of tympanic membrane

384.21/H72.0 Central perforation of tympanic membrane

384.22/H72.1 Attic perforation of tympanic membrane

384.23/H72.2X Other marginal perforations of tympanic membrane

384.24/H72.81 Multiple perforations of tympanic membrane

384.25/H72.82 Total perforations of tympanic membrane

—/S09.21XS Traumatic rupture of the right ear drum, sequela

—/S09.22XS Traumatic rupture of the left ear drum, sequela

Mastoid

383.1/H70.1 Chronic mastoiditis

383.32/H95.0 Recurrent cholesteatoma of postmastoidectomy cavity

383.33/H95.12 Granulations of postmastoidectomy cavity

383.81/H70.81 Postauricular fistula

385.33/H71.2 Cholesteatoma of mastoid

Vestibular Disorders

386.01/H81.0 Ménière's disease

386.40/H83.1 Labyrinthine fistula

386.8/H81.8X Other disorders of vestibular function

386.8/H82 Vertiginous syndromes in diseases classified elsewhere

386.8/H83.8X Other specified diseases of inner ear

Auditory Disorders

387.0/H80.0   Otosclerosis involving oval window, nonobliterative

387.1/H80.1   Otosclerosis involving oval window, obliterative

—/H80.2   Cochlear otosclerosis

387.9/H80.9   Unspecified otosclerosis

388.2/H91.2   Sudden idiopathic hearing loss

Facial Nerve

951.4/S04.50XS   Injury of facial nerve, unspecified side, sequela

Eustachian Tube/Nasopharynx

381.60/H68.10   Unspecified obstruction of Eustachian tube

381.7/H69.0   Patulous Eustachian tube

381.81/H69.8   Other specified disorders of Eustachian tube

Other

—/T16.1XX   Foreign body in right ear
(the applicable seventh character options are A for initial encounter, D for subsequent encounter, and S for sequela)

—/T16.2XX   Foreign body in left ear
(the applicable seventh character options are A for initial encounter, D for subsequent encounter, and S for sequela)

388.61/G96.0   Cerebrospinal fluid leak

Definition of Codes

The majority of ear codes are unilateral codes. Thus, a 50 modifier can be added if the procedure is done on both sides.

1. External Ear
   a. Examination
      i. Binocular microscopy (92504)—Do not append modifier 50 for bilateral procedures. This might be used when an ear is filled with keratin debris (not cerumen) and office ear debridement cannot be tolerated and it cannot be determined what the etiology is. The debris is removed and a cholesteatoma, or alternatively keratosis obturans is diagnosed. The definitive procedure can then be intelligently and accurately discussed, along with the concomitant risks.
      ii. Otolaryngic examination under general anesthesia (92502)—This should be used when an adequate examination is unattainable in an awake patient such as an uncooperative child or an adult with extreme pain. This involves a full otolaryngologic exam.
   b. Incision
      i. Drainage external ear, abscess or hematoma, simple (69000), complex (69005)—This should be used for incision and drainage of infectious and/or traumatic lesions of the auricle. Complex procedures involve the use of packing or a bolster, placement of a wick, or extensive debridement. Simple is typically done in the office.
      ii. Drainage external auditory canal, abscess (69020)—This should be used for incision and drainage of an external ear abscess medial to the concha.
   c. Excision
      i. Excision external ear, partial (69110), total (69120)—CPT 69110 includes *simple* repair. A simple repair generally requires only a single superficial layer closure. Intermediate or complex repairs/reconstructions such as multilayered closure, bolstering, or extensive undermining should be coded separately (12051–12057, 13150–13153) with 69110. The total auriculectomy code, includes closure, thus only 69120 should be billed.

ii. Excision exostosis, external auditory canal (69140)—This should be used for excision of either an exostosis or an osteoma of the external auditory canal.

iii. Excision soft tissue lesion, external auditory canal (69145) —This should be used for excision of lesions with a narrow margin and limited drilling. Skin grafting may be reported separately because the graft was obtained through a separate skin incision.

iv. Radical excision external auditory canal lesion (69150, 69155)—This should be used for excision of lesions of the external auditory canal including a wide margin of normal tissue without (69150) or with (69155) neck dissection. A resection extending medial to the tympanic membrane would be better reported as a temporal bone resection, external approach (69535).

d. Removal
   i. Removal foreign body from external auditory canal with general anesthesia (69205)—May be completed under direct visualization. Do not use for removal of ventilating tube. See (69424) for further details.

   ii. Removal impacted cerumen requiring instrumentation, unilateral (69210) —The patient must have cerumen impaction according to AAO-HNS and CPT guidelines, and the physician must use instrumentation during procedure. AAO-HNS and CPT defines a cerumen impaction as cerumen within the external auditory canal which causes symptoms or prevents necessary visualization of the ear. Proper instruments include curettes, wire loops, picks, and suction with or without an otoscope or microscope. The time and instrumentation used should be documented. Lavage alone should be included within the evaluation and manage ment (E/M) service and not reported

separately. Do not report 69210 for cerumen removal when performed as part of the approach for a more definitive otologic procedure. For example, do not report 69210 when removal of cerumen is performed prior to placing a tympanostomy tube (69436) or removing a tube (69424) under general anesthesia (69436) or prior to a tympanoplasty (eg, 69631). This code would be used in the operating room setting typically for a child or an adult who is unable to tolerate this in the office setting and thus anesthesia is required.

iii. Debridement mastoidectomy cavity, complex (69222)—Complex debridement is performed when more extensive cleaning is needed such as in the setting of infection, extensive debris, or when general anesthesia is required. This can thus be used as an office or OR-based code.

e. Repair
   i. Otoplasty, protruding ear, with or without size reduction (69300)—This is generally considered a cosmetic procedure and not reimbursed by payers unless the procedure is part of rehabilitating a functional hearing loss. Some payers may allow when there is a severe psychological component.

   ii. Reconstruction of external auditory canal (meatoplasty) due to acquired pathology (69310)—This should be used when soft tissue incisions and undermining are performed with or without bone removal. Note that this code includes the parenthetical term "separate procedure." This means that a meatoplasty may be billed unless it is an integral component of a total service or procedure. For example, a meatoplasty is an integral part of a modified radical and radical mastoidectomy (69505, 69511) and should not be reported separately.

   iii. Reconstruction external auditory canal for congenital atresia, single stage (69320)—When reconstruction involves the middle ear, then use tympanoplasty with or without mastoidectomy (69631–69646).

f. Unlisted procedure, external ear (69399)—An example is placement of osseointegrated implants for an auricular prosthesis.

2. Middle Ear

a. Incision

   i. Myringotomy including aspiration and/or Eustachian tube inflation with general anesthesia (69421)—Modifier 50 may be reported for bilateral procedures.

   ii. Ventilating tube removal requiring general anesthesia (69424)—Modifier 50 may be reported for bilateral procedures. Ventilating tube removal without general anesthesia can be included in E/M services or reported as *binocular microscopy* (92504) if a microscope is used. Generally, do not report if other otologic procedures are performed on the same ear. The CPT vignette for 69424 describes the ventilating tube as still in the tympanic membrane, not in the ear canal. Removal of a tube from the ear canal is included in the E/M code, or 92504 may be reported if a microscope (not an otoscope) was used for its removal.

   iii. Tympanostomy (requiring insertion of ventilating tube) with general anesthesia (69436)—Modifier 50 may be reported for bilateral procedures. Do not report with myringotomy (69420) as this is included within the procedure. Do not report separately with a more complex procedure on the same ear such as tympanoplasty as placement of the tympanostomy tube is considered included in the more complex procedure.

   iv. Middle ear exploration through post-auricular or ear canal incision (69440)—This should be used when a tympanomeatal flap is elevated to allow for complete middle ear inspec-

tion but no treatment is rendered at that time. Do not report 69440 with another procedure code on the same ear since all middle ear codes include an exploration.

   v. Tympanolysis, transcanal (69450)—This should be used when a tympano-meatal flap is elevated and adhesions to the tympanic membrane are lysed.

b. Excision

   i. Transmastoid antrotomy (simple mastoidectomy) (69501)—This is used for a cortical mastoidectomy typically performed to decompress acute infection. Drilling is limited to the cortex and antrum. The horizontal semicircular canal and facial nerve are not identified. The middle ear is not explored or treated.

   ii. Mastoidectomy; complete, primary (69502); revision (69601)—Mastoid air cells are drilled, and the horizontal semicircular canal, posterior canal wall, and facial nerve are identified. The middle ear is not explored or treated.

   iii. Mastoidectomy; modified radical, primary (69505); revision (69602)—This describes Bondy's procedure which is rarely indicated anymore. In addition to a complete mastoidectomy, the posterior canal wall down is removed to the level of the facial nerve, and a meatoplasty is performed. The middle ear is left unexplored. If the middle ear is explored and treated as in a tympanoplasty with canal wall down mastoidectomy, then report 69645 or 69646.

   iv. Mastoidectomy; radical, primary (69511); revision (69603)—In addition to a complete mastoidectomy, the posterior canal wall is removed to the level of the facial nerve, the tympanic membrane and some or all of the ossicles are removed, and a meatoplasty is performed.

   v. Petrous apicectomy including radical mastoidectomy, primary (69530);

revision (69605)—Radical mastoidectomy is not a required part of the procedure, but it is included if performed as part of the approach to the petrous apex.

vi. Resection temporal bone, external approach (69535)—Resection extending lateral to the tympanic membrane would be better reported as a radical excision external auditory canal lesion (69150, 69155). Parotidectomy, neck dissection, and complex reconstruction (eg, adjacent tissue transfer, skin grafting) are reported separately.

vii. Excision aural glomus tumor transcanal (69550); transmastoid (69552); extended (69554)—An extended procedure includes identification of cranial nerves exiting the jugular foramen and ligation of the internal jugular vein. Parotidectomy and complex reconstruction (eg, adjacent tissue transfer, skin grafting) are reported separately.

c. Repair

i. Tympanic membrane repair (69610)—This should be used when the perforation edges are freshened with or without application of a patch. Autogenous grafts are not used, and the middle ear is not explored. An example is a paper patch graft.

ii. Myringoplasty (69620)—This should be used when the perforation edges are freshened and an autogenous graft is used such as a fat plug or temporalis fascia graft. The middle ear is not explored. This code includes the graft harvest so do not code separately for it even when performed through a separate incision.

iii. Tympanoplasty without mastoidectomy (including canalplasty, atticotomy and/or middle ear surgery), initial or revision; *without* ossicular chain reconstruction (69631); *with* ossicular chain reconstruction (69632); *with* ossicular chain reconstruction and *synthetic prosthesis* (69633)—Tympanoplasty may be performed via a

transcanal or postauricular approach. These codes require middle ear exploration (ie, elevation of a tympanomeatal flap and inspection of the middle ear and ossicles). A graft does not have to be placed for the procedure to be coded as a tympanoplasty as long as the middle ear is explored. Graft harvesting is reported separately if it requires a separate incision such as temporalis fascia or tragal cartilage harvested (20926) for a transcanal approach. If the tragal cartilage is harvested for reconstruction of the ear canal and ossicular chain reconstruction, then 21235 may be reported since it is a reconstruction code and not just a graft harvest code. Placement of a tympanostomy tube (69436) is included when performed in the same ear and should not be separately billed.

iv. Tympanoplasty with antrotomy or mastoidotomy; *without* ossicular chain reconstruction (69635); *with* ossicular chain reconstruction (69636); *with* ossicular chain reconstruction and *synthetic prosthesis* (69637) (90-day global)—The guidelines are the same as for codes 69631–69632 except the procedures include "antrotomy or mastoidotomy." We interpret these terms to mean a limited mastoidectomy is performed with entrance into the mastoid antrum but without identification of deeper structures such as the horizontal semicircular canal, facial nerve, and incus. Clinically, this is an uncommon scenario, and codes 69641–69646 reflect the common practice when mastoid surgery is combined with tympanoplasty. Placement of a tympanostomy tube (69436) is included when performed in the same ear.

v. Tympanoplasty with mastoidectomy (including canalplasty, middle ear surgery, tympanic membrane repair) *without* ossicular chain reconstruction

(69641); *with* ossicular chain reconstruction (69642)—The guidelines are the same as for codes 69631–69632 except the procedures include mastoidectomy. The type of mastoidectomy is not specified, but we correlate this code clinically with a tympanoplasty with complete mastoidectomy. Placement of a tympanostomy tube (69436) is included when performed in the same ear.

vi. Tympanoplasty with mastoidectomy (including canalplasty, middle ear surgery, tympanic membrane repair) intact or reconstructed wall *without* ossicular chain reconstruction (69643); *with* ossicular chain reconstruction (69644)—The guidelines are the same as for codes 69631–69632 except the procedures include mastoidectomy intact or reconstructed wall. We use this code when the canal wall is reconstructed due to an acquired defect or after surgical removal. Placement of a tympanostomy tube (69436) is included when performed in the same ear.

vii. Tympanoplasty with mastoidectomy; radical or complete, *without* ossicular chain reconstruction (69645); *with* ossicular chain reconstruction (69646)—The guidelines are the same as for codes 69631–69632, except the procedures include radical or complete mastoidectomy. We correlate this code clinically with tympanoplasty with canal wall down mastoidectomy. Placement of tympanostomy tube (69436) is included when performed in the same ear.

viii. Stapes mobilization (69650)—This is used for congenital stapes fixation and, less frequently, tympanosclerosis patients.

ix. Stapedectomy or stapedotomy (69660) with footplate drillout (69661)—The standard stapedotomy technique using a microdrill to create a small fenestra in the footplate is not considered a drillout. Footplate drillout is used in cases of obliterative otosclerosis when a particularly thickened footplate requires extensive drilling.

x. Revision stapedectomy or stapedotomy (69662).

xi. Repair oval window fistula (69666)—Done when the patient has a high suspicion for a perilymphatic fistula and this is found as the site of the fistula during exploratory tympanotomy. If repaired, the definitive procedure would be billed alone and not with the middle ear exploration code (69440).

xii. Repair round window fistula (69667)—Similar to repair of the oval window fistula, but this is the identified site of the fistula.

xiii. Mastoid obliteration (69670)—Generally performed after a mastoidectomy for problems related to the cavity (eg, recurrent mastoid bowl infections, dizziness due to exposure of the semicircular canals or recurrent cholesteatoma).

xiv. Tympanic neurectomy (69676)—This might be performed in a patient experiencing chronic parotid sialectasis.

d. Other procedures
   i. Closure postauricular fistula, mastoid (69700)—This is an unusual complication but can occur in patients with poor wound healing (eg, diabetics, smokers) after a canal wall down tympmastoid, requiring a secondary closure.

   ii. Implantation or replacement or removal of electromagnetic bone conduction hearing device in temporal bone (69710).

   iii. Repair or removal of electromagnetic bone conduction hearing device in temporal bone (69711)—For example, removal of the old Audiant, or more recent Sophono implants.

   iv. Implantation or replacement of osseointegrated implant, temporal bone, with percutaneous attachment to external speech processor/cochlear stimulator (69714); with mastoidectomy (69715)—Use a 52 modifier (reduced services) if placing osseointegrated implant without an abutment as the first part of a staged procedure. Use the same code (69710) with modifiers 58 and 52 for the second-stage procedure when the abutment is attached.

v. Replacement (including removal of existing device), osseointegrated implant, temporal bone, with percutaneous attachment to external speech processor/cochlear stimulator (69717); with mastoidectomy (69718).

vi. Decompression facial nerve, intratemporal; lateral to the geniculate ganglion (69720); including medial to the geniculate ganglion (69725).

vii. Suture facial nerve, intratemporal, with or without graft or decompression; lateral to the geniculate ganglion (69740); including medial to the geniculate ganglion (69745)—For facial nerve neurorrhaphy distal to the stylomastoid foramen use suture of facial nerve; extracranial (64864); infratemporal (64865).

viii. Unlisted procedure, middle ear (69799) —An example is Eustachian tuboplasty or more recently Eustachian tube balloon dilatation should be coded as a miscellaneous procedure (69799). In the letter describing the procedure offer a comparison code such as balloon dilatation of the frontal sinus ostia (31296).

ix. Abdominal fat graft (20926)—This is a separately reportable procedure as a separate incision is required.

x. Temporalis fascia graft (20926)—It may be reported separately from the primary procedure if a separate incision is required as in transcanal tympanoplasty or when harvested from the contralateral side in a revision procedure.

xi. Graft ear cartilage (21235)—This is a separately reportable procedure if a separate incision is required and the graft is used for reconstruction of the ear canal and ossicular chain.

3. Inner Ear
   a. Incision and/or Destruction
      i. Labyrinthotomy, with perfusion of vestibuloactive drug(s); transcanal (69801)—Transcanal procedures include intratympanic injection of gentamicin or steroids for Ménière's or sudden sensorineural hearing loss. Do not report code more than once per day. This is typically done in the office but in select cases is done with anesthesia. The postoperative global period is 0 days so each injection on a separate day may be separately reported. Previously there was a code for labyrinthotomy with mastoidectomy (69802). This code has since been deleted.
      ii. Endolymphatic sac operation (69805); with shunt (69806).
      iii. Fenestration semicircular canal (69820); revision (69840).
   b. Excision
      i. Labyrinthectomy; transcanal (69905); with mastoidectomy (69910).
      ii. Vestibular nerve section, translabyrinthine approach (69915)—Use 61460 (Craniotomy, suboccipital; for section of 1 or more cranial nerves) when the vestibular nerve section is performed via a retrosigmoid approach. Use modifier 62 (two surgeons) on either code when this is performed with a neurosurgeon.
      iii. Cochlear device implantation (69930) —modifier 50 may be reported for bilateral procedures.
   c. Unlisted procedure, inner ear (69949)

Controversial Areas

Facial Nerve Monitoring

No area of coding operative otology has been more controversial in the last 20 years than intraoperative facial nerve monitoring. What is very clear now is that the operative surgeon cannot bill for the surgery and the facial nerve monitoring. The only way that facial nerve monitoring can be billed and appropriately reimbursed is to use a separate real-time monitoring physician, usually via remote access as economies of scale are necessary to make this viable. Not infrequently, the ambulatory surgery center or the hospital are bearing the costs of the monitoring service. Discussion of this model is beyond the scope of this chapter, but suffice it to say again, the operative surgeon cannot operate and monitor the facial nerve, from a coding and reimbursement standpoint, simultaneously. In surgical practice, most surgeons have the facial monitor running while they operate and use the real-time information to assist in patient safety, but do not bill for this service.

Eustachian Tube Procedures

Many surgeons are currently using sinus balloons to dilate the eustachian tube when patients have eustachian tube dysfunction alone or with sinus disease that warrants surgical treatment. Currently, there is a large multicenter randomized study to determine the efficacy of balloon dilatation of the eustachian tube. This balloon was specifically designed with safety features for dilatation of the eustachian tube. If efficacy is demon-

strated from this study and is US Food and Drug Administration (FDA) approval of the device is obtained, the arduous process of obtaining a new procedure code for balloon dilatation of the eustachian tube begins. Until a new code is developed, any procedures directly treating the eustachian tube must use the unlisted code, 69799.

Semicircular Canal Dehiscence

There currently is not a code to describe this procedure. This should be billed using an unlisted code or using 61304 (Craniectomy or craniotomy, exploratory; supratentorial). If using a skull base approach, the unlisted neurosurgical code, 64999, would be the most appropriate. Modifier 62 would be appended if performed with a neurosurgeon.

Endoscopic Ear Surgery

This is typically used as an adjunct to traditional ear surgery. Whether this is done in addition to the standard procedure or as a stand-alone procedure, yet the same procedure is done, only through a smaller incision, this will be billed using the traditional codes, as there are no separate procedure codes for endoscopic ear surgery. If the procedure is inherently changed from the standard procedure codes, then the unlisted middle ear code, 69799, should be used.

CHAPTER 27

Operative Facial Plastic Surgery

Rebecca E. Fraioli

Introduction

The most common codes for facial plastic surgery, as well as their indications and key points, are discussed below. It is important to remember that the procedure descriptions for many of these codes are somewhat ambiguous in that they could apply equally to functional or aesthetic surgery. It goes without saying that only functional procedures should be billed to the insurance company. However, because of the ambiguity of the procedure descriptions, the onus is on the surgeon to demonstrate clearly in the patient chart the symptoms and signs that necessitate the functional surgery in a particular patient. It is highly recommended for these ambiguous codes that insurance precertification or written predetermination be obtained well in advance of the surgery, even if the insurance company does not require this to be done.

Key Points

- A number of facial plastic surgery procedures do not have a specific unique *Current Procedural Terminology* (CPT) code; therefore, an unlisted code may need to be used.
- In other cases, there may be more than one code that could potentially apply (eg, osteotomies and placement of spreader grafts for a patient with a posttraumatic nasal deformity); in these cases, the

code that most closely fits the specific procedure components done should be chosen.
- Most operative facial plastic surgery codes have a 90-day global period. Exceptions to this are noted below.

Key Procedure Codes

Rhinoplasty and Nasal Airway Surgery

30400 Rhinoplasty, primary; lateral and alar cartilages and/or elevation of nasal tip
wRVU 10.86; Global 90

    30410 complete, external parts including bony pyramid, lateral and alar cartilages, and/or elevation of nasal tip
wRVU 14.00; Global 90

    30420 including major septal repair
wRVU 16.90; Global 90

30430 Rhinoplasty, secondary; minor revision (small amount of nasal tip work)
wRVU 8.24; Global 90

    30435 intermediate revision (bony work with osteotomies)
wRVU 12.73; Global 90

    30450 major revision (nasal tip work and osteotomies)
wRVU 19.66; Global 90

30465 Repair of nasal vestibular stenosis (eg, spreader grafting, lateral nasal wall reconstruction)
wRVU 12.36; Global 90

30630 Repair nasal septal perforation
wRVU 7.29; Global 90

Congenital Deformity

30460 Rhinoplasty for nasal deformity secondary to congenital cleft lip and/or palate, including columellar lengthening; tip only
wRVU 10.32; Global 90

    30462 tip, septum, osteotomies
wRVU 20.28; Global 90

40700 Plastic repair of cleft lip/nasal deformity; primary, partial or complete, unilateral
wRVU 14.17; Global 90

    40701 primary bilateral, 1-stage procedure
wRVU 17.23; Global 90

    40702 primary bilateral, 1 of 2 stages
wRVU 14.27; Global 90

    40720 secondary, by recreation of defect and reclosure
wRVU 14.72; Global 90

    40761 with cross lip pedicle flap (Abbe-Estlander type) includes sectioning and inserting of pedicle
wRVU 15.84; Global 90

69300 Otoplasty, protruding ear, with or without size reduction
wRVU 6.69; Global YYY

Skin Lesions and Neoplasms

11100 Biopsy of skin, subcutaneous tissue and/or mucous membrane (including simple closure), unless otherwise listed; single lesion
wRVU 0.81; Global 0

+11101 each separate/additional lesion (List separately in addition to code for primary procedure)
wRVU 0.41; Global ZZZ

11420 Excision, benign lesion including margins, except skin tag (unless listed elsewhere), scalp, neck, hands, feet, genitalia; excised diameter 0.5 cm or less
wRVU 1.03; Global 10

    11421 excised diameter 0.6 cm to 1.0 cm
wRVU 1.47; Global 10

    11422 excised diameter 1.1 cm to 2.0 cm
wRVU 1.68; Global 10

    11423 excised diameter 2.1 cm to 3.0 cm
wRVU 2.06; Global 10

    11424 excised diameter 3.1 cm to 4.0 cm
wRVU 2.48; Global 10

    11426 excised diameter over 4.0 cm
wRVU 4.09; Global 10

11440 Excision, other benign lesion including margins, except skin tag (unless listed elsewhere), face, ears, eyelids, nose, lips, mucous membrane; excised diameter 0.5 cm or less
wRVU 1.05; Global 10

    11441 excised diameter 0.6 cm to 1.0 cm
wRVU 1.53; Global 10

    11442 excised diameter 1.1 cm to 2.0 cm
wRVU 1.77; Global 10

    11443 excised diameter 2.1 cm to 3.0 cm
wRVU 2.34; Global 10

    11444 excised diameter 3.1 cm to 4.0 cm
wRVU 3.19; Global 10

    11446 excised diameter over 4.0 cm
wRVU 4.80; Global 10

11620 Excision, malignant lesion including margins, scalp, neck, hands, feet, genitalia; excised diameter 0.5 cm or less
wRVU 1.04; Global 10

11621 excised diameter 0.6 cm to 1.0 cm
wRVU 2.08; Global 10

11622 excised diameter 1.1 cm to 2.0 cm
wRVU 2.41; Global 10

11623 excised diameter 2.1 cm to 3.0 cm
wRVU 3.11; Global 10

11624 excised diameter 3.1 cm to 4.0 cm
wRVU 3.62; Global 10

11626 excised diameter over 4.0 cm
wRVU 4.61; Global 10

11640 Excision, malignant lesion including margins, face, ears, eyelids, nose, lips; excised diameter 0.5 cm or less
wRVU 1.67; Global 10

11641 excised diameter 0.6 cm to 1.0 cm
wRVU 2.17; Global 10

11642 excised diameter 1.1 cm to 2.0 cm
wRVU 2.62; Global 10

11643 excised diameter 2.1 cm to 3.0 cm
wRVU 3.42; Global 10

11644 excised diameter 3.1 cm to 4.0 cm
wRVU 4.34; Global 10

11646 excised diameter over 4.0 cm
wRVU 6.26; Global 10

Wound Repair

For complex repairs under 1.1 cm, use the appropriate simple or intermediate repair. Similarly, CPT 13150 has been removed.

12001 Simple repair of superficial wounds of scalp, neck, axillae, external genitalia, trunk and/or extremities (including hands and feet); 2.5 cm or less
wRVU 0.84; Global 0

12002 2.6 cm to 7.5 cm
wRVU 1.14; Global 0

12004 7.6 cm to 12.5 cm
wRVU 1.44; Global 0

12005 12.6 cm to 20.0 cm
wRVU 1.97; Global 0

12006 20.1 cm to 30.0 cm
wRVU 2.39; Global 0

12007 over 30.0 cm
wRVU 2.90; Global 0

12011 Simple repair of superficial wounds of face, ears, eyelids, nose, lips and/or mucous membranes; 2.5 cm or less
wRVU 1.07; Global 0

12013 2.6 cm to 5.0 cm
wRVU 1.22; Global 0

12014 5.1 cm to 7.5 cm
wRVU 1.57; Global 0

12015 7.6 cm to 12.5 cm
wRVU 1.98; Global 0

12016 12.6 cm to 20.0 cm
wRVU 2.68; Global 0

12017 20.1 cm to 30.0 cm
wRVU 3.18; Global 0

12018 over 30.0 cm
wRVU 3.61; Global 0

12031 Repair, intermediate, wounds of scalp, axillae, trunk and/or extremities (excluding hands and feet); 2.5 cm or less
wRVU 2.00; Global 10

12032 2.6 cm to 7.5 cm
wRVU 2.52; Global 10

12034 7.6 cm to 12.5 cm
wRVU 2.97; Global 10

12035 12.6 cm to 20.0 cm
wRVU 3.50; Global 10

12036 20.1 cm to 30.0 cm
wRVU 4.23; Global 10

12037 over 30.0 cm
wRVU 5.00; Global 10

12041 Repair, intermediate, wounds of neck, hands, feet and/or external genitalia; 2.5 cm or less
wRVU 2.10; Global 10

12042 2.6 cm to 7.5 cm
wRVU 2.79; Global 10

12044 7.6 cm to 12.5 cm
wRVU 3.19; Global 10

12045 12.6 cm to 20.0 cm
wRVU 3.75; Global 10

12046 20.1 cm to 30.0 cm
wRVU 4.30; Global 10

12047 over 30.0 cm
wRVU 4.95; Global 10

12051 Repair, intermediate, wounds of face, ears, eyelids, nose, lips and/or mucous membranes; 2.5 cm or less
wRVU 2.33; Global 10

12052 2.6 cm to 5.0 cm
wRVU 2.87; Global 10

12053 5.1 cm to 7.5 cm
wRVU 3.17; Global 10

12054 7.6 cm to 12.5 cm
wRVU 3.50; Global 10

12055 12.6 cm to 20.0 cm
wRVU 4.50; Global 10

12056 20.1 cm to 30.0 cm
wRVU 5.30; Global 10

12057 over 30.0 cm
wRVU 6.00; Global 10

13120 Repair, complex, scalp, arms, and/or legs; 1.1 cm to 2.5 cm
wRVU 3.23; Global 10

13121 2.6 cm to 7.5 cm
wRVU 4.00; Global 10

+13122 each additional 5 cm or less (List separately in addition to code for primary procedure)
wRVU 1.44; Global ZZZ

13131 Repair, complex, forehead, cheeks, chin, mouth, neck, axillae, genitalia, hands and/or feet; 1.1 cm to 2.5 cm
wRVU 3.73; Global 10

13132 2.6 cm to 7.5 cm
wRVU 4.78; Global 10

+13133 each additional 5 cm or less (List separately in addition to code for primary procedure)
wRVU 2.19; Global ZZZ

13151 Repair, complex, eyelids, nose, ears, and/or lips; 1.1 cm to 2.5 cm
wRVU 4.34; Global 10

13152 2.6 cm to 7.5 cm
wRVU 5.34; Global 10

+13153 each additional 5 cm or less (List separately in addition to code for primary procedure)
wRVU 2.38; Global ZZZ

14020 Adjacent tissue transfer or rearrangement, scalp, arms, and/or legs; defect 10 sq cm or less
wRVU 7.22; Global 90

14021 defect 10.1 sq cm to 30.0 sq cm
wRVU 9.72; Global 90

14040 Adjacent tissue transfer or rearrangement, forehead, cheeks, chin, mouth, neck, axillae, genitalia, hands and/or feet; defect 10 sq cm or less
wRVU 8.60; Global 90

14041 defect 10.1 sq cm to 30.0 sq cm
wRVU 10.83; Global 90

14060 Adjacent tissue transfer or rearrangement, eyelids, nose, ears and/or lips; defect 10 sq cm or less
wRVU 9.23; Global 90

14061 defect 10.1 sq cm to 30.0 sq cm
wRVU 11.48; Global 90

14301 Adjacent tissue transfer or rearrangement, any area; defect 30.1 sq cm to 60.0 sq cm
wRVU 12.65; Global 90

+14302 each additional 30.0 sq cm, or part thereof (List separately in addition to code for primary procedure)
wRVU 3.73; Global ZZZ

15004 Surgical preparation or creation of recipient site by excision of open wounds, burn eschar, or scar (including

subcutaneous tissues), or incisional release of scar contracture, face, scalp, eyelids, mouth, neck, ears, orbits, genitalia, hands, feet and/or multiple digits; first 100 sq cm or 1% of body area of infants and children
wRVU 4.58; Global 0

+15005   each additional 100 sq cm, or part thereof, or each additional 1% of body area of infants and children (List separately in addition to code for primary procedure)
wRVU 1.60; Global ZZZ

15120   Split-thickness autograft, face, scalp, eyelids, mouth, neck, ears, orbits, genitalia, hands, feet, and/or multiple digits; first 100 sq cm or less, or 1% of body area of infants and children (except 15050)
wRVU 10.15; Global 90

+15121   each additional 100 sq cm, or each additional 1% of body area of infants and children, or part thereof (List separately in addition to code for primary procedure)
wRVU 2.00; Global ZZZ

15240   Full thickness graft, free, including direct closure of donor site, forehead, cheeks, chin, mouth, neck, axillae, genitalia, hands, and/or feet; 20 sq cm or less
wRVU 10.41; Global 90

+15241   each additional 20 sq cm, or part thereof (List separately in addition to code for primary procedure)
wRVU 1.86; Global ZZZ

15260   Full thickness graft, free, including direct closure of donor site, nose, ears, eyelids, and/or lips; 20 sq cm or less
wRVU 11.64; Global 90

+15261   each additional 20 sq cm, or part thereof (List separately in addition to code for primary procedure)
wRVU 2.23; Global ZZZ

15570   Formation of direct or tubed pedicle, with or without transfer; trunk
wRVU 10.21; Global 90

15572   scalp, arms, or legs
wRVU 10.12; Global 90

15574   forehead, cheeks, chin, mouth, neck, axillae, genitalia, hands or feet
wRVU 10.70; Global 90

15576   eyelids, nose, ears, lips, or intraoral
wRVU 9.37; Global 90

15630   Delay of flap or sectioning of flap (division and inset); at eyelids, nose, ears, or lips
wRVU 4.08; Global 90

15781   Dermabrasion; segmental, face
wRVU 5.02; Global 90

Lip

40490   Biopsy of lip
wRVU 1.22; Global 0

40500   Vermilionectomy (lip shave), with mucosal advancement
wRVU 4.47; Global 90

40510   Excision of lip; transverse wedge excision with primary closure
wRVU 4.82; Global 90

40520   V-excision with primary direct linear closure
wRVU 4.79; Global 90

40525   full thickness, reconstruction with local flap (eg, Estlander or fan)
wRVU 7.72; Global 90

40527   full thickness, reconstruction with cross-lip flap (Abbe-Estlander)
wRVU 9.32; Global 90

40650   Repair lip, full thickness; vermilion only
wRVU 3.78; Global 90

40652 up to half vertical height
wRVU 4.43; Global 90

40654 over one-half vertical height, or complex
wRVU 5.48; Global 90

Facial Nerve Disorders

Rhytidectomy is a unilateral code and modifier 50 can be added if the procedure is performed on both sides.

15829 Rhytidectomy; superficial musculoaponeurotic system (SMAS) flap
wRVU 0; Global 0

15840 Graft for facial nerve paralysis; free fascia graft (including obtaining fascia)
wRVU 14.99; Global 90

    15841 free muscle graft (including obtaining graft)
wRVU 25.99; Global 90

    15842 free muscle flap by microsurgical technique
wRVU 41.01; Global 90

    15845 regional muscle transfer
wRVU 14.32; Global 90

64864 Suture of facial nerve; extracranial
wRVU 13.41; Global 90

64885 Nerve graft (includes obtaining graft), head or neck; up to 4 cm in length
wRVU 17.60; Global 90

    64886 more than 4 cm length
wRVU 20.82; Global 90

+69990 Microsurgical techniques, requiring use of operating microscope (List separately in addition to code for primary procedure
wRVU 3.46; Global ZZZ

Eyelid and Brow

15823 Blepharoplasty, upper eyelid, with excessive skin weighing down lid
wRVU 6.81; Global 90

21280 Medial canthopexy (separate procedure)
wRVU 7.13; Global 90

21282 Lateral canthopexy
wRVU 4.27; Global 90

67900 Repair of brow ptosis (supraciliary, mid-forehead or coronal approach)
wRVU 6.82; Global 90

67912 Correction of lagophthalmos, with implantation of upper lid load (eg, gold weight)
wRVU 6.36; Global 90

67914 Repair of ectropion; suture
wRVU 3.75; Global 90

    67915 thermocauterization
wRVU 2.03; Global 90

    67916 excision tarsal wedge
wRVU 5.48; Global 90

    67917 extensive (eg, tarsal strip operations)
wRVU 5.93; Global 90

67921 Repair of entropion; suture
wRVU 3.47; Global 90

    67922 thermocauterization
wRVU 2.03; Global 90

    67923 excision tarsal wedge
wRVU 5.48; Global 90

    67924 extensive (eg, tarsal strip or capsulopalpebral fascia repairs operation)
wRVU 5.93; Global 90

67950 Canthoplasty (reconstruction of canthus)
wRVU 5.99; Global 90

Trauma

Nose

21315 Closed treatment of nasal bone fracture; without stabilization
wRVU 1.83; Global 10

    21320 with stabilization
wRVU 1.88; Global 10

21325 Open treatment of nasal fracture; uncomplicated
wRVU 4.18; Global 90

    21330 complicated, with internal and/or external skeletal fixation
    wRVU 5.79; Global 90

    21335 with concomitant open treatment of fractured septum
    wRVU 9.02; Global 90

21336 Open treatment of nasal septal fracture, with or without stabilization
wRVU 6.77; Global 90

21337 Closed treatment of nasal septal fracture, with or without stabilization
wRVU 3.39; Global 90

Naso-Orbito-Ethmoid (NOE) Complex

21338 Open treatment of nasoethmoid fracture; without external fixation
wRVU 6.87; Global 90

    21339 with external fixation
    wRVU 8.50; Global 90

21340 Percutaneous treatment of nasoethmoid complex fracture, with splint, wire or headcap fixation, including repair of canthal ligaments and/or the nasolacrimal apparatus
wRVU 11.49; Global 90

Frontal Sinus

21343 Open treatment of depressed frontal sinus fracture
wRVU 14.32; Global 90

21344 Open treatment of complicated (eg, comminuted or involving posterior wall) frontal sinus fracture, via coronal or multiple approaches
wRVU 21.57; Global 90

LeFort I (Palatal or Maxillary) Fractures

21421 Closed treatment of palatal or maxillary fracture (LeFort I type), with interdental wire fixation or fixation of denture or splint
wRVU 6.02; Global 90

21422 Open treatment of palatal or maxillary fracture (LeFort I type);
wRVU 8.73; Global 90

    21423 complicated (comminuted or involving cranial nerve foramina), multiple approaches
    wRVU 10.85; Global 90

LeFort II (Nasomaxillary Buttress)

21345 Closed treatment of nasomaxillary complex fracture (LeFort II type), with interdental wire fixation or fixation of denture or splint
wRVU 9.06; Global 90

21346 Open treatment of nasomaxillary complex fracture (LeFort II type); with wiring and/or local fixation
wRVU 11.45; Global 90

    21347 requiring multiple open approaches
    wRVU 13.53; Global 90

    21348 with bone grafting (includes obtaining graft)
    wRVU 17.52; Global 90

LeFort III (Craniofacial Separation)

21431 Closed treatment of craniofacial separation (LeFort III type) using interdental wire fixation of denture or splint
wRVU 7.90; Global 90

21432 Open treatment of craniofacial separation (LeFort III type); with wiring and/or internal fixation
wRVU 8.82; Global 90

    21433 complicated (eg, comminuted or involving cranial nerve foramina), multiple surgical approaches
    wRVU 26.29; Global 90

    21435 complicated, utilizing internal and/or external fixation techniques (eg, head cap, halo device, and/or intermaxillary fixation)
    wRVU 20.26; Global 90

21436   complicated, multiple surgical approaches, internal fixation, with bone grafting (includes obtaining graft)
wRVU 30.30; Global 90

Zygomaticomaxillary Complex (ZMC)

21355   Percutaneous treatment of fracture of malar area, including zygomatic arch and malar tripod, with manipulation
wRVU 4.45; Global 10

21356   Open treatment of depressed zygomatic arch fracture (eg, Gillies approach)
wRVU 4.83; Global 10

21360   Open treatment of depressed malar fracture, including zygomatic arch and malar tripod
wRVU 7.19; Global 90

21365   Open treatment of complicated (eg, comminuted or involving cranial nerve foramina) fracture(s) of malar area, including zygomatic arch and malar tripod; with internal fixation and multiple surgical approaches
wRVU 16.77; Global 90

    21366   with bone grafting (includes obtaining graft)
wRVU 18.60; Global 90

Orbit

Orbital Blowout Fracture

21385   Open treatment of orbital floor blowout fracture; transantral approach (Caldwell-Luc type operation)
wRVU 9.57; Global 90

    21386   periorbital approach
wRVU 9.57; Global 90

    21387   combined approach
wRVU 10.11; Global 90

    21390   periorbital approach, with alloplastic or other implant
wRVU 11.23; Global 90

    21395   periorbital approach with bone graft (includes obtaining graft)
wRVU 14.70; Global 90

Orbit, not Blowout

21400   Closed treatment of fracture of orbit, except blowout; without manipulation
wRVU 1.50; Global 90

    21401   with manipulation
wRVU 3.68; Global 90

21406   Open treatment of fracture of orbit, except blowout; without implant
wRVU 7.42; Global 90

    21407   with implant
wRVU 9.02; Global 90

    21408   with bone grafting (includes obtaining graft)
wRVU 12.78; Global 90

Alveolar Ridge

21440   Closed treatment of mandibular or maxillary alveolar ridge fracture (separate procedure)
wRVU 3.44; Global 90

21445   Open treatment of mandibular or maxillary alveolar ridge fracture (separate procedure)
wRVU 6.26; Global 90

Mandible

21450   Closed treatment of mandibular fracture; without manipulation
wRVU 3.71; Global 90

    21451   with manipulation
wRVU 5.65; Global 90

21452   Percutaneous treatment of mandibular fracture, with external fixation
wRVU 2.40; Global 90

21453   Closed treatment of mandibular fracture with interdental fixation
wRVU 6.64; Global 90

21454 Open treatment of mandibular with external fixation
wRVU 7.36; Global 90

21461 Open treatment of mandibular fracture; without interdental fixation
wRVU 9.31; Global 90

    21462   with interdental fixation
    wRVU 11.01; Global 90

21465 Open treatment of mandibular condylar fracture
wRVU 13.12; Global 90

21470 Open treatment of complicated mandibular fracture by multiple surgical approaches including internal fixation, interdental fixation, and/or wiring of dentures or splints
wRVU 17.54; Global 90

Common Grafts in Facial Plastic Surgery

15760 Graft; composite (eg, full thickness of external ear or nasal ala), including primary closure, donor area
wRVU 9.86; Global 90

    15770   derma-fat-fascia
    wRVU 8.96; Global 90

20926 Tissue grafts, other (eg, paratenon, fat, dermis)
wRVU 5.79; Global 90

15275 Application of skin substitute graft to face, scalp, eyelids, mouth, neck, ears, orbits, genitalia, hands, feet, and/or multiple digits, total wound surface area up to 100 sq cm; first 25 sq cm or less wound surface area
wRVU 1.83; Global 0

    +15276   each additional 25 sq cm wound surface area, or part thereof (List separately in addition to code for primary procedure)
    wRVU 0.50; Global ZZZ

15277 Application of skin substitute graft to face, scalp, eyelids, mouth, neck, ears, orbits, genitalia, hands, feet, and/or multiple digits, total wound surface area greater than or equal to 100 sq cm; first 100 sq cm wound surface area, or 1% of body area of infants and children
wRVU 4.00; Global 0

    +15278   each additional 100 sq cm wound surface area, or part thereof, of each additional 1% of body area of infants and children, or part thereof (List separately in addition to code for primary procedure)
    wRVU 1.00; Global ZZZ

17999 Unlisted procedure, skin, mucous membrane and subcutaneous tissue
wRVU 0.00; Global YYY

20912 Cartilage graft; nasal septum
wRVU 6.54; Global 90

21208 Osteoplasty, facial bones; augmentation (autograft, allograft, or prosthetic implant)
wRVU 11.42; Global 90

21230 Graft; rib cartilage, autogenous, to face, chin, nose or ear (includes obtaining graft)
wRVU 11.17; Global 90

    21235   ear cartilage, autogenous, to nose or ear (includes obtaining graft)
    wRVU 7.50; Global 90

40818 Excision of mucosa of vestibule of mouth as donor graft
wRVU 2.83; Global 90

Key Modifiers

22   Increased Procedural Services
Use when the intensity, surgical time, or technical difficulty of the surgery is significantly more than usual for the chosen code.

51   Multiple Procedures
Use for additional procedures.

53 Discontinued Procedure
Use when a procedure must be aborted intraoperatively due to a medical problem that would threaten the patient's health if the surgery were continued.

58 Staged or Related Procedure or Service by the Same Physician or Other Qualified Health Care Professional During the Postoperative Period
This indicates that a second procedure performed during the postoperative period was anticipated from the outset.

59 Distinct Procedural Service
To use modifier 59, procedures must not normally be bundled together and must represent a separate anatomical site, separate lesion, or separate incision. If another code or modifier can be used, then that should be chosen over modifier 59.

76 Repeat Procedure or Service by Same Physician or Other Qualified Health Care Professional
This is a repeat procedure, with the same surgeon.

79 Unrelated Procedure or Service by the Same Physician or Other Qualified Health Care Professional During the Postoperative Period
This is placed on a procedure when done during the global period of a different procedure

Key ICD-9-CM/ICD-10-CM Codes

Rhinoplasty and Nasal Airway Surgery

470/J34.2 Deviated nasal septum

905.0/S02.2XXS Fracture of nasal bones, sequela

V15.51/Z87.81 Personal history of (healed) traumatic fracture

738.0/M95.0 Acquired deformity of nose

478.19/J34.89 Other specified disorders of nose and nasal sinuses

Congenital Deformity

380.32/H61.119 Acquired deformity of pinna, unspecified ear

744.01/Q16.0 Congenital absence of (ear) auricle

744.1/Q17.0 Accessory auricle

744.21/Q17.8 Other specified congenital malformations of ear

744.22/Q17.1 Macrotia

744.23/Q17.2 Microtia

744.81/Q18.6 Macrocheilia

744.82/Q18.7 Microcheilia

744.83/Q18.4 Macrostomia

744.84/Q18.5 Microstomia

744.9/Q18.9 Congenital malformation of face and neck, unspecified

749.11/Q36.9 Cleft lip, unilateral

749.12/Q36.9 Cleft lip, unilateral

749.13/Q36.0 Cleft lip, bilateral

749.14/Q36.0 Cleft lip, bilateral

749.21/Q37.9 Unspecified cleft palate with unilateral cleft lip

749.22/Q37.9 Unspecified cleft palate with unilateral cleft lip

749.23/Q37.8 Unspecified cleft palate with bilateral cleft lip

749.24/Q37.8 Unspecified cleft palate with bilateral cleft lip

Skin Lesions and Neoplasms

140.0/C00.0 Malignant neoplasm; of external upper lip

140.1/C00.1 of external lower lip

140.3/C00.3 of upper lip, inner aspect

140.4/C00.4 of lower lip, inner aspect

140.6/C00.6   of commissure of lip, unspecified

172.0/C43.0   of lip

172.0/D03.0   Melanoma in situ of lip

172.1/C43.10   Malignant melanoma; of unspecified eyelid, including canthus

172.2 /C43.20   of unspecified ear and external auricular canal

172.4/C43.4   of scalp and neck

172.4/D03.4   Melanoma in situ of scalp and neck

173.01/C44.01   Basal cell carcinoma of skin of lip

173.02/C44.02   Squamous cell carcinoma of skin of lip

173.09/C44.09   Other specified malignant neoplasm of skin of lip

701.4/L91.0   Hypertrophic scar

709.2/L90.5   Scar conditions and fibrosis of skin

906.0/S01.90XS   Unspecified open would of unspecified part of head, sequela

906.0/S11.90XS   Unspecified open wound of unspecified part of neck, sequela

906.5/T20.00XS   Burn of unspecified degree of head, face, and neck, unspecified site, sequela

Facial Nerve Disorders

351.8/G51.2   Melkersson's syndrome

351.8/G51.4   Facial myokymia

351.8/G51.8   Other disorders of facial nerve

351.9/G51.9   Disorder of facial nerve, unspecified

781.94/R29.810   Facial weakness

907.1/S04.9XXS   Injury of unspecified cranial nerve, sequela

951.4/S04.50XA   Injury of facial nerve, unspecified side, initial encounter

Eyelid and Brow

For eyelids, the sixth digit in *International Classification of Diseases, Tenth Revision, Clinical Modification* (ICD-10-CM) is for location.

1—Right upper eyelid

2—Right lower eyelid

3—Right, unspecified eyelid

4—Left upper eyelid

5—Left lower eyelid

6—Left, unspecified eyelid

9—Unspecified eye, unspecified eyelid

It is important to always use the most specific code. For description below, right upper eyelid is used.

374.11/H02.131   Senile ectropion of right upper eyelid

374.12/H02.121   Mechanical ectropion of right upper eyelid

374.13/H02.141   Spastic ectropion of right upper eyelid

374.14 /H02.111   Cicatricial ectropion of right upper eyelid

374.21/H02.231   Paralytic lagophthalmos of right upper eyelid

374.22/H02.221   Mechanical lagophthalmos of right upper eyelid

374.23/H02.211   Cicatricial lagophthalmos of right upper eyelid

374.31/H02.431   Paralytic ptosis of right eyelid

374.32/H02.421   Myogenic ptosis of right eyelid

374.33/H02.411   Mechanical ptosis of right eyelid

374.41/H02.531 Eyelid retraction right upper eyelid

374.86/H02.811 Retained foreign body in right upper eyelid

374.87/H02.831 Dermatochalasis of right upper eyelid

Trauma

In ICD-10-CM there are a number of codes that relate to trauma. This gets significantly more specific than *International Classification of Diseases, Ninth Revision, Clinical Modification* (ICD-9-CM). Facial fracture codes start with S02. The next two spaces tell the location of the trauma. The sixth character should either be a number or an X for a placeholder. The seventh character is especially important in respect to trauma and needs to be used. The following are the letters used for the seventh character:

A—Initial encounter for closed fracture

B—Initial encounter for open fracture

D—Subsequent encounter for fracture with routine healing

G—Subsequent encounter for fracture with delayed healing

K—Subsequent encounter for fracture with nonunion

S—Sequela

Below is a small example of various codes for trauma. Please consult a dedicated ICD-10-CM resource for a more comprehensive guide.

802.0/S02.2XXA Fracture of nasal bones, initial encounter for closed fracture

802.1/S02.2XXB Fracture of nasal bones, initial encounter for open fracture

802.4/S02.400A Malar fracture unspecified, initial encounter for closed fracture

802.4/S02.401A Maxillary fracture, unspecified, initial encounter for closed fracture

802.4/S02.402A Zygomatic fracture, unspecified, initial encounter for closed fracture

802.6/S02.3XXA Fracture of orbital floor, initial encounter for closed fracture

802.7/S02.3XXB Fracture of orbital floor, initial encounter for open fracture

802.21/S02.61XA Fracture of condylar process of mandible, initial encounter for closed fracture

802.31/S02.61XB Fracture of condylar process of mandible, initial encounter for open fracture

Definition of Codes

Rhinoplasty and Nasal Airway Surgery

1. Rhinoplasty (30400, 30410, 30420, 30430, 30435, 30450)
   a. *Indications*—Nasal valve compromise involving a septal deformity is the primary indication for this procedure when done for functional purposes. Because of this, CPT code 30420 (Rhinoplasty, primary including major septal repair) is the most appropriate code to bill in most cases. Specific indications may include deficiency or weakness of the caudal septum, a severe septal deviation within the caudal or dorsal L—strut, or a severe deviation of the bony pyramid that pulls the septum along with it.
   b. *Definition*—A complete rhinoplasty including osteotomies, lateral and alar cartilage work, and/or nasal tip adjustment, with the inclusion of major nasal septal repair.
   c. *Key points*—This code is different from other rhinoplasty codes because it includes major septal repair, which differentiates functional from purely aesthetic rhinoplasty. However, a few important notes should be made:
      i. A deviated septum alone does not make this a valid code. Rather, the sep-

tum must be deviated in such a way as to preclude correction by septoplasty alone (eg because the septal deviation involves the L-strut).

ii. For a nose with nasal valve compromise due to inward collapse of the upper lateral cartilages but a straight septal L-strut, CPT code 30465 (Repair of nasal vestibular stenosis [eg, spreader grafting, lateral nasal wall reconstruction]) would be a better choice.

iii. "Primary" means the procedure is the patient's first rhinoplasty. A "secondary" rhinoplasty means the patient has had a previous rhinoplasty. The terms are not related to whether the same surgeon has performed the procedures.

iv. Diagnosis codes more specific than, and in addition to that for deviated nasal septum should be used, such as ICD-10-CM code J34.89—Other specified disorders of nose and nasal sinuses—to indicate that there is nasal valve compromise as well as the septal deviation. If the patient has a history of nasal fracture that has caused the septonasal deformity, ICD-10-CM code S02.2XXS—Fracture of nasal bones, sequela—should be included as well as the primary disorder code such as nasal congestion (ICD-10-CM code R09.8). Finally, ICD-10-CM code M95.0—Acquired deformity of nose—should be used instead if the patient has not had any injury that has led to the septonasal deformity and nasal airway obstruction.

d. There is not uniform understanding among the insurance companies that this can be a functional code, and insurance pre-authorization should be obtained.

e. *Controversy*

i. Obtaining insurance approval for this code is often difficult, even in the most straightforward diagnostic case.

1. Patient photographs will be frequently be required by the insurance company prior to approval. In many cases, nasal endoscopy photos are more revealing than the external nasal photos. These are not required but may be sent in addition to document intranasal findings.

2. Documentation of the findings from the office visit is critical. It is important to document findings such as an absent or foreshortened caudal septum or a positive Cottle maneuver. It also may help to spell out in the assessment and plan of the note exactly why septoplasty will fail and rhinoplasty is required. For example, "The severe caudal septal deformity involves the supportive L-strut of the nose which cannot be adequately addressed with septoplasty alone. An open septorhinoplasty approach will be necessary in order to resect and rebuild the caudal septum."

3. Expect that in many cases the surgeon will need to speak directly with the medical director in order to explain the need for rhinoplasty rather than septoplasty alone.

ii. Patients often inquire about changes to their nasal appearance during functional rhinoplasty.

1. In many cases, these patients have a severely twisted nose with a post-traumatic dorsal hump; in these patients the surgery to correct the nasal airway has a good chance of also significantly improving the nasal appearance.

2. Other patients with a more subtle nasal deformity often wish for more subtle corrections (eg, narrowing a nose or refining a tip). In these cases, insurance may be billed for the functional surgery, but the patient must be charged separately for the surgeon's fee, anesthesia fee, and facility fee for the additional OR time spent performing the aesthetic portion of the procedure. Aesthetic rhinoplasty is not covered by the insurance company, even when it is

done in conjunction with functional rhinoplasty or septoplasty.

2. Repair of nasal vestibular stenosis (30465)
   a. *Indications*
      i. Most specifically, this code refers to nasal valve compromise caused by weakness and/or inward collapse of the upper and/or lower lateral cartilages.
      ii. In the absence of a more accurate code, this code can also be used to bill for repairing other forms of nasal vestibular stenosis such as that caused by facial paralysis or cicatricial scarring.
   b. *Definition*—The repair of vestibular stenosis caused by upper lateral cartilage weakness traditionally involves placement of cartilage spreader grafts. However, as noted above there is no better code for many newer techniques that have been described to address this problem.
      i. Other cartilage grafts such as the butterfly graft may also be used to relieve nasal vestibular stenosis due to upper lateral cartilage weakness and inward collapse.
      ii. External nasal valve collapse can also cause vestibular stenosis and is usually treated with alar batten or alar strut grafts.
      iii. Bone-anchored suture attached to the maxilla and passed through the nasal valve is especially useful in patients with nasal valve compromise caused by facial paralysis, and should also be billed using this code.
   c. *Key points*
      i. If performed along with a septoplasty, both codes can be billed. The rhinoplasty code should technically only be used if work is being done on the lateral or alar cartilages or work on the nasal tip or bony pyramid.
      ii. The code 30465 indicates a bilateral procedure. If unilateral repair is performed, modifier 52 (reduced services) should be added.
      iii. Harvest of a graft, if needed for this procedure, is not included in the code and may be billed separately.

3. Repair of nasal septal perforation (30630)
   a. *Indications*—Nasal septal perforation
   b. *Definitions*—Repair of nasal septal perforation
   c. *Key points*—This is the correct code to use for the repair, regardless of the method used for repair. This can be done by rotating a flap of local tissue, taking a graft from another location, using cadaveric tissue, or a combination of the above. However, in certain cases, these additional procedures may be able to be billed in addition to 30630. For further discussion on this topic, see the section, "Controversial Areas," below.

Congenital Deformity

1. Rhinoplasty for cleft nasal deformity (30460, 30462)—Similar to the other rhinoplasty codes, but has a distinct indication of cleft nasal deformity. This code should be chosen instead of 30420 in patients with a history of cleft lip or palate.

2. Plastic repair of cleft lip/nasal deformity (40700, 40701, 40702, 40720, 40761)—The specific code is determined by primary or secondary, unilateral or bilateral, and one or two stages.

3. Otoplasty (69300)
   a. *Indications*—Protruding ear
   b. *Definitions*—Setback ear
   c. *Key points*—Some insurance companies may consider this to be a cosmetic code; obtain insurance preapproval

Skin Lesions and Neoplasms

   a. *Indications*—These are excision codes and are coded based on the size and location and pathology of the lesion.
   b. *Definitions*
      i. 11100, +11101—Simple biopsy of skin with simple closure. Use 11100 for a single lesion and +11101 for each separate/ additional lesion. Note that biopsy of

lip is a special case and has a separate code (40490).

   ii. Excision of lesions—The choice of code is based on the widest diameters of the lesion plus the most narrow margins for excision.

   iii. The excision of skin lesion codes, 114xx and 116xx, include a simple repair. However, an intermediate or complex repair may be separately reported.

   iv. The adjacent tissue transfer codes, 14xxx, include the excision of benign (114xx) or malignant (116xx) skin lesion and should not be separately reported.

c. *Key points*

   i. If multiple lesions of different sites are removed through distinct excisions, these may be billed separately using modifier 51 or 59 depending on the circumstances. Refer to Chapter 11, "Demystifying Modifiers," for more information.

   ii. If multiple distinct lesions of the same site are removed that would all be correctly billed by identical excision codes, these may all be coded individually by adding the modifier 59 to the second and subsequent lesion codes.

Wound Repair

1. Wound repair is classified as simple, intermediate, or complex. Within each category, codes are based on size and location of the repaired wound.
2. For all wound closure codes, the repaired wounds should be measured in centimeters regardless of the shape of the wound.
3. In the case of multiple wounds repaired, add up the lengths of all wounds in the same depth classification (ie, superficial, intermediate, or complex) and in the same location classification, and bill for the total length closed.
4. Do not add lengths of wounds that are in a different location or classification that would necessitate a different code descriptor.
5. Note that in some cases, wound repair codes include various anatomical sites (eg, some

codes include wounds of the scalp, axillae, trunk, and/or extremities). In the code listings that follow, locations outside of the head and neck region have not been included in the code descriptor for simplicity.

6. When more than one classification of wounds is repaired, list the most complicated wound repair as the primary procedure and the less complicated as the secondary procedure, using modifier 59.
7. Debridement is considered a separate procedure only when it requires prolonged cleaning, removal of significant devitalized tissue, or when immediate wound closure is not performed.
8. Simple ligation and cautery of vessels in an open wound is considered part of the wound closure.

Code Descriptions for Wound Repair

1. Simple repair (12001–12007, 12011, 12013–12018)
   a. *Indications*—Use these codes for repair of a superficial wound (epidermis, dermis, subcutaneous tissues) that requires a simple one-layer closure.
   b. *Definitions*—Simple one-layer wound closure.
   c. *Key points*—Includes local anesthesia and cauterization.

2. Intermediate repair (12031–12037, 12041–12047, 12051–12057)
   a. *Indications*—This code is indicated for repair of wounds involving the subcutaneous tissue and fascia in addition to the skin closure.
   b. *Definitions*—This is for layered closure where one layer is in the skin and the deeper layer is in the subcutaneous tissue or fascia, but not within the muscle.
   c. *Key points*—This code may also be billed for simple closure of wounds that have required extensive cleaning or debridement.

3. Complex repair (13120–13122, 13131–13133, 13151–13153)
   a. *Indications*—Choose this code for wounds requiring more complex closure than an

intermediate wound closure. For example, scar revision, extensive debridement of a traumatic wound, extensive undermining, stents, or retention sutures.

b. *Key points*—In contrast to the adjacent tissue transfer codes (14xxx), the simple, intermediate, and complex closure codes do not include excision of benign or malignant lesions, excisional preparation of a wound bed, or debridement of an open fracture. However, simple closure is typically included in the codes for both benign and malignant lesions and thus cannot be separately billed. Often, if an intermediate or complex closure is required, this can be separately billed.

4. Adjacent tissue transfer—no pedicle (14020–14021, 14040–14041, 14060–14061, 14301–14302)
   a. *Indications*—Closure of a large or complex wound that requires elevation and movement of adjacent unaffected tissue into the defect.
   b. *Definitions*—Adjacent tissue transfer.
   c. Key points
      i. The area in square centimeters (sq cm) of both the primary and secondary defects should be documented in the operative note. The area of the primary defect is added to the area of the secondary defect created by the elevation and movement; the sum is used to report the total square centimeters for CPT code choice.
      ii. These codes are reported once per defect; not once per area of tissue moved. For example, bilateral adjacent tissue transfers to close a single primary defect is reported using one adjacent tissue transfer code.
      iii. In the case of adjacent tissue transfer where the flap is being immediately rotated to its final site (ie no delay or pedicle), the area listed refers to the recipient area (not the donor site). Note that the opposite is true for delayed or pedicled flaps.
      iv. Repair of a donor site is considered a separate procedure as long as it requires

harvesting graft material through a separate incision. Simple, intermediate, or complex closure of the primary and secondary defects for the adjacent tissue transfer codes are not separately reported.

Adjacent Tissue Transfer—Pedicled Flaps

1. Formation of direct or tubed pedicle (15572–15576)
   a. *Indication*—A large wound that cannot be closed primarily, but requires adjacent tissue with a pedicle to be moved in to the defect for closure.
   b. *Key points*
      i. Here, the listed body region corresponds to the donor site, not the recipient site as in non-pedicled adjacent tissue transfer.
      ii. Repair of a donor site is considered a separate procedure if is requires harvesting graft material through a separate incision. Otherwise, the primary closure of the surgical wound is included in 15572–15576.
      iii. The pedicled paramedian forehead flap is considered a separate code, as discussed below.

2. Pedicled paramedian forehead flap (15731)
   a. *Indication*—This is to cover open wounds or defects of the skin, often from skin cancer excision.
   b. *Definitions*—This involves elevation and inset of an axial skin flap from the forehead to a nearby location.
   c. *Key points*
      i. This code differs from a routine pedicled flap (15576) because it refers specifically to an axial paramedian forehead flap, where the supratrochlear vessels must be identified and included in the flap.
      ii. The forehead is the donor site for this flap, not the recipient site.
      iii. Primary closure of the donor and recipient sites are included in 15731. If harvest of graft material through a sep-

arate incision is required (eg, skin graft) then it may be separately reported.

3. Delay of flap or sectioning of flap—eyelids, nose, ears, or lips (15630)
   a. *Indications*—This is for either the delay of a flap or the later sectioning of a pedicled flap.
   b. *Definitions*
      i. Delay of flap—when a random skin flap (adjacent tissue transfer codes) is fully incised, undermined, and raised, but is then laid back into place and sutured down in position in order to interrupt the blood supply and allow for subsequent more robust blood supply to the flap.
      ii. Sectioning of pedicled flap—when a pedicled flap has previously been raised and transferred, and is finally being sectioned and inset into position after a time delay.
   c. *Key points*
      i. For a delayed flap which is elevated and replaced, the site listed refers to the donor site.
      ii. If a malignant lesion is excised and the defect closed with a delayed adjacent tissue transfer, at the initial surgery the lesion excision may be coded along with 15630 for raising and delaying the flap. In the second surgery, when the delayed flap is then raised and placed into position, the same code, 15630 appended with modifier 58 should be billed, if this occurs within the global period of the initial code.
      iii. If a pedicled flap is being used, the adjacent tissue transfer can be billed on the first surgical date, and then 15630 can be billed on the day of the flap division and inset, with modifier 58 (if within the global period).

Scar Revision

1. Complex repair codes generally apply for scar revision cases.

2. If adjacent tissue transfer is used (eg, Z-plasty), use the appropriate code from that section (14xxx).
3. Dermabrasion (15781) may be a billable code but requires separate additional work and documentation. This code should not be billed with all scar revisions. This is oftentimes not paid by insurance and should be prior authorized.
4. Some insurance carriers consider scar revision to be a cosmetic procedure.
5. Skin grafting:
   a. *Indications*—A skin graft may be used to close a defect when the location of the defect or other patient factors are not favorable to flap transfer.
   b. *Definitions*
      i. Split-thickness skin graft (15120, 15121) —includes only the epidermis and some of the dermis; this is a significantly thinner skin graft than the full-thickness graft.
      ii. Full-thickness skin graft (15240, 15260) —includes the entire epidermis and dermis down to the subcutaneous fat. The extra thickness often gives a superior cosmetic result when compared to a split-thickness graft. However, the full-thickness graft is used to resurface smaller defects than the split-thickness graft.
   c. *Key points*
      i. Code based on defect size and site.
      ii. A skin graft may be used to close the donor site which is created when an adjacent tissue transfer is used to close a defect. The skin graft to close the donor site may be billed in addition to the adjacent tissue transfer as long as the graft is harvested through a separate incision.

Lip

1. Biopsy of lip (40490)
   a. *Indications*—Lip lesion.
   b. *Definition*—Removal of a small piece of tissue for diagnosis.

c. *Key points*—Does not include full removal of the lesion or margins; if the entire lesion is removed, use an excision code (see below).

2. Excision of lip (40500, 40510, 40520, 40525, 40527)
   a. *Indications*—to fully excise a lip lesion. Do not use these codes for biopsy.
   b. Key points
      i. The lip codes above all include both excision of the lesion and the reconstruction.
      ii. The appropriate code should be based on the both the type of excision and the reconstruction used. If lip reconstruction is done without excision of the lesion, the appropriate skin closure code is included in 40500–40527 and should not be separately billed.
      iii. The most common reason for performing vermilionectomy with mucosal advancement is to treat actinic cheilitis.

3. Repair lip (40650, 40652, 40654)
   a. *Indications*—These codes are used to suture lacerations of the lip. For reconstruction of a surgical wound of the lip, use the appropriate lip closure code or simple, intermediate, complex, or adjacent tissue transfer code as indicated.
   b. *Key points*
      i. These codes all refer to a repair of a full-thickness laceration of the lip. For repair of a more superficial laceration, use the appropriate skin closure code discussed above (120xx, 1315x, 1406x).
      ii. CPT 40650 is used when the laceration involves only the vermilion of the lip. CPT 40652 is used for a more extensive laceration involving the vermilion and a portion of the cutaneous upper lip. CPT 40654 is for a larger or more complex laceration.

Facial Nerve Disorders

1. Nerve graft (64885, 64886)
   a. *Indications*—Facial nerve injury or paralysis requiring a nerve graft for an attempt to restore facial muscle function.
   b. *Key points*
      i. The great auricular and sural nerves are the most common donor nerves for graft.
      ii. Codes include harvest of the donor nerve and placement/suture of the nerve to the recipient site.
      iii. Closure of a separate incision for nerve harvest is included.

2. Suture facial nerve, extracranial (64864)
   a. *Indications*—Damage to the extracranial facial nerve (eg due to trauma or surgical excision for malignancy).
   b. *Definition*—Identification of the cut ends of the nerve, along with suturing of the nerve edges. A nerve graft may or may not be used (nerve graft code can be separately reported).
   c. *Key points*
      i. Includes CPT 69990 (microsurgical techniques requiring use of operating microscope) in addition to this code if an operating microscope was used.
      ii. Codes for harvest of nerve graft (above) may be billed in conjunction with this code if they were used.
      iii. CPT +64872 (suture of nerve, requiring secondary or delayed suture) may be used in addition to 64864 if circumstances such as wound infection or the patient's medical instability require a delayed repair. CPT 64872 is an add-on code, and must be used with an appropriate primary code.

3. Free fascia graft for facial paralysis (15840)
   a. *Indications*—Used when doing a static sling for facial suspension due to facial paralysis.
   b. *Definition*—An incision is made in the skin overlying the fascia to be harvested (ie fascia lata from the thigh), the fascia is harvested for use in the facial sling, and the wound is then closed.
   c. *Key points*—The code includes obtaining the fascia. CPT says modifier 50 may be used if a bilateral procedure is performed though payers may not recognize this modifier as CMS does not have the code set

up to accept modifier 50. In that instance, modifier 59 may be more appropriate on the second of the same code.

4. Free muscle graft for facial paralysis (15841)
   a. *Indications*—Muscle wasting secondary to long-standing facial nerve paralysis.
   b. *Definition*—A piece of muscle is harvested from a remote area of the body, and transferred to the face to reduce the facial deformity caused by muscle wasting from facial nerve paralysis.

5. Free muscle flap for facial paralysis—by microsurgical technique (15842)
   a. *Indications*—Long-standing facial nerve paralysis.
   b. *Definition*—A muscle distant from the face is harvested along with its supplying blood vessels and nerves, which are anastomosed in the recipient site using microsurgical techniques.
   c. *Key points*—Surgical microscope use is included with this code; 69990 may not be separately billed.

6. Regional muscle transfer for facial paralysis (15845)
   a. *Indications*—Facial nerve paralysis.
   b. *Definition*—A portion of the temporalis, masseter, or digastric muscle is rotated to the affected area of the face and sutured in place.
   c. *Key points*—No microsurgical techniques are used for this code.

7. Microsurgical techniques requiring use of operating microscope (69990)
   a. *Indications*—When an operating microscope is required to perform a procedure.
   b. *Definition*—Use of operating microscope for microdissection or microsurgical techniques. The code is not reported if the microscope is used only for magnification or illumination.
   c. *Key points*
      i. This code may be used in addition to the primary procedure code when necessary and documented appropriately in the procedure statement as well as in the body of the operative note.
      ii. CPT 69990 may only be added on once per surgical case even if used in during more than one billable procedure.
      iii. Some codes include the use of operating microscope; in these cases 69990 cannot be billed in addition to the primary code.

8. Rhytidectomy (15829)
   a. *Indications*—Primarily considered a cosmetic procedure code; however, in patients with severe skin laxity due to facial nerve paralysis, this code may be covered.
   b. *Definitions*—Skin and subcutaneous tissue as well as the superficial muscular aponeurotic system (SMAS) are raised, trimmed, and resutured to remove the excess laxity from the paralyzed side of the face and restore a more normal facial contour.
   c. *Key points*—Payment of this code will require extensive documentation in order for the insurer to not dismiss this as a cosmetic code.

Eyelid and Brow

1. Blepharoplasty—upper eyelid, with excessive skin weighing down lid (15823)
   a. *Indications*—Blepharoplasty may be billed to the insurance company when excess upper eyelid skin obscures the upper portion of the visual field. Follow payer specific medical policies.
   b. *Definitions*—Excision of excess upper eyelid skin and fat.
   c. *Key Points*—Visual field obstruction due to the redundant upper eyelid skin must be documented in order for this to be considered a medically necessary procedure that is covered by the insurance company.
      i. Visual field testing taped and untaped must demonstrate an improvement in visual field—check with provider for specific improvement necessary.
      ii. Photographs demonstrating excess upper eyelid skin (resting on or above eyelashes) are frequently requested and are helpful supporting documents.

2. Medial Canthopexy (21280)
   a. *Indications*—Lower eyelid laxity and poor drainage of lacrimal sec.
   b. *Definition*—Suspension of the medial canthal tendon using suture.
   c. *Key points*—If lateral canthopexy is done in the same setting, bill 21280 primarily and append modifier 51 to 21282.

3. Lateral Canthopexy (21282)
   a. *Indications*—Lower eyelid laxity, lagophthalmos.
   b. *Definition*—Resuspension of the lateral canthal tendon to the lateral orbital rim using sutures.
   c. *Key points*—If medial canthopexy is done in the same setting, bill 21280 primarily and append modifier 51 to 21282.

4. Canthoplasty (67950)
   a. *Indications*—Lower eyelid laxity, lagophthalmos.
   b. *Definition*—Reconstruction of canthus; includes lateral canthotomy with trimming and resuspension of excess length of lateral canthus.
   c. *Key points*—This code is included in repair codes such as 67917 and 67924, so it cannot be billed separately.

5. Correction of lagophthalmos with lid load (67912)
   a. *Indications*—Lagophthalmos with poor upper eyelid closure, most commonly due to facial nerve paralysis (paralytic lagophthalmos).
   b. *Definition*—Implantation of upper eyelid lid load (eg, gold weight).
   c. *Key points*—Most payers include the cost of the gold weight in the reimbursement for surgery, but if a payer does not include this, it may be billed separately using HCPCS code L8610, ocular implant, if you have incurred the expense for the implant. Otherwise, the cost is included in the facility's payment.

6. Ectropion (67914–67917)
   a. *Indications*—Symptomatic ectropion.

   b. *Key points*—Canthoplasty is included in CPT 67917, so 67950 cannot be billed in addition to this code.

7. Entropion (67921–67924)
   a. *Indications*—Symptomatic entropion.
   b. *Key points*—Canthoplasty is included in CPT 67924, so 67950 cannot be billed in addition to this code.

8. Repair of brow ptosis (67900)
   a. *Indication*—A ptotic brow due to facial paralysis.
   b. *Definition*—Elevation and resuspension of the frontalis muscle with excision of excess skin.
   c. *Key points*
      i. This procedure may be covered if the brow droop is causing visual field impairment. Taped and untaped visual fields will likely be required; the degree of improvement with taping necessary for approval will depend on the particular provider.

Trauma

1. Nasal fracture: Closed reduction of nasal fracture (21315, 21320)
   a. *Indications*—Displaced nasal bone fracture.
   b. *Definitions*—Reduction of nasal bone fracture without making incisions in nasal skin.
   c. *Key points*—CPT 21320 requires internal or external fixation; if no fixation is used then use 21315.

2. Nasal fracture: Closed reduction of nasal septal fracture (21337)
   a. *Indications*—To straighten a deviated nasal septum resulting from a nasal septal fracture.
   b. *Definition*—Manipulation of nasal septum, without any incision, in an attempt to mobilize the fractured septum back to midline.
   c. *Key points*—Code applies to fracture reduction with or without stabilization.

3. Nasal fracture: Open treatment of nasal fracture (21325, 21330, 21335, 21336)
   a. *Indications*—Nasal fracture that cannot be corrected with closed reduction alone.
   b. *Key points*
      i. If osteotomies alone correct the fracture, then this is considered an uncomplicated surgery. The use of wires, plates, screws, or grafts make this a complicated procedure.
      ii. There is controversy regarding when to use rhinoplasty codes and when to use open reduction of nasal fracture codes. This is discussed in more detail in the section, "Controversial Areas."

4. Naso-orbito-ethmoid (NOE) complex: open treatment of nasoethmoid fracture (21338–21340)
   a. *Indications*—Naso-orbito-ethmoid fracture.
   b. *Key points*—CPT 21340 includes repair of canthal ligaments and/or nasolacrimal apparatus.

5. Frontal sinus
   a. *Indications*—Frontal sinus fracture involving anterior or anterior and posterior.
   b. *Key points*—CPT 21344 indicates that a coronal or multiple approaches were used.

6. LeFort I (palatal or maxillary) fractures
   a. *Indications*—LeFort I fracture.
   b. *Key points*—LeFort fractures may not occur exactly along the textbook classification guidelines. In practice, choose the LeFort level that is most appropriate. The LeFort codes assume bilateral repair; therefore, modifier 50 is not used.

7. LeFort II (nasomaxillary buttress)
   a. *Indications*—Nasomaxillary complex fracture.
   b. *Key points*
      i. CPT 21348 includes obtaining the graft.
      ii. LeFort fractures may not occur exactly along the textbook classification guidelines. In practice, choose the LeFort level that is most appropriate.
      iii. The LeFort codes assume bilateral repair; therefore, modifier 50 is not used.

8. LeFort III (craniofacial separation)
   a. *Indications*—LeFort III fracture.
   b. *Key points*
      i. CPT 21436 includes obtaining bone graft.
      ii. LeFort fractures may not occur exactly along the textbook classification guidelines. In practice, choose the LeFort level that is most appropriate.
      iii. The LeFort codes assume bilateral repair; therefore, modifier 50 is not used.

9. Zygomaticomaxillary complex (ZMC)
   a. *Key points*—The correct code is determined based on fracture location, approach(es), degree of fixation necessary, and need for bone grafting.

10. Orbit—blowout fracture treatment
    a. *Key points*—The main determination of which code to choose is the approach used to reduce and fixate the fracture.

11. Orbit—non-blowout fracture treatment
    a. *Key points*—CPT 21400 is a management code but does not require manipulation. The remaining codes may be chosen based on open or closed treatment and with or without manipulation, implant, and bone grafting.

12. Alveolar ridge
    a. *Key points*—CPT 21440 is a separate procedure code—if this procedure is performed in the course of another, more extensive surgery, this code should not be used.

13. Mandible
    a. *Indications*—Mandible fracture.
    b. *Definitions*—This can be done open, closed, or percutaneous. Manipulation can be used, and the code will reflect this. Finally, the use of fixation can be part of the code.
    c. *Key points*
       i. CPT 21450 is an evaluation and management code without surgical manipulation
       ii. The remaining codes are determined based on the location of the fracture,

the type of fixation used, and the nature of the treatment (open vs closed).

   iii. *CPT Assistant*, November 2002, states this code is a unilateral procedure and may be reported with modifier 50 if separate right and left fractures are repaired.

Common Grafts in Facial Plastic Surgery

1. Composite graft harvest (15760)
   a. *Indications*—Need for a graft of skin and attached cartilage.
   b. *Definition*—Harvest of graft of skin with attached cartilage, often from ear, through a separate incision.
   c. *Key points*—Code includes closure of donor site.

2. Graft of dermis/fat/fascia (15770)
   a. *Indications*—To blend in blemishes or defects left behind by surgical excision, atrophy, or other fleshy "stand-outs."
   b. *Definition*—To restore the defect to its normal positioning as closely as possible by using multiple layers.
   c. *Key points*—The tissue used for the graft can be a continuous portion (containing all 3 of the layered components), individual parts (grafted layer by layer), or inserted in combination (such as fascia-fat layer, later covered by a dermal layer). (*CPT Assistant*, September 1997).

3. Tissue grafts, other (eg, paratenon, fat, dermis); (20926)
   a. *Indications*—Use when a single layer of tissue is harvested (eg, abdominal fat graft) through a separate incision.
   b. *Definition*—Removal of tissue for graft.
   c. *Key points*—Code includes the harvest and placement of the tissue as well as wound closure.

4. Acellular dermal replacement of the face (15275, 15276)
   a. *Indications*—When an acellular dermal replacement is necessary to act as skin

replacement in the face or neck up to the first 100 sq cm.
   b. *Definitions*—Acellular dermal replacement in face, scalp, eyelids, mouth, neck, ears, orbits (and some non-head and neck codes).
   c. *Key points*—For placement of a biologic implant for soft tissue reinforcement in the head and neck (ie, need for acellular dermal matrix as an inner layer during nasal septal perforation repair), an unlisted code, such as 17999, should be used. CPT 15777 may be reported only for a procedure in the breast or trunk.

5. Application of skin substitute graft to open wound (15277)
   a. *Indications*—This code is used when a skin substitute graft (eg, Oasis, Integra) is placed into an open wound to act as skin replacement. Used when the sum of the open wounds is 100 sq cm or greater. If the sum is less than 100 sq cm, then 15275 and 15276 should be used.
   b. *Definitions*—Application of skin substitute grafts to the face, scalp, eyelids, mouth, neck, ears, orbits (and some non-head and neck sites) to the first 100 sq cm or 1% of body area in children.
   c. *Key points*—This code applies when skin substitute is applied as a replacement for skin; it is not used when the biologic material is placed for soft tissue reinforcement.

6. Unlisted procedure, skin, mucous membranes, and subcutaneous tissue (17999)
   a. *Indications*—May be used when acellular dermal matrix is used as an implant for soft tissue reinforcement.
   b. *Definitions*—Unlisted procedure, skin, mucous membrane, and subcutaneous tissue.
   c. *Key points*—Although 15777 describes most closely the use of acellular dermal matrix as an implant for soft tissue reinforcement as used during repair of nasal septal perforation, the code description is used to describe reinforcement of only the breast and trunk. For the intranasal use,

the unlisted procedure code 17999 may be used, and 15777 may be given as a comparison code.

7. Nasal septal cartilage harvest for graft (20912)
   a. *Indications*—Need for cartilage for graft for use in another procedure.
   b. *Definitions*—Harvest of nasal septal cartilage for graft, through a separate incision, to another site.
   c. *Key points*
      i. The technique used is similar to that for septoplasty, but the goal is to harvest cartilage for use as graft material rather than to correct the nasal airway.
      ii. Nasal septal cartilage harvest is separately billable if a rhinoplasty (30410) is billed as the primary code, but not if septorhinoplasty (30420) or septoplasty (30520) is billed.

8. Osteoplasty, Facial bones; augmentation (autograft, allograft, or prosthetic implant); (21208)
   a. *Indications*—Facial deformity requiring surgical augmentation.
   b. *Definitions*—Augmentation of the facial skeleton using autograft, allograft, or prosthetic implant.
   c. *Key points*—This code applies whether graft is an autograft, allograft, or even a prosthetic implant.

9. Graft; rib cartilage, autogenous, to face, chin, nose or ear (includes obtaining graft (21230)
   a. *Indications*—Need for cartilage graft for reconstruction of a different facial site, frequently the nose.
   b. *Definitions*—Harvest of autogenous rib cartilage and use of that cartilage to reconstruct a portion of the face (eg, nose, ear).
   c. *Key points*—Clearly document why the rib cartilage harvest is necessary for functional and not just cosmetic reasons. Code includes harvest of graft and placement of it for reconstruction.

10. Ear cartilage harvest for graft (21235)
    a. *Indications*—Need for cartilage for a separate procedure.
    b. *Definitions*—A separate incision is used for the sole purpose of harvesting ear cartilage to be used as a graft in a distinct procedure.
    c. *Key points*—Operative report must clearly document that the cartilage is necessary for a functional, and not cosmetic, procedure. This code includes the harvest of the graft and the placement of it into the donor area.

11. Excise oral mucosa for graft (40818)
    a. *Indications*—Need for oral mucosal as graft material.
    b. *Definitions*—Excision of vestibule of mouth as donor graft.
    c. *Key points*—A buccal mucosal graft is an example of a procedure that would fit this code.

Controversial Areas

Rhinoplasty

Much of the problem stems from the fact that the available codes tend to match aesthetic rhinoplasty more than they match functional rhinoplasty. Another problem is that functional rhinoplasty is quite variable, with different parts of the procedure necessary in different patients. For example, 30400 covers cartilage and tip work, 30410 represents "complete" rhinoplasty with osteotomies, upper lateral cartilage, and tip work, and 30420 represents a "complete" rhinoplasty plus a major septal repair. The difficulty is that patients requiring functional rhinoplasty may not need tip work, but need major septal repair and spreader grafts. In general, however, if a patient requires a septorhinoplasty rather than a septoplasty to improve airway function, this frequently involves some modification of the tip (at least a columellar strut graft), and so 30420 is most appropriate for the majority of these cases.

A related controversy is the scenario where spreader grafts are placed and a septoplasty is performed in order to open a patient's nasal airway. In many cases where both procedures are necessary to improve the airway, this will require a septorhinoplasty, and the correct code will be 30420. However, in the event that nasal vestibular stenosis is repaired without rhinoplasty, report the septoplasty code (30520) and 30465. However, if septal cartilage is harvested for spreader grafts during the septoplasty, then do not separately report the graft harvest (20912). Separate reporting of the graft harvest, 20912, harvest of cartilage graft from the nasal septum, in addition to 30465 requires no separate work on the septum.

The final controversy (or confusion) related to nasal surgery is of when to bill for open treatment of nasal bone fracture (21325, 21330, 21335) and when to bill for rhinoplasty when it is done to correct the late effects of nasal bone fracture. In general, the fracture codes should be used for an acute or recent fracture. If the patient has a remote history of fracture that caused the deformity, this is important to document for the insurance coverage of functional rhinoplasty, but the correct codes to choose would be the rhinoplasty rather than the fracture codes. Also, note that the fracture codes do not permit separate billing of septoplasty (30520). Rather, if an open nasal septal fracture is treated concomitantly with an open nasal bone fracture, the correct code is 21335.

Closure of Nasal Septal Perforation

Surgical closure of nasal septal perforation (30630) includes the local tissue advancement used to close the defect. However, in the case of large septal perforations (>1 cm), this local tissue is likely to be inadequate to close the defect. In such cases, more extensive surgery must be performed and tissue recruited from elsewhere to close the defect. For these cases, the Medicare RVUs assigned to 30630 do not accurately reflect the time and effort needed to close the defect. This can be somewhat overcome by adding modifier 22 (increased procedural services) appended to the original code 30620. When using modifier 22, the surgeon must document the actual time spent on the repair, as well as the complex nature of the repair.

Conclusion

Coding for facial plastic surgery may be challenging due to the fact that complex reconstructive surgeries may not always fit cleanly into a single CPT code. The guidelines above should help to clarify scenarios in which a given code should be used, and also suggestions for when and how to use an unlisted code. Even with proper coding, reimbursement may be difficult in the case of many facial plastic surgery procedures, which insurance carriers tend to view as cosmetic unless strong proof otherwise is provided. It is essential to obtain insurance preapproval and work out ahead of time with the insurance carrier which codes will be submitted for a particular case. In addition, in order to prove that the surgery is functional or reconstructive and not aesthetic, expect to submit photographs and written justification for the planned procedure. With proper coding and documentation, reimbursement for these procedures can be achieved.

CHAPTER 28

Operative Head and Neck Surgery

Andrew M. Hinson and Brendan C. Stack, Jr.

Introduction

This chapter describes coding for head and neck oncologic surgery including lymphatic neck dissection, laryngectomy, glossectomy, parotidectomy, thyroidectomy, parathyroidectomy, and skull base surgery. Coding and billing procedures with their respective medical indication(s) is generally intuitive based on the definitions provided in the *Current Procedural Terminology*[1] (CPT) and International Classification of Diseases[2] (ICD) handbooks. However, the services described in this chapter are rather complex and often performed in various combinations with one another. When multiple surgeons are involved in the procedure, each surgeon should only code for the procedure that he or she was involved in. Thus, it is appropriate for these codes to be unbundled in these situations unless the 2 surgeons were co-surgeons (then use modifier 62). Special attention is thus given to billing comprehensive versus component codes when it comes to codes that include a radical neck dissection (eg, parotidectomy, glossectomy, laryngectomy), and how/when it is appropriate to append modifiers in the context of National Correct Coding Initative[3] (NCCI) edits. Finally, some novel surgical techniques are not yet described by current CPT codes, and reimbursement depends on unlisted codes.

Key Points

- The comprehensive head and neck CPT codes often include a radical neck dissection (RND) with the resection, but not modified radical neck dissection (MRND). NCCI edits bundles some (but not all) comprehensive codes with a MRND. As a result, when performing a resection with a MRND, and there is an option for a code that includes a radical neck dissection, one must use the resection code without the neck dissection and bill the MRND separately with a 59 modifier.
- Laryngectomy (31360–31395) and total glossectomy (41140–41153) include a planned tracheostomy (31600).
- Thyroidectomy with a limited neck dissection (60252) includes removal of lymph nodes in the perithyroid region and a central neck dissection, which is not considered to have laterality—modifier 50 does *not* apply.
- Autotransplantation of a parathyroid gland during the course of a partial or total thyroidectomy is appended with modifier 22 to the primary procedure code and not separately reported with the add-on code, 60512.

303

- Parathyroid autotransplantation is reported as the add-on code 60512 after parathyroidectomy and is never reported independently.
- It is not accurate to use existing open skull base codes for endonasal endoscopic procedures because the existing codes describe an open procedure involving skin incision(s) and lengthy inpatient care (see Chapter 30, "Skull Base Surgery," for more details).
- Medical indications for using computer-assisted navigational guidance (61782, cranial, extradural) should be supported in both the clinical and operative documentation (eg, extradural skull base tumor resection).
- Some otolaryngologists provide exposure to the cervical spine for spine surgeons (eg, anterior cervical discectomy, decompression, and fusion). The approach to the cervical spine is included in all spine surgery codes such as 22551 and 63081. There are no separate approach codes; therefore, the otolaryngologist would report the spine surgeon's primary procedure code with modifier 62 (2 surgeons).
- Intraoperative nerve monitoring (IONM) add-on codes (95940, 95941, or G0453) are not coded separately unless a qualified provider is solely dedicated to the service.

Key Procedure Codes

Head/Maxillofacial

21011 Excision, tumor, soft tissue of face or scalp, subcutaneous; less than 2 cm
wRVU 2.99; Global 90

   21012 2 cm or greater
   wRVU 4.45; Global 90

21034 Excision of malignant tumor of maxilla or zygoma
wRVU 17.38; Global 90

21040 Excision of benign tumor or cyst of mandible, by enucleation and/or curettage
wRVU 4.91; Global 90

21044 Excision of malignant tumor of mandible:
wRVU 12.80; Global 90

   21045 radical resection
   wRVU 18.37; Global 90

21046 Excision of benign tumor or cyst of mandible; requiring intra-oral osteotomy (eg, locally aggressive or destructive lesion[s])
wRVU 14.21; Global 90

   21047 requiring extra-oral osteotomy and partial mandibulectomy (eg, locally aggressive or destructive lesion[s])
   wRVU 20.07; Global 90

21048 Excision of benign tumor or cyst of maxilla; requiring intra-oral osteotomy (eg, locally aggressive or destructive lesion[s])
wRVU 14.71; Global 90

   21049 requiring extra-oral osteotomy and partial maxillectomy (eg, locally aggressive or destructive lesion[s])
   wRVU 19.32; Global 90

21198 Osteotomy, mandible, segmental
wRVU 15.71; Global 90

21206 Osteotomy, maxilla, segmental (eg, Wassmund or Schuchard)
wRVU 15.59; Global 90

21299 Unlisted craniofacial and maxillofacial procedure
wRVU 0.00; Global YYY

21499 Unlisted musculoskeletal procedure, head
wRVU 0.00; Global YYY

31040 Pterygomaxillary fossa surgery, any approach
wRVU 9.77; Global 90

31225 Maxillectomy; without orbital
exenteration
wRVU 26.70; Global 90

> **31230** with orbital exenteration
> (en bloc)
> *wRVU 30.82; Global 90*

Respiratory

31360 Laryngectomy; total, without radical
neck dissection
wRVU 29.91; Global 90

> **31365** total, with radical neck
> dissection
> *wRVU 38.81; Global 90*
>
> **31367** subtotal supraglottic, without
> radical neck dissection
> *wRVU 30.57; Global 90*
>
> **31368** subtotal supraglottic, with
> radical neck dissection
> *wRVU 34.19; Global 90*

31370 Partial laryngectomy
(hemilaryngectomy); horizontal
wRVU 27.57; Global 90

> **31375** laterovertical
> *wRVU 26.07; Global 90*
>
> **31380** anterovertical
> *wRVU 25.57; Global 90*
>
> **31382** antero-latero-vertical
> *wRVU 28.57; Global 90*

31390 Pharyngolaryngectomy, with radical
neck dissection; without reconstruction
wRVU 42.51; Global 90

> **31395** with reconstruction
> *wRVU 43.80; Global 90*

31420 Epiglottidectomy
wRVU 11.43; Global 90

31525 Laryngoscopy, direct, with or without
tracheoscopy; diagnostic, except
newborn
wRVU 2.63; Global 0

31599 Unlisted procedure, larynx
wRVU 0.00; Global YYY

31600 Tracheostomy, planned (separate
procedure)
wRVU 7.17; Global 0

31603 Tracheostomy, emergency procedure;
transtracheal
wRVU 4.14; Global 0

> **31605** cricothyroid membrane
> *wRVU 3.57; Global 0*

31610 Tracheostomy, fenestration procedure
with skin flaps
wRVU 9.38; Global 90

31613 Tracheostoma revision; simple, without
flap rotation
wRVU 4.71; Global 90

> **31614** complex, with flap rotation
> *wRVU 8.63; Global 90*

31622 Bronchoscopy, rigid or flexible, including
fluoroscopic guidance, when performed;
diagnostic, with cell washing, when
performed (separate procedure)
wRVU 2.78; Global 0

31785 Excision of tracheal tumor or carcinoma;
cervical
wRVU 18.35; Global 90

Lymphatics

38500 Biopsy or excision of lymph node(s);
open, superficial
wRVU 3.79; Global 10

> **38505** by needle, superficial (eg,
> cervical, inguinal, axillary)
> *wRVU 1.14; Global 0*
>
> **38510** open, deep cervical node(s)
> *wRVU 6.74; Global 10*
>
> **38520** open, deep cervical node(s) with
> excision of scalene fat pad
> *wRVU 7.03; Global 90*

38542 Dissection, deep jugular node(s)
wRVU 7.95; Global 90

38550 Excision of cystic hygroma, axillary or cervical; without deep neurovascular dissection
wRVU 7.11; Global 90

  38555 with deep neurovascular dissection
  wRVU 15.59; Global 90

38700 Suprahyoid lymphadenectomy
wRVU 12.81; Global 90

38720 Cervical lymphadenectomy (complete)
wRVU 21.95; Global 90

38724 Cervical lymphadenectomy (modified radical neck dissection)
wRVU 23.95; Global 90

38999 Unlisted procedure, hemic or lymphatic system
wRVU 0.00; Global YYY

Digestive Tract

41112 Excision of lesion of tongue with closure; anterior two-thirds
wRVU 2.83; Global 90

  41113 posterior one-third
  wRVU 3.29; Global 90

41120 Glossectomy; less than one-half tongue
wRVU 11.14; Global 90

  41130 hemiglossectomy
  wRVU 15.74; Global 90

  41135 partial, with unilateral radical neck dissection
  wRVU 30.14; Global 90

  41140 complete or total, with or without tracheostomy, without radical neck dissection
  wRVU 29.15; Global 90

  41145 complete or total, with or without tracheostomy, with unilateral radical neck dissection
  wRVU 37.93; Global 90

41150 composite procedure with resection floor of mouth and mandibular resection, without radical neck dissection
wRVU 29.86; Global 90

  41153 composite procedure with resection floor of mouth, with suprahyoid neck dissection
  wRVU 33.59; Global 90

  41155 composite procedure with resection floor of mouth, mandibular resection, and radical neck dissection (Commando type)
  wRVU 44.30; Global 90

41559 Unlisted procedure, tongue, floor of mouth
wRVU 0.00; Global YYY

41830 Alveolectomy, including curettage of osteitis or sequestrectomy
wRVU 3.45; Global 10

41899 Unlisted procedure, dentoalveolar structures
wRVU 0.00; Global YYY

42104 Excision, lesion of palate, uvula; without closure
wRVU 1.69; Global 90

42120 Resection of palate or extensive resection of lesion
wRVU 11.86; Global 90

42140 Uvulectomy, excision of uvula
wRVU 1.70; Global 90

42299 Unlisted procedure, palate, uvula
wRVU 0.00; Global YYY

42808 Excision or destruction of lesion of pharynx, any method
wRVU 2.35; Global 10

42842 Radical resection of tonsil, tonsillar pillars, and/or retromolar trigone; without closure
wRVU 12.23; Global 90

42890 Limited pharyngectomy
wRVU 10.13; Global 90

42892 Resection of lateral pharyngeal wall or pyriform sinus, direct closure by advancement of lateral and posterior pharyngeal walls
wRVU 26.03; Global 90

43100 Excision of lesion, esophagus, with primary repair; cervical approach
wRVU 9.66; Global 90

43191 Esophagoscopy, rigid, transoral; diagnostic, including collection of specimen(s) by brushing or washing when performed (separate procedure)
wRVU 2.49; Global 0

43200 Esophagoscopy, flexible, transoral; diagnostic, including collection of specimen(s) by brushing or washing, when performed (separate procedure)
wRVU 1.52; Global 0

Salivary Glands

42400 Biopsy of salivary gland; needle
wRVU 0.78; Global 0

> **42405** incisional
> *wRVU 3.34; Global 10*

42408 Excision of sublingual salivary cyst (ranula)
wRVU 4.66; Global 90

42409 Marsupialization of sublingual salivary cyst (ranula)
wRVU 2.91; Global 90

42410 Excision of parotid tumor or parotid gland; lateral lobe, without nerve dissection
wRVU 9.57; Global 90

> **42415** lateral lobe, with dissection and preservation of facial nerve
> *wRVU 17.16; Global 90*

> **42420** total, with dissection and preservation of facial nerve
> *wRVU 19.53; Global 90*

> **42425** total, en bloc removal with sacrifice of facial nerve
> *wRVU 13.42; Global 90*

> **42426** total, with unilateral radical neck dissection
> *wRVU 22.66; Global 90*

42440 Excision of submandibular (submaxillary) gland
wRVU 6.14; Global 90

42450 Excision of sublingual gland
wRVU 4.74; Global 90

42699 Unlisted procedure, salivary glands or ducts
wRVU 0.00; Global YYY

Thyroid and Parathyroid Glands

60210 Partial thyroid lobectomy, unilateral; with or without isthmusectomy
wRVU 11.23; Global 90

> **60212** with contralateral subtotal lobectomy, including isthmusectomy
> *wRVU 16.43; Global 90*

60220 Total thyroid lobectomy, unilateral; with or without isthmusectomy
wRVU 11.19; Global 90

> **60225** with contralateral subtotal lobectomy, including isthmusectomy
> *wRVU 14.79; Global 90*

60240 Thyroidectomy, total or complete
wRVU 15.04; Global 90

60252 Thyroidectomy, total or subtotal for malignancy; with limited neck dissection
wRVU 22.01; Global 90

> **60254** with radical neck dissection
> *wRVU 28.42; Global 90*

60260 Thyroidectomy, removal of all remaining thyroid tissue following previous removal of a portion of thyroid
wRVU 18.26; Global 90

60270 Thyroidectomy, including substernal thyroid; sternal split or transthoracic approach
wRVU 23.20; Global 90

60271 cervical approach
wRVU 17.62; Global 90

60500 Parathyroidectomy or exploration of parathyroid(s);
wRVU 15.60; Global 90

60502 re-exploration
wRVU 21.15; Global 90

60505 with mediastinal exploration, sternal split or transthoracic approach
wRVU 23.06; Global 90

+60512 Parathyroid autotransplantation (List separately in addition to code for primary procedure)
wRVU 4.44; Global ZZZ

60520 Thymectomy, partial or total; transcervical approach (separate procedure)
wRVU 17.16; Global 90

60521 sternal split or transthoracic approach, with radical mediastinal dissection (separate procedure)
wRVU 19.18; Global 90

60699 Unlisted procedure, endocrine system
wRVU 0.00; Global YYY

Neck

21555 Excision, tumor, soft tissue of neck or anterior thorax, subcutaneous; less than 3 cm
wRVU 3.96; Global 90

#21552 3 cm of greater
wRVU 6.49; Global 90

21556 Excision, tumor, soft tissue of neck or anterior thorax, subfascial (eg, intramuscular); less than 5 cm
wRVU 7.66; Global 90

#21554 5 cm or greater
wRVU 11.13; Global 90

21557 Radical resection of tumor (eg, sarcoma), soft tissue of neck or anterior thorax; less than 5 cm
wRVU 14.75; Global 90

21558 5 cm or greater
wRVU 21.58; Global 90

42810 Excision branchial cleft cyst or vestige, confined to skin and subcutaneous tissues
wRVU 3.38; Global 90

42815 Excision branchial cleft cyst, vestige, or fistula, extending beneath subcutaneous tissues and/or into pharynx
wRVU 7.31; Global 90

60600 Excision of carotid body tumor; without excision of carotid artery
wRVU 25.09; Global 90

60605 with excision of carotid artery
wRVU 31.96; Global 90

Skull and Skull Base

(See Chapter 30, "Skull Base Surgery," for more details.)

61575 Transoral approach to skull base, brain stem or upper spinal cord for biopsy, decompression or excision of lesion,
wRVU 36.56; Global 90

61576 requiring splitting of tongue and/or mandible (including tracheostomy)
wRVU 55.31; Global 90

61580 Craniofacial approach to anterior cranial fossa; extradural, including lateral rhinotomy, ethmoidectomy, sphenoidectomy, without maxillectomy or orbital exenteration
wRVU 34.51; Global 90

62165 Neuroendoscopy, intracranial; with excision of pituitary tumor, transnasal or transphenoidal approach
wRVU 23.23; Global 90

69150 Radical excision external auditory canal lesion; without neck dissection
wRVU 13.61; Global 90

69155 with neck dissection
wRVU 23.35; Global 90

69535 Resection temporal bone, external approach
wRVU 37.42; Global 90

69960 Decompression internal auditory canal
wRVU 29.42; Global 90

69970 Removal of tumor, temporal bone
wRVU 32.41; Global 90

Special Topics

36500 Venous catheterization for selective organ blood sampling blood sampling
wRVU 3.51; Global 0

+61781 Stereotactic computer-assisted (navigational) procedure; cranial, intradural (List separately in addition to code for primary procedure)
wRVU 3.75; Global ZZZ

+61782 cranial, extradural (List separately in addition to code for primary procedure)
wRVU 3.18; Global ZZZ

+69990 Microsurgical techniques, requiring use of operating microscope (List separately in addition to code for primary procedure)
wRVU 3.46; Global ZZZ

78808 Injection procedure for radiopharmaceutical localization by non-imaging probe study, intravenous (eg, parathyroid adenoma)
wRVU 0.18; Global XXX

92585 Auditory evoked potentials for evoked response audiometry and/or testing of the central nervous system; comprehensive
wRVU (26) 0.50 (TC) 0.00; Global XXX

95867 Needle electromyography; cranial nerve supplied muscle(s), unilateral
wRVU (26) 0.79 (TC) 0.00; Global XXX

#+95887 Needle electromyography, non-extremity (cranial nerve supplied or axial) muscle(s) done with nerve conduction, amplitude and latency/velocity study (List separately in addition to code for primary procedure)
wRVU (26) 0.71 (TC) 0.00; Global ZZZ

#+95940 Continuous intraoperative neurophysiology monitoring in the operating room, one on one monitoring requiring personal attendance, each 15 minutes (List separately in addition to code for primary procedure)
wRVU 0.60; Global XXX

#+95941 Continuous intraoperative neurophysiology monitoring, from outside the operating room (remote or nearby) or for monitoring of more than one case while in the operating room, per hour (List separately in addition to code for primary procedure)
wRVU 0.00; Global XXX

G0453 Continuous intraoperative neurophysiology monitoring, from outside the operating room (remote or nearby), per patient, (attention directed exclusively to one patient) each 15 minutes (list in addition to primary procedure)
wRVU 0.60; Global XXX

Key Modifiers

22 Increased Procedural Services
This could be used when additional non-lymphatic structures are removed during a neck dissection besides those listed for a RND or MRND. Thus modifier 22 would be appended to 38720 or 38724.

50 Bilateral Procedure
This would be used for a bilateral neck dissection; modifier 50 is appended to 38720 or 38724.

59 Distinct Procedural Service
At times this is needed to inform the payer that 2 procedures are done at the same time and should

not be bundled. This can occur when performing both laryngoscopy and bronchoscopy at the same setting. Often both procedures are required for thorough examination of the upper airway for pathology. Modifier 59 should thus be added to 31622, the lower valued code, in these situations when 31525 and 31622 are appropriately billed together.

Key ICD-9-CM/ICD-10-CM Codes

140.5/C00.5   Malignant neoplasm; of lip, unspecified, inner aspect

140.9/C00.2   of external lip, unspecified

141.0/C01   of base of tongue

141.4/C02.3   of anterior two-thirds of tongue, part unspecified

142.0/C07   of parotid gland

142.1/C08.0   of submandibular gland

142.2/C08.1   of sublingual gland

143.0/C03.0   of upper gum

143.1/C03.1   of lower gum

144.9/C04.9   of floor of mouth, unspecified

145.0/C06.0   of cheek mucosa

145.2/C05.0   of hard palate

145.3/C05.1   of soft palate

145.6/C06.2   of retromolar area

145.8/C06.89   of overlapping sites of other parts of mouth

145.9/C06.9   of mouth, unspecified

146.0/C09.9   of tonsil, unspecified

146.1/C09.0   of tonsillar fossa

146.2/C09.1   of tonsillar pillars (anterior) (posterior)

146.3/C10.0   of vallecula

146.4/C10.1   of anterior aspect of epiglottis

146.5/C10.8   of overlapping sites of oropharynx

146.7/C10.3   of posterior wall of oropharynx

146.8/C10.4   of branchial cleft

146.8/C10.8   of overlapping sites of oropharynx

147.0/C11.0   of superior wall of nasopharynx

147.1/C11.1   of posterior wall of nasopharynx

147.2/C11.2   of lateral wall of nasopharynx

147.3/C11.3   of anterior wall of nasopharynx

147.8/C11.8   of overlapping sites of nasopharynx

148.0/C13.0   of postcricoid region

148.1/C12   of pyriform sinus

148.2/C13.1   of aryepiglottic fold, hypopharyngeal aspect

148.3/C13.2   of posterior wall of hypopharyngeal

148.8/C13.8   of overlapping sites of hypopharynx

150.0/C15.3   of upper third of esophagus

160.0/C30.0   of nasal cavity

160.2/C31.0   of maxillary sinus

160.3/C31.1   of ethmoidal sinus

160.4/C31.2   of frontal sinus

160.5/C31.3   of sphenoid sinus

160.8/C31.8   of overlapping sites of accessory sinuses

161.0/C32.0   of glottis

161.1/C32.1   of supraglottis

161.2/C32.2   of subglottis

161.3/C32.3   of laryngeal cartilage

161.8/C32.8   of overlapping sites of larynx

170.0/C41.0   of bones of skull and face

170.1/C41.1   of mandible

171.0/C49.0   of connective and soft tissue of head, face and neck

173.00/C44.00   Unspecified malignant neoplasm of skin of lip

173.02/C44.02   Squamous cell carcinoma of skin; of lip

173.22/C44.221   of unspecified ear and external auricular canal

173.42/C44.42   of scalp and neck

193/C73   Malignant neoplasm of thyroid gland

196.0/C77.0   Secondary and unspecified malignant neoplasm of lymph nodes of head, face and neck

210.2/D11.9   Benign neoplasm; of major salivary gland, unspecified

210.4/D10.30   of unspecified part of mouth

210.4/D10.39   of other parts of mouth

212.0/D14.0   of middle ear, nasal cavity and accessory sinuses

225.1/D33.3   of cranial nerves

225.2/D32.0   of cerebral meninges

225.2/D32.9   of meninges, unspecified

226/D34   of thyroid gland

227.3/D35.2   of pituitary gland

227.3/D35.3   of craniopharyngeal duct

235.0/D37.030   Neoplasm of uncertain behavior; of the parotid salivary glands

235.0/D37.031   of the sublingual salivary glands

235.0/D37.032   of the submandibular salivary glands

235.0/D37.039   of the major salivary glands, unspecified

235.1/D37.01   of lip

235.1/D37.02   of tongue

235.1/D37.04   of the minor salivary glands

235.6/D38.0   of larynx

238.2/D48.5   of skin

239.0/D49.0   of digestive system

239.1/D49.1   of respiratory system

239.7/D49.7   of endocrine glands and other parts of nervous system

241.0/E04.1   Nontoxic single thyroid nodule

241.1/E04.2   Nontoxic multinodular goiter

242.00/E05.00   Thyrotoxicosis with diffuse goiter without thyrotoxic crisis or storm

242.20/E05.20   Thyrotoxicosis with toxic multinodular goiter without thyrotoxic crisis or storm

252.00/E21.3   Hyperparathyroidism, unspecified

252.02/E21.1   Secondary hyperparathyroidism, non-renal

259.3/E34.2   Ectopic hormone secretion, not elsewhere classified

275.5/E83.81   Hungry bone syndrome

351.0/G51.0   Bell's palsy

478.31/J38.01   Paralysis of vocal cords and larynx, unilateral

478.32/J38.01   Paralysis of vocal cords and larynx, unilateral

Definition of Codes

1. Panendoscopy
   a. *Indications*—Mucosal malignancies (squamous cell carcinoma [SCC]), of the head and neck. Advanced diagnostic imaging and in-office evaluation using fiberoptic scopes with biopsy channels has decreased the value for routine panendoscopy under general anesthesia.
   b. *Definitions*—Upper aerodigestive tract endoscopic examination. Diagnostic endoscopy codes are bundled into surgical endoscopy

codes; code the surgical endoscopy with higher relative value units (RVU). The primary operative endoscopies include

   i. Direct laryngoscopy (31525)
   ii. Bronchoscopy (31622)
   iii. Esophagoscopy (43191, 43200)

c. Billing laryngoscopy and bronchoscopy with modifier 59—NCCI bundles laryngoscopy and bronchoscopy codes (*modifier 1* status). Both laryngoscopy and bronchoscopy are often required for thorough examination of the upper airway for pathology. These scopes often require separate and distinct instrumentation and/or anesthetic management. Modifier 59 (distinct procedural services) is appropriate because laryngoscopy and bronchoscopy are complimentary and cannot be billed under a single code. According to the American Academy Otolaryngology-Head and Neck Surgery (AAO-HNS), denial of payment for 31525 and 31622 on the basis of unbundling is inaccurate.[4]

d. Billing esophagoscopy separately—esophagoscopy (eg, 43191, 43200) is considered separate and distinct from either laryngoscopy or bronchoscopy. Append modifier 59 to the esophagoscopy, since CCI edits bundle it into the laryngoscopy procedure, when performed as described by the new CPT 2015 guideline: "Esophagoscopy includes examination from the cricopharyngeus muscle (upper esophageal sphincter) to and including the gastroesophageal junction. It may also include examination of the proximal region of the stomach via retroflexion when performed." Therefore, the documentation should support examination of these anatomic areas to support reporting a separate esophagoscopy code and modifier 59 may be appended to the esophagoscopy code. If only a cervical esophagoscopy is performed, then it is included in the laryngoscopy or bronchoscopy code reported."

e. Billing triple endoscopy with a neck dissection separately—NCCI edits do *not* bundle neck dissection codes (38720, 38724) with

codes such as 31525, 31622, or 43200. Code these procedures separately with normal multiple surgery parameters.

f. A surgical procedure such as a laryngectomy includes a diagnostic laryngoscopy at the same operative session; a glossectomy includes a diagnostic esophagoscopy at the same operative session. An exception is when a diagnostic laryngoscopy is performed (eg, for biopsy) and there is a waiting period for pathology results to be received and the remainder of the procedure is performed based on the pathology results. The diagnostic laryngoscopy may then be reported with modifier 59 as it is considered a separate procedure; while not a common scenario in otolaryngology, it can occur. However, the diagnostic laryngoscopy procedure may not be separately reported if the laryngoscopy is performed and the laryngectomy (or definitive procedure) is performed without waiting for pathology results for procedure planning purposes.

2. Neck Dissection
a. *Indications*—Primary head and neck malignancy confirmed by biopsy or prior surgery; enlarging or persisting neck mass with history of regional primary malignancy; neck mass malignancy proven by biopsy or fine needle aspiration with unknown primary malignancy.

b. *Definitions*—Unilateral resection of cervical lymphatic tissue.

c. Radical neck dissection (RND) (38720)—Comprehensive removal of lymphatic tissue (levels I–V) including sacrifice of the ipsilateral spinal accessory nerve, sternocleidomastoid muscle, and internal jugular vein.

d. Modified radical neck dissection (MRND) (38724)—Comprehensive removal of lymphatic tissue (levels I–V) with preservation of at least one nonlymphatic structure listed for RND. This code can be used if less than all the levels are removed but more then what is done in a suprahyoid neck dissection. For instance, if a suprahyoid neck dissection is completed (removal of levels I–III).

e. Suprahyoid neck dissection (38700)—Dissection limited to lymphatic tissue in the submental and submandibular triangles (level Ia/b); Nonlymphatic structures are commonly spared but removal is not exclusionary. Do *not* report with 38720 or 38724.

f. Extended neck dissection—If additional nonlymphatic structures are removed besides those listed for RND (eg, deep cervical musculature, digastric muscle, cranial nerves), append modifier 22 (increased procedural services) to 38720 or 38724.

g. Billing global, or comprehensive, procedures that include a neck dissection—NCCI edits bundle 38720 and 38724 into several (but not all) primary procedure codes such as a laryngectomy, glossectomy, parotidectomy, or thyroidectomy. This requires reviewing the latest NCCI edits (updated quarterly) and determining whether the primary procedure code bundles, or includes, 38724. If not bundled, the primary procedure code and 38724 are payable separately, and no modifier is necessary to show the 2 are separate procedures. Bilateral neck dissections are reported with modifier 50. For example, if a laryngectomy with bilateral modified radical neck dissections is performed then report the unbundled laryngectomy code (31360) and the MRND code (38724-50, 59), as there is no code for a laryngectomy with MRND. Modifier 59 is necessary on 38724 because NCCI edits include the MRND in the laryngectomy code (31360). However, there is a code for a laryngectomy and unilateral RND and thus use 31365, and not unbundle, when performing a RND with a laryngectomy. See *Controversial Topics* at the end of the chapter for a history and detailed discussion of modifier 59 for this purpose.

3. Billing tracheostomy with a neck dissection separately—A neck dissection does not include a tracheostomy (31600), and the tracheostomy is reported separately.

4. Laryngectomy

a. *Indications*—Malignancy with invasion into the larynx. Various organ preservation techniques are performed for a wide spectrum of tumor stages with the goal of maximizing oncologic results and maintaining organ function.

b. *Definition*—Surgical removal of the larynx and separation of the airway from the mouth, nose, and esophagus; includes surrounding soft tissue and cartilage. Laryngectomy *always* includes a planned tracheostomy and thus cannot be billed separately. A thyroidectomy is included in a laryngectomy code when performed for access. However, if there is disease in the thyroid then the removal is separately reported.

c. Total laryngectomy (31360)
   i. With RND (31365)—Commonly performed prior to the laryngectomy but at the same operative session. Anterior belly of digastric muscle and/or strap muscles may be involved; if resected, report modifier 22 (increased procedural services). For total laryngectomy with bilateral RND, also code 38720-59 for the second side.
   ii. With MRND—NCCI edits bundle 38724 with 31365 and 31360. For a total laryngectomy with unilateral MRND, code 31360 and 38724-59. For a total laryngectomy with bilateral MRND, code 31360 and 38724-50-59. Carriers may request that LT/RT modifiers be used for clarification (eg, 31360, 38724-59-LT [or –RT]).

d. Subtotal supraglottic laryngectomy (31367)—Operation to remove epiglottis, false vocal cords and superior half of the thyroid cartilage. Report supracricoid laryngectomy as 31599 (unlisted procedure, larynx). Use 31367 as a base code for determining a reasonable fee.
   i. With RND (31368)—For bilateral RND, code 31368 and 38720-59.
   ii. With MRND—NCCI edits bundle 38724 with both 31368 and 31367. For supraglottic laryngectomy with unilateral

MRND, code 31367 and 38724-59. For supraglottic laryngectomy with bilateral MRND, code 31367 and 38724-50-59.

e. Partial laryngectomy (hemilaryngectomy) (31370, 31375, 31380, 31382)—CPT and NCCI do *not* bundle these codes with 38720 or 38724 as none of these codes including a neck dissection. Indicate bilateral neck dissections with modifier 50 (*not* modifier 59).

f. Pharyngolaryngectomy with RND (31390) —Total laryngopharyngectomy is performed for hypopharyngeal carcinoma.
   i. For bilateral RND, code 31390 and 38720-59.
   ii. With MRND—There is not a single code for a pharyngolaryngectomy with MRND and NCCI bundles 38724 with 31390. For pharyngolaryngectomy with unilateral MRND, code either 31599 (unlisted code) and the MRND code(s) or consider appending 31390 with a 52 modifier.

5. Glossectomy
   a. *Indications*—Primary or secondary malignancy with tongue involvement.
   b. *Definition*—Partial or total removal of the tongue. Glossectomy (41140–41153) includes a planned tracheostomy (31600) and placement of a naso- or orogastric feeding tube (43752). Oral tongue refers to the anterior two-thirds of the tongue and base of tongue refers to the posterior one-thrid of the tongue.
   c. Partial glossectomy (41120)—Resection of less than one-half of the tongue. This includes robotic base of tongue (BOT) resections (see Chapter 31, "Robotic Surgery," for more details).
      i. With RND (41135)—For partial glossectomy with bilateral RND, code 41135 and 38720-59.
      ii. With MRND—NCCI edits do *not* bundle 38724 with 41120. For MRND, code 38724 and 41120-51. For bilateral MRND, code 38724-50 and 41120-51. CPT 38724 has a higher total RVU than

41120; therefore, 41120 is appended with modifier 51.
   d. Hemiglossectomy (41130)—Resection of at least one-half of the tongue. The mandible may be split to allow access to the floor of mouth (included in the global package; do *not* report separately). CPT and NCCI edits do *not* bundle 38720 or 38724 with 41130. For RND, code 41130 and 38720. For bilateral RND, code 41130 and 38720-50. For MRND, code 41130-51 with 38724. For bilateral MRND, code 41130-51 and 38724-50. The RND and MRND codes have a higher total RVU than 41130; therefore, modifier 51 (multiple procedures) is appended to the lower code, 41130. Closure or repair of the mandible, if split for access to the floor of mouth) is included in 41130.
   e. Total glossectomy (41140)
      i. With RND (41145)—For total glossectomy with bilateral RND, code 41145 and 38720-59.
      ii. With MRND—NCCI bundles 38724 with 41145 and 41140. For total glossectomy with MRND, code 41140 and 38724-59. For total glossectomy with bilateral MRND, code 41140 and 38724-50-59.
   f. Total glossectomy with floor of mouth and mandibular resection (41150)—composite resection indicated for malignancy of the tongue and oropharynx with mandibular involvement. Reconstruction of the mandible is included in 41150 and 41155 and not separately reported with a code such as 21244.
      i. With suprahyoid neck dissection (41153) —For bilateral level I dissection, code 41153 and 38700-59.
      ii. With RND (41155)—Composite procedure including glossectomy, resection of floor of mouth, and RND (also called a "Commando" procedure). For bilateral RND, code 41155 and 38720-59.
      iii. With MRND—NCCI bundles 38724 with 41155 and 41150. For MRND, code 41150 and 38724-59. For bilateral MRND, code 41150 and 38724-50-59.

6. Thyroidectomy
   a. *Indications*—Large mass in the thyroid gland, difficulties with breathing/swallowing related to thyroid mass, suspected or confirmed thyroid cancer, hyperthyroidism, history of medullary carcinoma in the family with positive RET ("rearranged during transfection") oncogene, increased calcitonin, or positive stimulation test for calcitonin.
   b. *Definition*—CPT generally uses "thyroidectomy" in reference to total thyroidectomies and anything less is referred to as a "lobectomy." Many codes still listed in CPT have fallen out of use, especially by high-volume thyroid surgeons. Subtotal removal of thyroid tissue (60225) is generally discouraged due to bleeding and obliteration of view of the recurrent laryngeal nerve (RLN). Usually complete lobectomy (60220) or total thyroidectomy (60240) is performed. See Figure 28–1.
   c. Hemithyroidectomy (60220)—Excision of entire lobe on one side with or without the isthmus. Most surgeons agree that the minimum amount of thyroid tissue removed should be a lobectomy with isthmectomy for suspected thyroid carcinoma (<10 mm diameter).
   d. Subtotal thyroid lobectomy (60210)—Not routinely performed as an isolated procedure. Partial (60210) or total thyroid lobectomy (60220) may be combined with excision of part of the contralateral lobe and isthmus (60212, 60225).
   e. Total thyroidectomy (60240)—Complete removal of both thyroid lobes and isthmus. Total thyroidectomy without neck dissection should be coded 60240 regardless of whether the indication is for benign or malignant disease.
      i. With RND (60254)—Rarely required in the context of thyroid cancer.
      ii. With MRND—NCCI does *not* bundle 38724 with 60250. For MRND, code 60240 and 38724-51. For bilateral MRND, code 60240 and 38724-50. This is not considered unbundling, as there

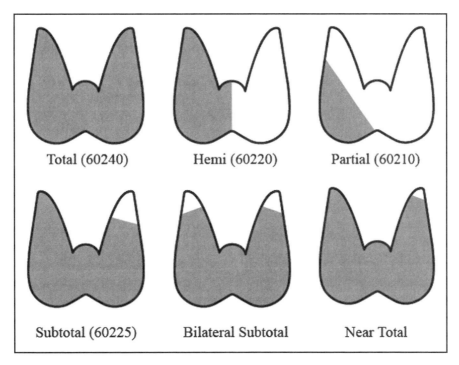

Figure 28–1. Thyroidectomy types with procedure codes. Original illustration provided by Andrew M. Hinson.

is no code for a total thyroidectomy with MRND.

 iii. Limited neck dissection (60252)—Includes all lymph nodes in the perithyroid region and central neck dissection (Delphian, paratracheal, upper mediastinal lymph nodes). Central neck dissection is not considered to have laterality and modifier 50 does not apply. NCCI edits do not bundle 38724 with 60252, therefore, for central compartment and MRND, code 60252 and 38724. For central compartment and bilateral MRND, code 60252 and 38724-50. Note that some payers incorrectly ask for the reduced services modifier (52) because the limited neck dissection is included in 60252. However, the central compartment lymph nodes are excised in the operative field of the thyroidectomy, and this zone should not be considered part of the MRND. The operative documentation should clearly specify the differences between the dissections.

f. Completion thyroidectomy (60260)—Amount of resected thyroid tissue depends on the amount of remaining thyroid tissue after previous resection. If thyroid tissue is resected from both sides of the neck, code 60260-50. Append modifier 58 (staged procedure) to 60260 if performed in the global period, as a completion procedure, of a previous thyroid lobectomy procedure.

g. Substernal thyroidectomy (60270-60271)—CPT uses only the "thyroidectomy" language in reference to coding for substernal thyroid tumors. This makes accurate coding for a unilateral substernal thyroid resection (lobectomy) ambiguous. In general, 60271 is reported despite only one of the lobectomies being substernal. Some carriers may request modifier 52 (reduced services) for unilateral resection.

h. Hemi, possible total thyroidectomy—The surgeon performs a frozen section that influences how the procedure proceeds. If cancer is called on the frozen section, the contralateral lobe is removed. In this sce-

nario, code 60240 (total). If frozen shows no malignancy, the surgeon completes the partial thyroidectomy and closes the wound. In this scenario, code for the procedure performed. Use 60260 (completion) when remaining tissue is removed in an already operated field (at a second operative session). If final pathology describes malignancy, the contralateral lobe is resected at a later time; if the procedure is performed within the global period (90 days), use code 60260-58 (staged procedure modifier).

7. Parathyroidectomy
 a. *Indications*—Symptomatic primary hyperparathyroidism (pHPT); asymptomatic pHPT with hypercalcemia, hypercalciuria, decreased creatinine clearance, nephrolithiasis, young age, osteoporosis); medical refractory secondary hyperparathyroidism.
 b. *Definition*—Exploration and potential resection of one or more parathyroid glands.
 c. Parathyroidectomy or exploration of parathyroid(s) (60500)—Standard, all-encompassing code for resection of one or more parathyroid glands. The procedure can only be only reported once independent of the number of glands resected. Use 60502 for reexploration. Use 60505 when a sternal split or transthoracic approach is required.
 d. Parathyroid autotransplantation (list separately in addition to code for primary procedure) (60512)—Following removal of all parathyroid glands, the surgeon may dissect normal parathyroid tissue into millimeter slices and implant the tissue into the sternocleidomastoid, forearm muscle, or another location. If the transplant site is in the neck and approached through the same neck incision as the primary procedure into the adjacent tissue, then 60512 may not be separately reported. CPT 60200, 60210, and 60220 are not listed as separately reportable with 60512 because the 2 parathyroids associated with the nonexcised lobe or portion of gland would not be at risk. Autotransplantation of a parathyroid gland during the course of a partial or total

thyroidectomy may be reported with 22 modifier added to the appropriate thyroid code instead. Parathyroid autotransplantation (60512) after total parathyroidectomy should be used as an add-on code with 60500. CPT 60512 is an add-on code that may be reported in conjunction with 60500, 60502, 60505, 60212, 60225, 60240, 60252, 60254, 60260, 60270, and 60271 when clinically indicated.

e. Intraoperative PTH assay (36500, venous catheterization for selective organ blood sampling)—After resection, a ≥50% decrease from baseline preoperative PTH values (and into the reported normal range) has traditionally been considered indicative of successful resection of all hyperactive parathyroid tissue. CPT 36500 is a one-time charge regardless of the number of blood draws and assays performed if performed by another provider; this is not billable for the surgeon.

f. Radioguided parathyroidectomy—A handheld gamma probe detects radiotracer that accumulates in hyperactive parathyroid tissue. CPT 78808 is not separately billable by the surgeon when performed intraoperatively. However, it may be reported by the provider, typically a radiologist, who performs the service and documents the radiographic findings. CPT 78808 has separate professional (modifier 26) and technical components (modifier TC) so the provider should bill accordingly.

g. Intraoperative ultrasonography (US)—High-resolution intraoperative US may help localize radiographically identified, nonpalpable thyroid and parathyroid lesions within the thyroid bed or nodal basins or in reexploration cases for hyperparathyroidism where there is significant surgical fibrosis. At present, intraoperative US guidance is not billed separately by the surgeon in either thyroidectomy or parathyroidectomy or any other head and neck procedures.

h. Methylene blue injection—Used in primary and reoperation parathyroidectomy. The blue color aids in identifying parathy-roid tissue that may be hidden by edema and seroma fluid. Methylene blue injection is not a recognized procedure code and the respective Healthcare Common Procedure Coding System (HCPCS) code (A9535) was removed in 2010. This service is included in the global surgical package for the procedure code billed by the surgeon.

8. Skull Base Surgery (see Chapter 30, "Skull Base Surgery," for more information)
   a. *Indications*—Benign and malignant neoplasms involving the skull base.
   b. *Definitions*—Single-stage surgery (distinct codes) consisting of 3 primary components including an approach, resection, and reconstruction.
   c. Open (traditional) skull base surgery—Nonendoscopic technique that involves skin incisions, removal of bone and brain retraction to access the skull base. The lesion is subsequently resected with or without use of an operating microscope. Skull base surgery often combines otolaryngology and neurosurgery services. Each surgeon reports only the procedures he or she actually performed. Modifier 51 does not apply if procedures were performed independently by separate providers. Modifier 51 does apply if one surgeon performs both the approach and the resection.
   d. Endonasal endoscopic assisted (EEA) surgery—Enhanced endoscopic equipment and image guidance have facilitated novel endonasal approaches to the anterior skull base and brain, which increases surgical exposure, reduces brain retraction, and minimizes damage to nerves. According to the AAO-HNS, it is not appropriate to use the existing skull base codes (except 62165) for endonasal/endoscopic procedures because the current codes describe an open procedure involving skin incision(s) and involve length postoperative inpatient care.
   e. CPT 62165 (endoscopic pituitary surgery)—Currently the only existing endoscopic transnasal skull base/brain surgery code. The otolaryngologist traditionally performs

the endonasal approach, and then assists the neurosurgeon who opens the dura and resects the pituitary mass. The otolaryngologist then closes the defect with a local flap. CPT 62165 includes the approach, resection, and closure. Append modifier 62 (two surgeons) to 62165 when performed by both the otolaryngologist and neurosurgeon.

f. Unlisted codes—Before new codes are added, the surgeon(s) must employ an unlisted code to accurately document the procedure performed. For EEA surgery,[5]

  i. It is often recommended that the surgeon performing the approach uses code 31299 (unlisted procedure, accessory sinuses). The surgeon performing the resection uses code 64999 (unlisted procedure, nervous system). Modifiers are usually not used with unlisted codes (eg, 64999-62). Note that payers frequently deny claims where 2 surgeons report the same unlisted code.

  ii. Both surgeons then designate a second and separate code that most closely approximates the procedure they independently performed (ie, a base code). This determines the charged fee. If assisting, the otolaryngologist's reimbursement includes his or her work on the neurosurgeon's base code (modifier 80, 82). Depending on the base code chosen, the unlisted code may be assigned either a 0- or 90-day global period.

g. Intraoperative navigation, extracranial or intracranial (61781, 61782)—This is an add-on service that combines imaging with navigational software to provide intraoperative assistance in complex sinus and skull base surgery. The navigation code is reported once per operative session, and reimbursement depends on clinical and operative documentation supporting its medical indication. According to AAO-HNS,[6] this should include one or more of

the following: revision sinus surgery; distorted sinus anatomy; extensive sinonasal polyposis; significant pathology involving frontal, posterior ethmoid, and sphenoid sinuses; disease abutting the skull base, orbit, optic nerve, or carotid artery; skull base defects with CSF rhinorrhea; and/or benign and malignant sinonasal neoplasms. The surgeon should carefully document all preincision work of loading scans, registration, calibration, confirmation of accuracy, planning the procedure, and specific usage of the navigation during the case. Note, since 61782 and 61781 are add-on codes, they cannot be billed as the sole procedure and must always accompany an appropriate primary procedure code.

Controversial Areas

Billing Intraoperative Nerve Monitoring (IONM) (95940, 95941, or G0453*)

IONM are add-on codes used for complex surgical procedures involving cranial nerves. If the surgeon or anesthesiologist performs the service, the CPT code is included in the primary procedure code (eg, thyroidectomy, laryngectomy) and is not separately billable. To bill for IONM, another qualified provider solely dedicated to the service must always be available either locally (95940) or remotely (95941 or G0453) to intervene. Additionally, these services are *not* stand-alone codes and must be linked to the appropriate neurophysiologic monitoring code. If the physician performs only the interpretation and does not own the equipment, he or she should append modifier 26 (professional component). The provider performing the monitoring must report the intraoperative findings and record the precise level of involvement to obtain reimbursement. See the following examples:

---

*In 2013, Centers of Medicare and Medicaid Services (CMS) did not accept the CPT Editorial Panel's addition of 95941. They instead created G0453 (continuous intraoperative neurophysiology monitoring, from outside the operating room) remote or nearby, **per patient**, each 15 minutes).

1. The auditory nerve is at risk during resection of acoustic neuromas and skull base procedures involving the posterior cranial fossa. An audiologist (or other qualified provider) continuously monitors for waveform changes and then differentiates whether the changes are related to surgical dissection or background noise. The audiologist codes the diagnostic procedure 92585-26 (modifier 26 is necessary because the audiologist does not own the equipment used) and the add-on code 95940 under their national provider identifier (NPI). This clearly indicates to the payer that the monitoring was both continuous and a provider other than the operating surgeon performed the service.

2. The facial nerve courses through the parotid gland, and may lie in intimate contact with a benign or malignant parotid neoplasm. The qualified provider (not the surgeon) codes 95867 (EMG) and the add-on code, 95887. The surgeon will not bill for intraoperative nerve monitoring because this service is included in the global surgical package of the primary procedure (eg, parotidectomy) for the surgeon. Note that the majority of carriers consider nerve monitoring with automated devices as integral components to the surgery and do not reimburse these services separately.

3. The recurrent laryngeal nerve lies within the operative field and is subject to injury during thyroid and parathyroid surgery. Routine IONM for thyroid and parathyroid surgery is controversial but may be clinically justified especially in the presence of large tumors, paratracheal node disease, and excessive scar tissue with altered surgical planes. That said, the surgeon may not bill for IOMN. Note that there is not a code for reporting surface electrode EMG monitoring for recurrent laryngeal nerve monitoring during thyroid or parathyroid surgery,[7] because this activity is also included in the surgeon's code as part of prepping the patient for the procedure.

Use of Modifier 59 (Distinct Procedural Services) and Neck Dissections

Modifier 59 is presently defined by CPT as indicating a different procedure, different site or organ system, separate excision, or separate lesion not ordinarily encountered or performed during the same session by the same person. In 1997, the NCCI introduced modifier 59 to specifically separate 2 head and neck codes—14040 and 11642 (excision of basal cell of forehead with flap reconstruction; excision of basal cell of cheek). Recall that 14040 includes 11642 (or any lesion removal) at the same site. Before modifier 59, the surgeon could not bill these codes simultaneously without a payer's computer software automatically denying 11642 as inclusive to 14040 when the lesion was actually separate. NCCI edits, updated quarterly, gradually expanded over the next decade. In 2004, NCCI (version 9.0) changed the modifier indicator from 0 to 1 for a number of primary procedures in order to allow the surgeon to bill the contralateral neck dissection.[†] Some coders are appending modifier 59 to NCCI edits that bundle neck dissections (38720, 38724) into primary procedure codes in order to indicate that a MRND (rather than a RND) was performed. Compared to a RND, a MRND is a more delicate procedure and requires longer operating times and hospital resources. Although MRND (wRVU 23.95) pays only slightly more than a RND (wRVU 21.95), the difference (approximately $75–$100) may be significant in high-volume head and neck centers. Thus, surgeons often argue that the NCCI edits are unfair and at odds with CPT descriptors. To overcome this problem, some expert coders suggest instead reporting the primary procedure code (without the included RND) and MRND code because this accurately reflects the procedure performed. However, some institutions do not allow physicians to bill CPT code combinations that defy Medicare's NCCI edits. Refer to Chapter 11, "Demystifying Modifiers," for more information.

[†]The NCCI separate HCPCS/CPT code pairs into 2 columns. If 2 paired codes are reported during the same operative session, codes in *Column 1* are eligible for payment but codes in *Column 2* are not—*unless* appended with a modifier. Each edit is assigned a modifier status of 0 or 1; 0 indicates that an edit *cannot* be bypassed even if a modifier is assigned, and 1 indicates that a modifier is allowed to bypass the edit but may not necessarily be appropriate.

Interestingly, Medicare has historically reimbursed a majority of modifier 59 claims (both appropriate and inappropriate) because the modifier bypasses initial programming filters that otherwise automatically reject code pairs that are not allowed (*status 0*) and unmodified (*status 1*). Thus, some physicians who have received reimbursement from both Medicare (follows NCCI edits) and private payers (do not always follow all NCCI edits) may often report modifier 59 incorrectly. Payers have recognized this trend and some are increasingly scrutinizing operative documentation to ensure coding compliance and prevent any further abuse. In summary, the safest billing practice is staying up-to-date with NCCI edits, despite their antiquity and clinical irrelevance, and billing safely within CPT and NCCI parameters. It is imperative that operative documentation always state the precise indication(s) for appending modifier 59 in order to avoid reimbursement delay, rejection, denial, and/or potential audit.

References

1. American Medical Association. CPT 2014 Professional Edition. Chicago, IL: AMA; 2014.
2. World Health Organization. International Classification of Diseases (ICD) Information Sheet. http://www.who.int/classifications/icd/factsheet/en/. Accessed October 3, 2014.
3. National Correct Coding Initiative Policy Manual for Medicare and Medicaid Services (Coding Policy Manual). http://www.cms.gov/Medicare/Coding/NationalCorrectCodInitEd/index.html. Accessed November 8, 2014.
4. American Academy of Otolaryngology-Head and Neck Surgery. Laryngoscopy and bronchoscopy—Position statement, reimbursement. http://www.entnet.org/?q=node/927. Updated September 28, 2013. Accessed November 4, 2014.
5. Pollock K, LeGrand M. Coding and reimbursement strategies: using an unlisted code for endoscopic skull base surgery. *American Academy of Otolaryngology-Head and Neck Surgery Bulletin*. April 2013; 32(4):39–40. http://bulletin.entnet.org/wp-content/uploads/2013/10/Bulletin_April_2013.pdf. Accessed January 31, 2016.
6. American Academy of Otolaryngology-Head and Neck Surgery. Intra-Operative Use of Computer Guided Surgery: Position statement, reimbursement. http://www.entnet.org/content/intra-operative-use-computer-aided-surgery. Revised March 2, 2014. Accessed November 8, 2014.
7. American Academy of Otolaryngology-Head and Neck Surgery. What is intraoperative neurophysiology coding and can I bill for it? CPT for ENT: Intraoperative neurophysiology testing. Coding, CPT for ENT, Reimbursement. http://www.entnet.org/content/cpt-ent-intraoperative-neurophysiology-testing. Accessed November 10, 2014.

CHAPTER 29

Reconstructive Head and Neck Surgery

Babak Givi, Adam S. Jacobson, and Neal D. Futran

Introduction

This chapter describes coding and billing for head and neck reconstructive procedures performed in the operating room. Each code is associated with distinct relative value units (RVUs) that can be determined by looking at the Centers for Medicare and Medicaid Services (CMS) website, American Medical Association (AMA) publications, or through the American Academy of Otolaryngology-Head and Neck Surgery. Each *Current Procedural Terminology* (CPT) code is associated with specific *International Classification of Diseases, Ninth Revision, Clinical Modification* (ICD-9-CM)/ *International Classification of Diseases, Tenth Revision, Clinical Modification* (ICD-10-CM) diagnosis codes. When performing these procedures, the CPT codes can be modified with a variety of different modifiers to reflect specific situations.

Because many of these reconstructive procedures are long and intense surgeries, many surgeons employ the 2-team or 2-surgeon models. If 2 distinct surgeons perform different portions of a procedure, the surgeons can then determine which codes represent the unique procedures they performed and independently bill for these codes (eg, the ablative procedure(s) is performed and billed by surgeon A while the reconstruction is performed and billed by surgeon B). If the surgeons perform the entire surgery together, the codes can be appended with modifiers such as 62

(co-surgeons) or 80/82 (assistant surgeon). Refer to Chapter 11, "Demystifying Modifiers," for more information.

Key Points

- Repair of a donor site requiring a skin graft, an adjacent tissue transfer, or extensive immobilization is considered an additional separate procedure and should be coded separately.
- Do not report the use of an operating microscope (69990) separately for a microvascular procedure, as this is already included in the procedure code.
- The harvest of autogenous bone, cartilage, tendon, fascia lata grafts, or other tissues through separate incisions is to be reported only when a graft is not already listed as part of the basic procedure.
- The harvest of a vein graft is not reported separately when using code 35231 (Repair blood vessel with vein graft; neck).
- Report a carotid artery/neck exploration only if no other service is performed. If the carotid artery is examined through the same incision used for a procedure during the same operative session, the exploration is not reported. If the

carotid artery is examined and a defect is discovered and repaired, report the repair, not the exploration.

Key Procedure Codes

Similar to other discussions in reconstructive surgery, we follow the concept of the reconstructive ladder to describe different procedures used in reconstruction in increasing order of complexity. We start by primary repairs, followed by adjacent tissue transfers, free grafts, regional flaps, and finish with free tissue transfer procedures.

Skin Repair

Primary repairs are classified into 3 categories: simple, intermediate, and complex.

Simple Repairs

Superficial repairs that require only one layer closure are considered simple repair. The head and neck area is divided into 2 sections: scalp/neck and face (including eyelids, nose, ear). Codes are classified by the length of the repair. If multiple wounds of the same nature and anatomic location are repaired, add the length of all wounds and report the code that corresponds to the total length. These codes apply when surgical glue or staples are used, even if no sutures are placed; however, they do not apply when using adhesive strips. If closing a superficial wound dehiscence, then a separate code is used. Debridement of the wound is also not part of these codes.

12001   Simple repair of superficial wounds of scalp, neck, axillae, external genitalia, trunk and/or extremities (including hands and feet); 2.5 cm or less
wRVU 0.84; Global 0

     12002   2.6 cm to 7.5 cm
wRVU 1.14; Global 0

     12004   7.6 cm to 12.5 cm
wRVU 1.44; Global 0

     12005   12.6 cm to 20.0 cm
wRVU 1.97; Global 0

     12006   20.1 cm to 30.0 cm
wRVU 2.39; Global 0

     12007   over 30.0 cm
wRVU 2.90; Global 0

12011   Simple repair of superficial wounds of face, ears, eyelids, nose, lips and/or mucous membranes; 2.5 cm or less
wRVU 1.07; Global 0

     12013   2.6 cm to 5.0 cm
wRVU 1.22; Global 0

     12014   5.1 cm to 7.5 cm
wRVU 1.57; Global 0

     12015   7.6 cm to 12.5 cm
wRVU 1.98; Global 0

     12016   12.6 cm to 20.0 cm
wRVU 2.68; Global 0

     12017   20.1 cm to 30.0 cm
wRVU 3.18; Global 0

     12018   over 30.0 cm
wRVU 3.61; Global 0

12020   Treatment of superficial wound dehiscence; simple closure
wRVU 2.67; Global 0

Intermediate Repair

Intermediate repair involves closing the wound in multiple layers. When deeper tissues are closed with absorbable sutures, in addition to skin closure, these codes are used. The head and neck area is divided into 3 sections: scalp, neck, and face. Similar to simple repairs, measure the length of repair to find the most suitable code. If more than one wound of same complexity is repaired, add the length and report one code that corresponds with the total length. Repair of tendons, blood vessels, and nerves should be reported separately under appropriate codes. The codes for blood vessel repair, nerves, and tendons include intermediate closure; therefore, do not add these codes to those repairs. For the majority of flaps, intermediate closure of the donor site is part of the code for the flap procedure; do not report it separately. Major debridement is not covered under these codes.

12031   Repair, intermediate, wounds of scalp, axillae, trunk and/or extremities (excluding hands or feet); 2.5 cm or less
wRVU 2.00; Global 10

    12032   2.6 cm to 7.5 cm
wRVU 2.52; Global 10

    12034   7.6 cm to 12.5 cm
wRVU 2.97; Global 10

    12035   12.6 cm to 20.0 cm
wRVU 3.50; Global 10

    12036   20.1 cm to 30.0 cm
wRVU 4.23; Global 10

    12037   30.0 cm
wRVU 5.00; Global 10

12041   Repair, intermediate, wounds of neck, hands, feet and/or external genitalia; 2.5 cm or less
wRVU 2.10; Global 10

    12042   2.6 cm to 7.5 cm
wRVU 2.79; Global 10

    12044   7.6 cm to 12.5 cm
wRVU 3.19; Global 10

    12045   12.6 cm to 20.0 cm
wRVU 3.75; Global 10

    12046   20.1 cm to 30.0 cm
wRVU 4.30; Global 10

    12047   over 30.0 cm
wRVU 4.95; Global 10

12051   Repair, intermediate, wounds of face, ears, eyelids, nose, lips and/or mucous membranes; 2.5 cm or less
wRVU 2.33; Global 10

    12052   2.6 cm to 5.0 cm
wRVU 2.87; Global 10

    12053   5.1 cm to 7.5 cm
wRVU 3.17; Global 10

    12054   7.6 cm to 12.5 cm
wRVU 3.50; Global 10

    12055   12.6 cm to 20.0 cm
wRVU 4.50; Global 10

    12056   20.1 cm to 30.0 cm
wRVU 5.30; Global 10

    12057   over 30.0 cm
wRVU 6.00; Global 10

Complex Repair

These codes apply when a deep wound contains crushed, torn, or deeply lacerated tissues and requires trimming of the edges or extensive undermining the tissues and closed in layers. The wound closure is more complicated than an intermediate, or layered closure. For example, repairing blast injuries or gunshot wounds that require removing foreign objects or debridements. These added steps have to be documented in the operative report. The head and neck is divided into 3 sections: (1) scalp; (2) forehead, cheek, chin, mouth, neck; and (3) and eyelids, nose, ear, and lips. If repair of the blood vessels, nerves, or tendons were performed and then the wound closed in a complex fashion, use the appropriate codes for the repair first and then use the complex closure code appended with modifier 59. While CPT states it is appropriate to also report the complex repair code, most payers consider it inclusive to the primary procedure. If the closure is less than 1.1 cm then use the appropriate code for simple or intermediate repair as the codes for complex repairs of small wounds have been deleted.

13100   Repair, complex, trunk; 1.1 cm to 2.5 cm
wRVU 3.00; Global 10

    13101   2.6 cm to 7.5 cm
wRVU 3.50; Global 10

    +13102   each additional 5 cm or less (List separately in addition to code for primary procedure)
wRVU 1.24; Global ZZZ

13120   Repair, complex, scalp, arms, and/or legs; 1.1 cm to 2.5 cm
wRVU 3.23; Global 10

    13121   2.6 cm to 7.5 cm
wRVU 4.00; Global 10

+13122   each additional 5 cm or less (List separately in addition to code for primary procedure)
wRVU 1.44; Global ZZZ

13131   Repair, complex, forehead, cheeks, chin, mouth, neck, axillae, genitalia, hands and/or feet; 1.1 cm to 2.5 cm
wRVU 3.73; Global 10

13132   2.6 cm to 7.5 cm
wRVU 4.78; Global 10

+13133   each additional 5 cm or less (List separately in addition to code for primary procedure)
wRVU 2.19; Global ZZZ

13151   Repair, complex, eyelids, nose, ears, and/or lips; 1.1 cm to 2.5 cm
wRVU 4.34; Global 10

13152   2.6 cm to 7.5 cm
wRVU 5.34; Global 10

+13153   each additional 5 cm or less (List separately in addition to code for primary procedure)
wRVU 2.38; Global ZZZ

Secondary Repair

13160   Secondary closure of surgical wound or dehiscence, extensive or complicated
wRVU 12.04; Global 90

Repair of Arteries and Veins

Repair of arteries and veins include intermediate closure. If the wound requires extensive debridement, complex wound closure or adjacent tissue transfer, report those separately. If the operative microscope was used for these repairs it could be reported separately (69990). These codes are reported when the vessel repair is the primary procedure performed. If a vessel is repaired as part of another procedure, such as a microvascular free flap, then the repair code is not used.

35201   Repair blood vessel, direct, neck
wRVU 16.93; Global 90

35231   Repair blood vessel with vein graft; neck
wRVU 21.16; Global 90

35701   Exploration (not followed by surgical repair), with or without lysis of artery; carotid artery
wRVU 9.19; Global 90

(This code cannot be used if another procedure was performed during the same operative session through the same incision.)

35761   other vessels
wRVU 5.93; Global 90

Nerve Repair

Nerve repair codes are quite specific and are based on each individual nerve, region, and the type of repair. If the operative microscope was used for these repairs, it should be reported separately (69990). Nerve suture codes include wound closure but do not include reconstruction; code this procedure separately. If a secondary nerve suture was performed (64872, 64874) report those in addition to the code for suturing the nerve; secondary means at a different operative session.

64861   Suture of; brachial plexus
wRVU 20.89; Global 90

64864   Suture of facial nerve; extracranial
wRVU 13.41; Global 90

64865   infratemporal, with or without grafting
wRVU 16.09; Global 90

64866   Anastomosis; facial-spinal accessory
wRVU 16.83; Global 90

64868   facial-hypoglossal
wRVU 14.90; Global 90

+64872   Suture of nerve; requiring secondary or delayed suture (List separately in addition to code for primary neurorrhaphy)
wRVU 1.99; Global ZZZ

+64874   requiring extensive mobilization, or transposition of nerve (List separately in addition to code for nerve suture)
wRVU 2.98; Global ZZZ

64885 Nerve graft (includes obtaining graft), head and neck; up to 4 cm in length
wRVU 17.60; Global 90

    64886 more than 4 cm length
    wRVU 20.82; Global 90

+69990 Microsurgical techniques, requiring use of operating microscope (List separately in addition to code for primary procedure)
wRVU 3.46; Global ZZZ

Bone Repair (Mandible)

These codes could be used if for example a second physician repairs the mandible after segmental resection (21215) or the mandible is put together after a mandibulotomy approach for posterior oral cavity and pharyngeal resections. Depending on the primary procedure code reported for the resection of the lesion, a separate reconstruction code may be warranted separate from harvest of a free flap (by a second surgeon). Typically, any CPT code that requires an osteotomy includes the internal fixation as part of the usual closure. The osteocutaneous flap codes do include mandibular reconstruction.

21215 Graft, bone; mandible (includes obtaining graft)
wRVU 12.23; Global 90

21244 Reconstruction of mandible, extraoral, with transosteal bone plate (eg, mandibular staple bone plate)
wRVU 13.62; Global 90

Adjacent Tissue Transfer

These codes apply when adjacent tissues are transferred or rearranged to close a surgical or traumatic wound. They are commonly known as local flaps but should not be confused with the complex repair codes. The adjacent tissue transfer codes cover most of common local flaps such as advancement, rotational, interposition, V-Y, random island flaps, and others. Please note that wide undermining alone is not considered an adjacent tissue transfer. These codes require addi-

tional incisions to be made. When these codes are used to report the repair of a benign or malignant lesion excisional defect, the excision should not be reported separately. Include the total area of the excision (the primary defect) and the secondary defect due to rearrangement in reporting the size. Common flaps that are reported under these codes are rhomboid, bilobed, melolabial, cervicofacial, and palatal island flap, among others. Different codes exist for forehead paramedian flap (see under regional flaps).

14000 Adjacent tissue transfer or rearrangement, trunk; defect 10 sq cm or less
wRVU 6.37; Global 90

    14001 defect 10.1 sq cm to 30.0 sq cm
    wRVU 8.78; Global 90

14020 Adjacent tissue transfer or rearrangement, scalp, arms and/or legs; defect 10 sq cm or less
wRVU 7.22; Global 90

    14021 defect 10.1 sq cm to 30.0 sq cm
    wRVU 9.72; Global 90

14040 Adjacent tissue transfer or rearrangement, forehead, cheeks, chin, mouth, neck, axillae, genitalia, hands and/or feet; defect 10 sq cm or less
wRVU 8.60; Global 90

    14041 defect 10.1 sq cm to 30.0 sq cm
    wRVU 10.83; Global 90

14060 Adjacent tissue or rearrangement, eyelids, nose, ears and/or lips; defect 10 sq cm or less
wRVU 9.23; Global 90

    14061 defect 10.1 sq cm to 30.0 sq cm
    wRVU 11.48; Global 90

14301 Adjacent tissue transfer or rearrangement, any area; defect 30.1 sq cm to 60.0 sq cm
wRVU 12.65; Global 90

    +14302 each additional 30.0 sq cm, or part thereof (List separately in addition to code for primary procedure)
    wRVU 3.73; Global ZZZ

Free Grafts

Free grafts are divided based on the type and the composition of the tissue being transferred. They include 2 broad categories: simple (when only one type of tissue is transferred) and composite (multiple tissue types are harvested and transferred). The closure of the donor site is again included in these codes, unless the donor site was skin grafted or an adjacent tissue transfer was performed.

Simple Grafts

20900 Bone graft, any donor area; minor or small (eg, dowel or button)
wRVU 3.00; Global 0

> **20902** major or large
> *wRVU 4.58; Global 0*

20910 Cartilage graft; costochondral
wRVU 5.53; Global 90

> **20912** nasal septum
> *wRVU 6.54; Global 90*

20920 Fascia lata graft; by stripper
wRVU 5.51; Global 90

> **20922** by incision and area exposure, complex or sheet
> *wRVU 6.93; Global 90*

20924 Tendon graft, from a distance (eg, palmaris, toe extensor, plantaris)
wRVU 6.68; Global 90

20926 Tissue grafts, other (eg, paratenon, fat, dermis)
wRVU 5.79; Global 90

Composite Grafts

In these procedures, multiple types of tissue are transferred and grafted. The tissues do not have to be a continuous piece. The graft can contain individual pieces of tissues harvested separately and laid in, layer by layer, in the recipient bed. These codes should be reported once per graft.

15760 Graft; composite (eg, full thickness of external ear or nasal ala), including primary closure, donor area
wRVU 9.86; Global 90

15770 derma-fat-fascia
wRVU 8.96; Global 90

Skin Grafts

Skin grafts are commonly used in repair of primary or secondary wounds of head and neck or free flap donor sites. When skin grafts are done, they are always reported separately. The reporting is based on the recipient site, not the donor. Preparation of the recipient site should be reported separately when appropriate. These codes are subject to multiple procedures rule and adding a 51 modifier is not required.

Split-Thickness Grafts

15100 Split-thickness autograft, trunk, arms, legs; first 100 sq cm or less, or 1% of body area of infants and children (except 15050)
wRVU 9.90; Global 90

> **+15101** each additional 100 sq cm, or each additional 1% of body area of infants and children, or part thereof (List separately in addition to code for primary procedure)
> *wRVU 1.72; Global ZZZ*

15120 Split-thickness autograft, face, scalp, eyelids, mouth, neck, ears, orbits, genitalia, hands, feet, and/or multiple digits; first 100 sq cm or less, or 1% of body area of infants and children (except 15050)
wRVU 10.15; Global 90

> **+15121** each additional 100 sq cm, or each additional 1% of body area of infants and children, or part thereof (List separately in addition to code for primary procedure)
> *wRVU 2.00; Global ZZZ*

Full-Thickness Grafts. Same rules as split-thickness skin graft applies. The closure of the donor site is included, unless a split-thickness skin graft is performed through a separate incision or adjacent tissue transfer (additional incisions to cover the donor site).

15200 Full thickness graft, free, including direct closure of donor site, trunk; 20 sq cm or less
wRVU 9.15; Global 90

> **+15201** each additional 20 sq cm, or part thereof (List separately in addition to code for primary procedure)
> *wRVU 1.32; Global ZZZ*

15220 Full thickness graft, free, including direct closure of donor site, scalp, arms, and/or legs; 20 sq cm or less
wRVU 8.09; Global 90

> **+15221** each additional 20 sq cm, or part thereof (List separately in addition to code for primary procedure)
> *wRVU 1.19; Global ZZZ*

15240 Full thickness graft, free, including direct closure of donor site, forehead, cheeks, chin, mouth, neck, axillae, genitalia, hands, and/or feet; 20 sq cm or less
wRVU 10.41; Global 90

> **+15241** each additional 20 sq cm, or part thereof (List separately in addition to code for primary procedure)
> *wRVU 1.86; Global ZZZ*

15260 Full thickness graft, free, including direct closure of donor site, nose, ears, eyelids, and/or lips; 20 sq cm or less
wRVU 11.64; Global 90

> **+15261** each additional 20 sq cm, or part thereof (List separately in addition to code for primary procedure)
> *wRVU 2.23; Global ZZZ*

Allograft

These codes are used when allografts such as acellular dermis is placed as a skin substitute, not when placed below the skin or for soft tissue reinforcement. Currently, there is not a code for placement of acellular dermis as soft tissue reinforcement in the head and neck. Add-on code, 15777 is reported only when placed in the breast or trunk but not in the head or neck. Use an unlisted code, such as 17999 and compare it to 15777 for a head and/or neck procedure if the biologic is placed below the skin for soft tissue reinforcement.

15275 Application of skin substitute graft to face, scalp, eyelids, mouth, neck, ears, orbits, genitalia, hands, feet, and/or multiple digits, total wound surface area up to 100 sq cm; first 25 sq cm or less wound surface area
wRVU 1.83; Global 0

> **+15276** each additional 25 sq cm wound surface area, or part thereof (List separately in addition to code for primary procedure)
> *wRVU 0.50; Global ZZZ*

15277 Application of skin substitute graft to face, scalp, eyelids, mouth, neck, ears, orbits, genitalia, hands, feet, and/or multiple digits, total wound surface area greater than or equal to 100 sq cm; first 100 sq cm wound surface area, or 1% of body area of infants and children
wRVU 4.00; Global 0

> **+15278** each additional 100 sq cm wound surface area, or part thereof, or each additional 1% of body area of infants and children, or part thereof (List separately in addition to code for primary procedure)
> *wRVU 1.00; Global ZZZ*

+15777 Implantation of biologic implant (eg, acellular dermal matrix) for soft tissue reinforcement (ie, breast, trunk) (List separately in addition to code for primary procedure)
wRVU 3.65; Global ZZZ

17999 Unlisted procedure, skin, mucous membrane and subcutaneous tissue
wRVU 0.00; Global YYY

Regional Flaps

Regional flap codes are unique in that they are always identified by the donor site, not the recipient. In general, they are divided into 2 large categories: flaps that involve skin transfer only and flaps that involve transfer of fascia and muscle independently or in addition to the skin. The codes that involve transfer of deeper tissues are usually assigned higher RVUs. The closure of the donor site is included in the code for the harvest of the flap, unless more than a primary closure was performed (eg, skin graft, adjacent tissue transfer). When deciding which code to use, consider the type of the tissues being transferred.

Forehead Flap

Paramedian forehead flap has its own unique code. If the donor site was repaired with skin graft, that should be reported separately.

15731 Forehead flap with preservation of vascular pedicle (eg, axial pattern flap, paramedian forehead flap)
wRVU 14.38; Global 90

If the pedicle is divided later, use general code for dividing the pedicle (eg, 15630—as final division and inset is report for the defect site—see next section for more details).

Regional Flap That Involves Transfer of Skin Only

15570 Formation of direct or tubed pedicle, with or without transfer; trunk
wRVU 10.21; Global 90

   15572   scalp, arms, or legs
wRVU 10.12; Global 90

   15574   forehead, cheeks, chin, mouth, neck, axillae, genitalia, hands or feet
wRVU 10.70; Global 90

   15576   eyelids, nose, ears, lips, or intraoral
wRVU 9.37; Global 90

15600 Delay of flap or sectioning of flap (division and inset); at trunk
wRVU 2.01; Global 90

   15610   at scalp, arms, or legs
wRVU 2.52; Global 90

   15620   at forehead, cheeks, chin, neck, axillae, genitalia, hands, or feet
wRVU 3.75; Global 90

   15630   at eyelids, nose, ears, or lips
wRVU 4.08; Global 90

15740 Flap; island pedicle requiring identification and dissection of an anatomically named axial vessel
wRVU 11.80; Global 90

Regional Flaps With Transfer of Muscle or Fascia

15732 Muscle, myocutaneous, or fasciocutaneous flap; head and neck (eg, temporalis, masseter muscle, sternocleidomastoid, levator scapulae)
wRVU 16.38; Global 90

   15734   trunk
wRVU 19.86; Global 90

   15736   upper extremity
wRVU 17.04; Global 90

   15750   Flap; neurovascular pedicle
wRVU 12.96; Global 90

Free Flaps

Free tissue transfers involve harvest of the tissue with its blood supply and transfer and reestablishing the blood supply at a remote location. These procedures are usually quite complex, lengthy and considered high risk. The majority of cases involve more than one surgical team; therefore, it is important for the operating surgeons to code these procedures accurately. All these codes include the use of operative microscope; do not report use of operative microscope separately (69990). These codes include the closure of the donor site (eg, intermediate and complex closure). If the donor site needs to be skin grafted or adjacent tissue transfer needs to be done (additional incisions), then closure should be reported separately. Extensive immobilization should be reported separately (codes 15570–15738 do not include extensive mobilization so casting and other immobilizing devices may be separately reported). Additionally, repair of the donor site requiring harvest of graft through a separate incision (eg, skin graft, adjacent tissue transfer) may also be separately reported.

These codes are classified based on the type of the tissue being transferred. Please note that when an osseous flap is performed, the codes are different based on the presence or absence of a skin paddle. If additional vessels have to be harvested, this is included in the free flap code; however, it is reasonable to add a 22 modifier to the code under these circumstances, as this increases the work and complexity of the case.

Soft Tissue

15756 Free muscle or myocutaneous flap with microvascular anastomosis
wRVU 36.94; Global 90

15757 Free skin flap with microvascular anastomosis
wRVU 37.15; Global 90

15758 Free fascial flap with microvascular anastomosis
wRVU 36.90; Global 90

43496 Free jejunum transfer with microvascular anastomosis
wRVU 0.00; Global 90

49906 Free omental flap with microvascular anastomosis
wRVU 0.00; Global 90

Osseous Flaps

These codes include the harvest of the donor graft and placement into the recipient site. The primary closure (eg, intermediate or complex repair, plate for internal fixation) of both defects is also

included. A separate graft to close the donor defect site may be reported (eg, skin graft).

20955 Bone graft with microvascular anastomosis; fibula
wRVU 40.26; Global 90

20956 iliac crest
wRVU 41.18; Global 90

20962 other than fibula, iliac crest, or metatarsal
wRVU 39.21; Global 90

20969 Free osteocutaneous flap with microvascular anastomosis; other than iliac crest, metatarsal, or great toe
wRVU 45.43; Global 90

20970 iliac crest
wRVU 44.58; Global 90

Key Modifiers

22 Increased Procedural Services
This should be added when the work is above and beyond what is typically required for the code selected. An example would be if during a free flap an additional vessel has to be harvested through another incision as a donor vessel.

58 Staged or Related Procedure or Service by the Same Physician or Other Qualified Health Care Professional During the Postoperative Period
This would be used when a planned procedure occurs during the global period; for instance if a paramedian forehead flap was performed and then divided and inset during the 90-day global period. Modifier 58 is appended to the code(s) for the second procedure.

59 Distinct Procedural Service
This is used when multiple procedures are done at the same setting that are distinct from each other. For example, the harvest of a radial forearm free flap with a need to repair the donor site with a skin graft. The lower-valued code, skin graft, is appended with modifier 59 because Medicare's

Correct Coding Initiative (CCI) edits bundle the 2 procedures together.

62   Two Surgeons
Used when 2 surgeons perform an entire procedure, CPT code, together in equal amounts (co-surgeons).

80   Assistant Surgeon
Use when a second surgeon assists the primary surgeon with the procedure.

82   Assistant Surgeon (When Qualified Resident Surgeon Not Available)
Used in academic facilities when a resident is not available and a second surgeon is required to assist the primary surgeon.

Key ICD-9-CM/ICD-10-CM Codes

All procedure codes should be accompanied by an appropriate diagnosis code. Below is a list of some of the commonly used codes, broken down by anatomic site, with a description of the code.

Neck

874.8/S11.80XA   Unspecified open wound; of other specified part of neck, initial encounter

874.8/S11.90XA   of unspecified part of neck, initial encounter

Head/Face

873.0/S01.00XA   Unspecified open wound; of scalp, initial encounter

873.42/S01.80XA   of other part of head, initial encounter

870.9/S01.109   of unspecified eyelid and periocular area, initial encounter

872.00/S01.309A   of unspecified ear, initial encounter

873.41/S01.409A   of unspecified cheek and temporomandibular area, initial encounter

170.0/C41.0   Malignant neoplasm; of bones of skull and face

170.1/C41.1   of mandible

171.0/C49.0   of connective and soft tissue of head, face and neck

173.30/C44.300   Unspecified malignant neoplasm; of skin of unspecified part of face

173.30C44.301   of skin of nose

173.30/C44.309   of skin of other parts of face

173.31/C44.310   Basal cell carcinoma; of skin of unspecified parts of face

173.31/C44.311   of skin of nose

173.31/C44.319   of skin of other parts of face

173.32/C44.320   Squamous cell carcinoma; of skin of unspecified parts of face

173.32/C44.321   of skin of nose

173.32/C44.329   of skin of other parts of face

173.40/C44.40   Unspecified malignant neoplasm of skin of scalp and neck

173.41/C44.41   Basal cell carcinoma of skin of scalp and neck

173.42/C44.42   Squamous cell carcinoma of skin of scalp and neck

173.49/C44.49   Other specified malignant neoplasm of skin of scalp and neck

195.0/C76.0   Malignant neoplasm of head, face and neck

Nose

160.0/C30.0   Malignant neoplasm; of nasal cavity

160.2/C31.0   of maxillary sinus

160.3/C31.1   of ethmoid sinus

160.4/C31.2   of frontal sinus

160.5/C31.3   of sphenoidal sinus

160.8/C31.8   of overlapping sites of accessory sinuses

160.9/C31.9   of accessory sinus, unspecified

738.0/M95.0   Acquired deformity of nose

Oral Cavity

873.53/S01.521A   Laceration with foreign body of lip, initial encounter

873.60/S01.502A   Unspecified open wound of oral cavity, initial encounter

873.61/S01.512A   Laceration without foreign body of oral cavity, initial encounter

210.0/D10.0   Benign neoplasm; of lip

210.1/D10.1   of tongue

210.3/D10.2   of floor of mouth

210.4/D10.30   of unspecified part of mouth

210.4/D10.39   of other parts of mouth

141.0/C01   Malignant neoplasm; of base of tongue

141.1/C02.0   of dorsal surface of tongue

141.2/C02.1   of border of tongue

141.3/C02.2   of ventral surface of tongue

141.4/C02.3   of anterior two-thirds of tongue, part unspecified

141.5/C02.8   of overlapping sites of tongue

141.6/C02.4   of lingual tonsil

141.8/C02.8   of overlapping sites of tongue

141.9/C02.9   of tongue, unspecified

143.0/C03.0   of upper gum

143.1/C03.1   of lower gum

143.9/C03.9   of gum, unspecified

144.0/C04.0   of anterior floor of mouth

144.1/C04.1   of lateral floor of mouth

144.8/C04.8   of overlapping sites of floor of mouth

144.9/C04.9   of floor of mouth, unspecified

145.0/C06.0   of cheek mucosa

145.1/C06.1   of vestibule of mouth

145.2/C05.0   of hard palate

145.3/C05.1   of soft palate

145.4/C05.2   of uvula

145.5/C05.8   of palate, unspecified

145.6/C06.2   of retromolar area

145.8/C06.89   of overlapping sites of other parts of mouth

170.0/C41.0   of bones of skull and face

170.1/C41.1   of mandible

526.89/M27.8   Other specified diseases of jaws

V10.01/Z85.810   Personal history of malignant neoplasm; of tongue

V10.02/Z85.818   of other sites of lip, oral cavity, and pharynx

V10.02/Z85.819   of malignant neoplasm of unspecified site of lip, oral cavity, and pharynx

Pharynx

874.4/S11.20XA   Unspecified open wound of pharynx and cervical esophagus, initial encounter

210.5/D10.4   Benign neoplasm; of tonsil

210.6/D10.5   of other parts of oropharynx

210.7/D10.6   of nasopharynx

210.8/D10.7   of hypopharynx

210.9/D10.9   of pharynx, unspecified

146.0/C09.9   Malignant neoplasm of tonsil, unspecified

146.1/C09.9   of tonsillar fossa

146.2/C09.1   of tonsillar pillar (anterior) (posterior)

146.3/C10.0   of vallecula

146.4/C10.1   of anterior aspect of epiglottis

146.5/C10.8   of overlapping sites of oropharynx

146.6/C10.2   of lateral wall of oropharynx

146.7/C10.3   of posterior wall of oropharynx

146.8/C10.4   of branchial cleft

146.8/C10.8   of overlapping sites of oropharynx

147/C11.0   of superior wall of nasopharynx

147.1/C11.1   of posterior wall of nasopharynx

147.2/C11.2   of lateral wall of nasopharynx

147.3/C11.3   of anterior wall of nasopharynx

147.8/C11.8   of overlapping sites of nasopharynx

147.9/C11.9   of nasopharynx, unspecified

148.0/C13.0   of postcricoid region

148.1/C12   of pyriform sinus

148.2,148.3/C13.1   of aryepiglottic fold, hypopharyngeal aspect

148.8/C13.8   of overlapping sites of hypopharynx

148.9/C13.9   of hypopharynx, unspecified

V10.02/Z85.818   Personal history of malignant neoplasm; of other sites of lip, oral cavity, and pharynx

V10.02/Z85.819   of malignant neoplasm of unspecified site of lip, oral cavity, and pharynx

Larynx

874.01/S11.019A   Unspecified open wound of larynx, initial encounter

212.1/D14.1   Benign neoplasm of larynx

161.0/C32.0   Malignant neoplasm; of glottis

161.1/C32.1   of supraglottis

161.2/C32.2   of subglottis

161.3/C32.2   of laryngeal cartilage

161.8/C32.8   of overlapping sites of larynx

161.9/C32.9   of larynx, unspecified

V10.21/Z85.21   Personal history of malignant neoplasm of larynx

Salivary Gland

210.2/D11.9   Benign neoplasm of major salivary gland, unspecified

142.0/C07   Malignant neoplasm; of parotid gland

142.1/C08.0   of submandibular gland

142.2/C08.1   of sublingual gland

142.8, 142.9/C08.9   of major salivary gland, unspecified

V10.02/Z85.818   Personal history of malignant neoplasm; of other sites of lip, oral cavity, and pharynx

V10.02/Z85.819   of unspecified site of lip, oral cavity, and pharynx

Miscellaneous

453.89/I82.890   Acute embolism and thrombosis of other specified veins

998.11/L76.22   Hemorrhage complicating a procedure

998.13/T88.8XXA   Other specified complications of surgical and medical care, not elsewhere classified, initial encounter

998.31/T81.32XA   Disruption of internal operation (surgical) wound, not elsewhere classified, initial encounter

998.6/T81.83XA   Persistent postprocedural fistula, initial encounter

Definition of Procedure Codes

Commonly Used Regional Flaps in Head and Neck Reconstruction

Be sure that the documentation supports the code reported.

CODE	FLAP
15570	Deltopectoral
15572	Scalp
15732	Sternocleidomastoid muscle
	Trapezius (superior and lower)
	Temporalis fascia or temporalis muscle
15734	Pectoralis major
	Latissimus dorsi
15740	Supraclavicular island
	Submental island

Commonly Used Free Flaps in Head and Neck Reconstruction

Be sure that the documentation supports the code reported.

CODE	FLAP
15756	Rectus abdominis
	Latissmus dorsi
	Gracillis
15757	Radial forearm
	Ulnar forearm
	Anterolateral thigh
	Lateral arm
	Parascapular
15758	Temporoparietal fascia
20955	Fibula without skin paddle
20956	Iliac crest without skin paddle
20962	Scapula without skin paddle
20969	Osteocutaneous radial forearm
	Fibula with skin paddle
	Scapula with skin paddle
20970	Iliac crest with skin

Controversial Areas

1. Co-surgeon modifier for free flaps (15756–15758)—In general, the co-surgeon modifier and assistant surgeon codes are accepted modifiers for all free flaps. Payers may not allow the co-surgeons to be of the same specialty (eg, ear, nose, and throat [ENT]). If one ENT surgeon performs the ablative surgery (tumor removal) and another ENT performs the reconstruction, then the co-surgery modifier (62) does not apply as each surgeon will report his or her own CPT codes. See Chapter 11, "Demystifying Modifiers," for more information.

2. Co-surgeon modifier for regional flaps (15732–15738)—In general, the co-surgeon modifier is paid for regional flaps with documentation. The assistant surgeon modifier is accepted as well.

3. Patients with satisfactory remaining dentition and dentoalveolar architecture can be rehabilitated with conventional non-implant-retained prostheses. More commonly, osseointegrated implants are required for adequate prosthetic stability. Insurance preauthorization should be sought in all potential osseointegrated implant candidates, but this will only be successful in a small portion of patients. Those patients whose insurance does not reimburse for implant rehabilitation will have to bear the costs on their own. This is separate from the actual prosthetic reconstruction, which is almost always a significant out-of-pocket expense. There are no specific CPT codes for placement of osseointegrated implants, and this is a separate negotiated situation with the payer and/or patient.

CHAPTER 30

Skull Base Surgery

Belachew Tessema and Jack A. Shohet

Introduction

This chapter focuses on otolaryngologic procedures that involve the skull base and upper spine. It is divided into regions (anterior, middle, lateral, posterior, spine) and separated into 3 stages: approach, resection, and reconstruction. Coding and billing for these procedures can be confusing as skull base surgery often involves multiple disciplines, including neurosurgery, head and neck oncology, neurotology, rhinology, plastic and reconstructive surgery, and others. The otolaryngologist may be involved in all 3 or only 1 of the aforementioned stages. Each interdisciplinary surgical team should delineate the surgical responsibilities in any manner they find appropriate; therefore, a multitude of coding options exist. Common, but not exclusive, scenarios for a team approach to skull base surgery coding are included in the examples below. For all cases, each operative report and subsequent coding/billing should clearly reflect each physician's involvement. Understanding appropriate modifiers can allow for accurate co-surgeon billing. *Current Procedural Terminology* (CPT) codes covered below will include both open and endoscopic techniques for skull base surgery.

Unlike other areas of otolaryngology, accurate skull base coding typically depends more on the disease location than the pathology. For approach codes, skull base regions are divided anatomically into the anterior, middle, and posterior cranial fossa. Similarly, resection codes are also catego-rized anatomically and further refer to intra- or extradural locations. It is important to note that approach and resection codes refer to the region of the pathology; therefore, identical codes can be correctly applied to a variety of pathologies. In those cases where disease- or pathology-specific codes do exist, they are listed and described below. Additionally, in highly complex cases where the approach or resection involves multiple skull base regions, it is appropriate to use codes that refer each involved regions. In these rare cases, there may be multiple approach and resection codes for a single procedure.

Operative management of skull base disease is challenging and complex. Surgical approach, resection, and reconstruction are influenced by a myriad of clinical and pathologic factors that are beyond the scope of this chapter. For example, pathology of the internal auditory canal (such as a vestibular schwannoma) can be approached via the middle or posterior fossa. Operative approach is dependent on a variety of factors, including but not limited to tumor size, hearing and facial nerve status, patient age, comorbid disease, and so on. Each surgeon or surgical team must weigh the clinical factors that influence approach and ultimately choose the code that best represents the procedure performed. Although the procedure may be performed at the skull base, that does not guarantee the use of the skull base surgery CPT codes. CPT provides some single, stand-alone codes for skull base procedures that would preclude the use of the skull base surgery codes. The anatomic boundaries highlighted below are offered only to assist with code categorization; each surgeon is responsible for matching his or her intimate knowledge of the patient's anatomy with the appropriate code.

Key Points

- In many cases, coding should be separated into approach, resection, and reconstruction. However, reconstruction is often included in the resection code, and in these instances, cannot be billed separately, unless performed by an additional surgeon (rare) or at a different operative session.
- When co-surgeons use modifier 62 each surgeon must dictate a separate operative report specifying their level of involvement.
- Endoscopic procedures may not be reported with an open existing CPT code. An unlisted code must be used when an appropriate endoscopic code does not exist. The only existing endoscopic skull base surgery codes are for an endoscopic resection of a pituitary tumor (62165) and endoscopic cerebrospinal fluid leak repair (31290, 31291).
- Acoustic neuroma (also known as vestibular schwannoma) surgery has specific stand-alone codes for standardized approaches (eg, translabyrinthine approach, retrosigmoid approach), and these codes include the approach, tumor removal, and closure; thus, these codes (61520, 61526) should be billed in most cases and not the newer skull base codes.
- CPT guidelines specifically state that surgeons cannot bill for intraoperative monitoring, including auditory and facial nerve monitoring, as this service is included in all surgical CPT codes.
- Additional procedures such as harvest of an abdominal fat graft (20926), use of the operating microscope for microdissection (69990), and placement of a lumbar drain

(62272) may be separately reported. CPT 69990 is an add-on code and should not be appended with modifier 51 (multiple procedures), and other reported stand-alone codes (eg, 20926, 62272) would be appended with modifier 51.

Key Procedure Codes

Approach

The skull base approach codes are divided into 3 anatomic locations: anterior cranial fossa, middle cranial fossa, and posterior cranial fossa.

Anterior Cranial Fossa

The anterior cranial fossa is bordered by the posterior wall of the frontal sinus (anteriorly), the clinoid processes and planum sphenoidale (posteriorly), and the frontal bones (laterally). Approaches that involve this anatomic region should use the codes below. Presently, this area can be accessed endoscopically or through an open approach. However, the codes in this section all describe open access surgery and should not be used if a purely endoscopic (endonasal) approach is performed.

61580 Craniofacial approach to anterior cranial fossa; extradural, including lateral rhinotomy, ethmoidectomy, sphenoidectomy, without maxillectomy or orbital exenteration
wRVU 34.51; Global 90

    61581 extradural, including lateral rhinotomy, orbital exenteration, ethmoidectomy, sphenoidectomy and/or maxillectomy
wRVU 39.13; Global 90

    61582 extradural, including unilateral or bifrontal craniotomy, elevation of frontal lobe(s), osteotomy of base of anterior cranial fossa
wRVU 35.14; Global 90

61583 intradural, including unilateral or bifrontal craniotomy, elevation or resection of frontal lobe, osteotomy of base of anterior cranial fossa
wRVU 38.50; Global 90

61584 Orbitocranial approach to anterior cranial fossa, extradural, including supraorbital ridge osteotomy and elevation of frontal and/or temporal lobe(s); without orbital exenteration
wRVU 37.70; Global 90

61585 with orbital exenteration
wRVU 42.57; Global 90

61586 Bicoronal, transzygomatic and/or LeFort I osteotomy approach to anterior cranial fossa with or without internal fixation, without bone graft
wRVU 27.48; Global 90

Middle Cranial Fossa

The middle fossa is bounded by the greater wing of the sphenoid (anteriorly and laterally), the petrous temporal bone and clivus (posteriorly), the parietal bone, and squamous portion of the temporal bone (laterally). Currently, this region is primarily accessed through an open approach via a pre- or postauricular craniotomy. The most common pathology in this region involves the internal auditory canal (IAC)/cerebellopontine angle (CPA) and floor of the temporal bone. However, the craniotomy for IAC/CPA tumors (eg, 61520, 61526) should be used instead of these skull base surgery codes and are mentioned in the section under cerebellopontine angle surgery.

The skull base codes were implemented in 1994 to report resection of tumors by newer techniques that had not previously been removed. Removal of an acoustic neuroma (vestibular schwannoma) at the IAC/CPA by translabyrinthine (61526) and retrosigmoid (61520) approaches was performed prior to the introduction of skull base codes; therefore, these existing codes are to be used for these procedures. However, a true middle cranial fossa approach is a newer technique to the IAC/CPA. This approach did not exist prior

to the time when the 61520 and 61526 codes were proposed; therefore, it falls out of their purview and may be reported using the skull base codes.

61590 Infratemporal pre-auricular approach to middle cranial fossa (parapharyngeal space, infratemporal and midline skull base, nasopharynx), with or without disarticulation of the mandible, including parotidectomy, craniotomy, decompression and/or mobilization of the facial nerve and/or petrous carotid artery
wRVU 47.04; Global 90

61591 Infratemporal post-auricular approach to middle cranial fossa (internal auditory meatus, petrous apex, tentorium, cavernous sinus, parasellar area, infratemporal fossa) including mastoidectomy, resection of sigmoid sinus with or without decompression and/or mobilization of contents of auditory canal or petrous carotid artery
wRVU 47.02; Global 90

61592 Orbitocranial zygomatic approach to middle cranial fossa (cavernous sinus and carotid artery, clivus, basilar artery or petrous apex) including osteotomy of zygoma, craniotomy, extra- or intradural elevation of temporal lobe
wRVU 43.08; Global 90

Posterior Cranial Fossa

The posterior fossa is bounded by the posterior surface of the petrous temporal bone (anteriorly), the clivus and greater wing of the sphenoid bones (anterio-medially), and the occipital bone (laterally and posteriorly). A variety of pathologies can occur in this region, including that related to the internal auditory canal/CPA, foramen magnum, and clivus. Two common approaches to the IAC/CPA—specifically, the translabyrinthine and retrosigmoid approaches—use the same code (61595). However, again, the craniotomy for IAC/CPA tumors (eg, 61520, 61526) should be used instead of these skull base surgery codes. These approaches differ drastically in application and technique, but they are represented by the same code. Also, as specified below, codes in this category include the entirety of the approach and, therefore, may not be combined with additional mastoid or temporal bone codes (eg, 69644).

61595   Transtemporal approach to posterior cranial fossa, jugular foramen or midline skull base, including mastoidectomy, decompression of sigmoid sinus and/or facial nerve, with or without mobilization
wRVU 33.74; Global 90

61596   Transcochlear approach to posterior cranial fossa, jugular foramen or midline skull base, including labyrinthectomy, decompression, with or without mobilization of facial nerve and/or petrous carotid artery
wRVU 39.43; Global 90

61597   Transcondylar (far lateral) approach to posterior cranial fossa, jugular foramen or midline skull base, including occipital condylectomy, mastoidectomy, resection of C1-C3 vertebral body(s), decompression of vertebral artery, with or without mobilization
wRVU 40.82; Global 90

61598   Transpetrosal approach to posterior cranial fossa, clivus or foramen magnum, including ligation of superior petrosal sinus and/or sigmoid sinus
wRVU 36.53; Global 90

Spine

The following 2 codes are stand-alone codes and include the approach, tumor resection, and closure.

61575   Transoral approach to skull base, brain stem or upper spinal cord for biopsy, decompression or excision of lesion
wRVU 36.56; Global 90

61576   requiring splitting of tongue and/or mandible (including tracheostomy)
wRVU 55.31; Global 90

Resection

As with approach, skull base resection codes refer to the location of the pathology. Specifically, whether the resection is extra- or intradural. The codes below are not disease specific and can used for a variety of pathologies, including neoplastic, vascular, or infectious.

Base of Anterior Cranial Fossa

61600   Resection or excision of neoplastic, vascular or infectious lesion of base of anterior cranial fossa; extradural
wRVU 30.01; Global 90

61601   intradural, including dural repair, with or without graft
wRVU 31.14; Global 90

Base of Middle Cranial Fossa

61605   Resection or excision of neoplastic, vascular or infectious lesion of infratemporal fossa, parapharyngeal space, petrous apex; extradural
wRVU 32.57; Global 90

61606   intradural, including dural repair, with or without graft
wRVU 42.05; Global 90

61607   Resection or excision of neoplastic, vascular or infectious lesion of parasellar area, cavernous sinus, clivus or midline skull base; extradural
wRVU 40.93; Global 90

61608   intradural, including dural repair, with or without graft
wRVU 45.54; Global 90

Base of Posterior Cranial Fossa

61615   Resection or excision of neoplastic, vascular or infectious lesion of base of posterior cranial fossa, jugular foramen, foramen magnum, or C1-C3 vertebral bodies; extradural
wRVU 35.77; Global 90

61616 intradural, including dural repair, with or without graft
wRVU 46.74; Global 90

Cerebellopontine Angle

The following 2 codes are stand-alone codes and include the approach, tumor resection, and closure.

61520 Craniectomy for excision of brain tumor, infratentorial or posterior fossa; cerebellopontine angle tumor
wRVU 57.09; Global 90

61526 Craniectomy, bone flap craniotomy, transtemporal (mastoid) for excision of cerebellopontine angle tumor
wRVU 54.08; Global 90

Repair and/or Reconstruction

This includes reconstruction above and beyond that which is included in the resection codes. All of the definitive procedure or resection codes include dural reconstruction as part of the procedure. For instance, a pericranial flap is often used for reconstruction of the dura. If this is done as part of the primary procedure through the same incision, this is not to be reported separately. For a more detailed discussion of reconstruction, specifically flap reconstruction, please see Chapter 29, "Reconstructive Head and Neck Surgery."

Secondary Dural Repair

These codes are used when the dura repair is performed at a separate operative session. All intradural tumor resection codes include the primary (same operative session) dural repair.

61618 Secondary repair of dura for cerebrospinal fluid leak, anterior, middle or posterior cranial fossa following surgery of the skull base; by free tissue graft (eg, pericranium, fascia, tensor fascia lata, adipose tissue, homologous or synthetic grafts)
wRVU 18.69; Global 90

61619 by local or regionalized vascularized pedicle flap or myocutaneous flap (including galea, temporalis, frontalis or occipitalis muscle)
wRVU 22.10; Global 90

Other codes that might be used for a secondary dural repair include

62100 Craniotomy for repair of dural/cerebrospinal fluid leak, including surgery for rhinorrhea/otorrhea
wRVU 23.53; Global 90

62120 Repair of encephalocele, skull vault, including cranioplasty
wRVU 24.59; Global 90

62121 Craniotomy for repair of encephalocele, skull base
wRVU 23.03; Global 90

Grafts

On occasion graft material may need to be harvested through a separate skin incision to close the operative wound. Examples include

15120 Split-thickness autograft, face, scalp, eyelids, mouth, neck, ears, orbits, genitalia, hands, feet and/or multiple digits; first 100 sq cm or less, or 1% of body area of infants and children (except 15050)
wRVU 10.15; Global 90

+15121 each additional 100 sq cm, or each additional 1% of body area of infants and children, or part thereof (list separately in addition to code for primary procedure)
wRVU 2.00; Global ZZZ

20926 Tissue grafts, other (eg paratenon, fat, dermis)
wRVU 5.79; Global 90

This code is typically used for harvest of abdominal fat. Graft material obtained through the same incision (eg, temporalis fascia) is not separately reported.

20902 Bone graft, any donor area; major or large
wRVU 4.58; Global 0

An example is a split calvarial bone graft that is harvested through a separate incision; bone harvested and grafted from the same cranial bone flap is not separately reported.

Flaps

15750 Flap; neurovascular pedicle
wRVU 12.96; Global 90

The physician forms a neurovascular pedicle flap and covers the defect by rotating it into a nearby but not immediately adjacent defect through a subcutaneous tunnel and sutured into position. This code includes not only skin but also a functional motor or sensory nerve(s). The flap serves to reinnervate a damaged portion of the body dependent on touch or movement (eg, thumb). Therefore, this code is not appropriate to be used for a nasoseptal flap performed for skull base reconstruction after endonasal/endoscopic skull base surgery. This is discussed in more detail later in this chapter.

Diagnosis or Structure-Specific CPT Codes

These codes refer to the treatment of a specific disorder. When appropriate, these codes are more specific and preferred to the general skull base codes listed earlier in this chapter.

Cerebrospinal Fluid Leak/ Encephalocele Repair

62100 Craniotomy for repair of dural/ cerebrospinal fluid leak, including surgery for rhinorrhea/otorrhea
wRVU 23.53; Global 90

62121 Craniotomy for repair of encephalocele, skull base
wRVU 23.03; Global 90

31290 Nasal/sinus endoscopy, surgical, with repair of cerebrospinal fluid leak; ethmoid region
wRVU 18.61; Global 10

31291 sphenoid region
wRVU 19.56; Global 10

Pituitary Tumors

62165 Neuroendoscopy, intracranial; with excision of pituitary tumor, transnasal or trans-sphenoidal approach
wRVU 23.23; Global 90

61548 Hypophysectomy or excision of pituitary tumor, transnasal or transseptal approach, nonstereotactic
wRVU 23.37; Global 90

Note that this code, 61548, includes use of the operating microscope; therefore, it is not appropriate to separately report 69990.

Glomus Tumors

This section includes only the code for an extended approach. There are separate codes for transcanal and transmastoid approaches. See Chapter 26, "Operative Otology," for more information.

69554 Excision aural glomus tumor extended (extratemporal)
wRVU 35.97; Global 90

Facial Nerve

69960 Decompression internal auditory canal
wRVU 29.42; Global 90

This code is typically used for facial nerve decompression as is done for idiopathic facial paralysis or facial nerve injuries; this code is included in all IAC/CPA tumor removal codes such as 61520, 61526, 61595, 61696.

64864 Suture of facial nerve; extracranial
wRVU 13.41; Global 90

64866 Anastomosis; facial-spinal accessory
wRVU 16.83; Global 90

64868   facial-hypoglossal
wRVU 14.90; Global 90

64885   Nerve graft (includes obtaining graft), head or neck; up to 4 cm in length
wRVU 17.60; Global 90

64886   more than 4 cm length
wRVU 20.82; Global 90

Orbital Decompression

61330   Decompression of orbit only, transcranial approach
wRVU 25.30; Global 90

31292   Nasal/sinus endoscopy, surgical; with medial or inferior orbital wall decompression
wRVU 15.90; Global 10

31293   with medial orbital wall and inferior orbital wall decompression
wRVU 17.47; Global 10

31294   with optic nerve decompression
wRVU 20.31; Global 10

Intraoperative Monitoring

This includes facial nerve electromyography, auditory brainstem response testing, evoked potentials, and so on. CPT codes 95940, 94941, 92516, and 95868 are not billable by the surgeon, assistant surgeon, co-surgeon, or anesthesiologist. Intraoperative monitoring performed by any of the above providers is included in his or her primary service code(s) and should not be separately submitted. These CPT codes can be billed by another qualified individual, such as an electrophysiologist or audiologist, who performs and documents the intraoperative testing/monitoring.

Operating Microscope

+69990 Microsurgical techniques, requiring use of operating microscope (List separately in addition to code for primary procedure)
wRVU 3.46; Global ZZZ

Use of the operating microscope should be billed when microdissection and microsurgical techniques are utilized, not when the microscope is used for magnification or illumination. The operative report must specify the appropriate use of the operating microscope. While both the otolaryngologist and neurosurgeon may report 69990, payers may not reimburse both surgeons so an appeal may be necessary. CPT 69990 is an add-on code so modifier 51 does not apply. It should be reimbursed the full allowable by payers.

Many CPT codes include use of the operating microscope, including procedures requiring microvascular anastomosis (eg, free flaps such as 15756–15758), transnasal/transeptal excision of pituitary tumor (61548), and the anterior cervical spine decompression surgery (eg, 22551, 63075). Even when billed appropriately according to CPT guidelines, Medicare's correct coding initiative (CCI) edits do not allow for reimbursement on 69990 such as when reported with complex ear procedure codes. Reimbursement from other insurance carriers varies.

Intraoperative Navigation

Intraoperative stereotactic navigation enables the surgeon to better identify anatomy for surgical removal and may reduce the likelihood of injury to vital structures. The use of computer-assisted navigation is separately billable and should be coded according to whether the pathology is extradural or intradural. Navigation codes are considered "add-on" codes, which implies that they are never billed as the sole procedure. When used, navigation codes are billed full-fee (even in cases performed with a co-surgeon, although modifier 62 on the navigation code is never acceptable), should be listed in rank order of all procedures billed and without a modifier. Add-on codes should be reimbursed by payers at the full allowable. Typically payers will only pay either the neurosurgeon or otolaryngologist on a navigation code, as the majority of the value of these codes is for the setup and not for the use of this equipment. Therefore, if each surgeon bills a navigation code, there needs to be good documentation that each surgeon did his or her own setup, planning, and registration.

+61781 Stereotactic computer-assisted (navigational) procedure; cranial, intradural (List separately in addition to code for primary procedure)
wRVU 3.75; Global ZZZ

> **+61782** cranial, extradural (List separately in addition to code for primary procedure)
> *wRVU 3.18; Global ZZZ*

CPT 61781 and 61782 are never reported by the same provider during the same operative session. Documentation must include, according to CPT, the following: "The documentation for the use of one of these codes should include the physician work of image-based planning, description of the image acquisition, attachment of a reference frame, registration and review of the image data sets, and verification of the accuracy. The physician work of image-based planning must also be included when reporting these codes."

Other

31299 Unlisted procedure, accessory sinuses
wRVU 0.00; Global YYY

64999 Unlisted procedure, nervous system
wRVU 0.00; Global YYY

Key Modifiers

22 Increased Procedural Services
Surgeries for which services performed are significantly greater than usually required. The operative report must specifically support this modifier with a separate complexity paragraph.

58 Staged or Related Procedure or Service by the Same Physician or Other Qualified Health Care Professional During the Postoperative Period
This could be used if the physician was resecting an esthesioneuroblastoma and required a 2-stage procedure due to the patient's health which precludes a lengthy anesthesia. The endonasal, extradural procedure is done on day 1 and several days later a craniotomy is done for the secondary pro-

cedure. Modifier 58 would then go on the intradural resection code (the second procedure). This is not appropriate for a complication during the global period, such as repair of a CSF leak in the postoperative period.

62 Two Surgeons
This is when 2 surgeons work together as primary surgeons performing distinct parts of a procedure. For this, both surgeons submit the same CPT code, appended by the 62 modifier. Typically, a co-surgeon brings different expertise to the procedure and must have pre- and postop responsibilities. This modifier requires separate operative reports by each primary surgeon specifying their level of involvement as it pertains to each code they submit. It should not be appended to all codes billed for a specific procedure, but only to the code(s) that both surgeons performed together. There are a multitude of scenarios for coding of interdisciplinary skull base procedures, a few of which are covered below.

78 Unplanned Return to the Operating/Procedure Room by the Same Physician or Other Qualified Health Care Professional Following Initial Procedure for a Related Procedure During the Postoperative Period
This is used if a surgeon takes a patient back to the operating room during the global period. This is often used for a complication requiring reoperation (eg, CSF leak following a skull base procedure).

80 Assistant Surgeon
This is used when an assistant surgeon (MD or DO) provides full assistance to the primary surgeon. The primary surgeon dictates the operative report and specifies the role of the assistant. This modifier cannot be used in academic centers where residents are available.

82 Assistant Surgeon (when qualified resident surgeon not available)
This is used only in academic centers when a qualified resident is unavailable and another surgeon (MD or DO) assists the primary surgeon. This is used when a resident may be available from a different specialty or a junior resident that is not capable of being the assistant.

Key ICD-9-CM/ICD-10-CM Codes

160.0/C30.0   Malignant neoplasm; of nasal cavity

160.1/C30.1   of middle ear

160.2/C31.0   of maxillary sinus

160.3/C31.1   of ethmoidal sinus

160.4/C31.2   of frontal sinus

160.5/C31.3   of sphenoid sinus

160.8/C31.8   of overlapping sites of accessory sinuses

170.0/C41.0   of bones of skull and face

191.0/C71.0   of cerebrum, except lobes and ventricles

191.1/C71.1   of frontal lobe

194.3/C75.1   of pituitary gland

194.3/C75.2   of craniopharyngeal duct

212.0/D14.0   Benign neoplasm of middle ear, nasal cavity and accessory sinuses

216.2/D23.20   Other benign neoplasm; of skin of unspecified ear and external auricular canal

225.0/D23.30   of skin of unspecified part of face

225.0/D23.39   of skin of other parts of face

225.1/D33.3   Benign neoplasm; of cranial nerves

225.2/D32.0   of cerebral meninges

225.2/D32.9   of meninges, unspecified

227.3/D35.2   of pituitary gland

227.3/D35.3   of craniopharyngeal duct

237.0/D44.3   Neoplasm of uncertain behavior; of pituitary gland

237.0/D44.4   of craniopharyngeal duct

237.3/D44.6   of carotid body

237.3/D44.7   of aortic body and other paraganglia

237.5/D43.2   of brain, unspecified

237.5/D43.4   of spinal cord

237.6/D42.0   of cerebral meninges

237.6/D42.1   of spinal meninges

237.6/D42.9   of meninges, unspecified

239.7/D49.7   of endocrine glands and other parts of nervous system

239.1/D49.1   of respiratory system

253.0/E22.0   Acromegaly and pituitary, gigantism

253.1/E22.8   Other hyperfunction of pituitary gland

253.1/E22.9   Hyperfunction of pituitary gland, unspecified

349.81/G96.0   Cerebrospinal fluid leak

376.01/H05.019   Cellulitis of unspecified orbit

376.21/H05.89   Other disorders of orbit

376.30/H05.20   Unspecified exophthalmos

376.32/H05.239   Hemorrhage of unspecified orbit

385.82/H74.8X9   Other specified disorders of middle ear and mastoid, unspecified ear

388.61/G96.0   Cerebrospinal fluid leak

742.0/Q01.9   Encephalocele, unspecified

950.0/S04.019A   Injury of optic nerve, unspecified eye, initial encounter

951.4/S04.50XA   Injury of facial nerve, unspecified site, initial encounter

Controversial Areas

Endoscopic Skull Base Surgery

Endoscopic skull base surgery has evolved rapidly over the past decade with unique advantages when compared to open skull base surgery. However, the CPT codes have not been properly updated to describe the breadth and complexity of the work performed in these cases. With the exception of pituitary tumor surgery (62165) and cerebrospinal leak repair (31290, 31291), there are no CPT codes for endoscopic skull base procedures.

Similar to open skull base surgery, endoscopic procedures can include the components of approach, resection, and reconstruction. However, many of the components of open skull base surgery CPT codes including open incisions do not apply to endoscopic approaches. Therefore, physicians have been using different and nonstandardized ways to code for these cases. A recent survey by the American Rhinologic Society highlights the controversy in the different methods their members code for endoscopic skull base surgery. In the study, 32% reported coding endoscopic skull base procedures using open codes, 29% used unlisted endoscopic codes, 24% used sinus codes, and 15% used the unlisted nervous system code.[1]

Currently, there are task forces around the country working on developing coding consensus for these cases. At the time of this publication none of these were published or accepted by a society. That said, here are some general guidelines for billing endoscopic skull base surgery procedures other than pituitary tumor removal (62165):

1. Open codes (61580–61619) cannot be used to code for an endoscopic skull base procedure.
2. Endoscopic sinus surgery codes (31254–31288) should not be used as a substitute for approach codes or replacement for this complex work performed.
3. Typically the unlisted accessary sinus code, 31299, is the unlisted code the otolaryngologist submits for his or her service (eg, the approach, assisting with the tumor resection, closure) in an endoscopic skull base procedure.
4. Typically the unlisted nervous system code, 64999, is the unlisted code the neurosurgeon submits for his or her service (eg, tumor resection, dural closure) in an endoscopic skull base procedure.
5. A detailed letter should be written to the claims department of the insurance provider explaining the rationale behind the use of the unlisted code. The CPT code(s) that best approximates the service provided should be

listed in the letter to approximate the value (eg, RVU, fee) with or without additional charges for complexity of the case. Typically the approximate code(s) is an open skull base code. The full operative report(s) should also be included.

6. Do not append modifiers 62 or 80/82 to unlisted codes. Rather, consider including the value of assisting or being a co-surgeon (or assistant) in your fee determination for the single unlisted code you bill.
7. Technically unlisted codes do not have a postoperative global period although some payers may apply the global period that corresponds to the comparison code used to determine your fee.
8. If possible, preauthorization of these unlisted codes can reduce the amount of time for reimbursement. Some payers will not preauthorize unlisted codes, and thus the comparison codes can be preauthorized, even if they are not subsequently billed.
9. Postoperative endoscopic sinus debridement (31237) should be considered as a staged/related procedure and preauthorized. It can be billed with modifier 58 when a global period does exist. Some payers may consider the service part of the postoperative global care and may not provide reimbursement.

Reconstruction With Intranasal Flaps

Perhaps the most controversial area currently is the reconstructive component of the endoscopic skull base surgery. Initially, most endoscopic procedures involved abdominal fat (20926) placement or grafting with fascia lata (20920, 20922) or tissue substitutes (no separate codes). The harvest of these grafts through a separate incision is billable; however, the dural reconstruction is included in the open skull base intradural resection codes. All of the intradural resection codes say, "including dural repair, with or without graft." Recently, intranasal flaps (eg, nasoseptal flap) have become more popular for reconstruction. This requires time and expertise to harvest and inset this flap. This is beyond the typical procedure performed and may be considered outside the standard resection. Flaps are traditionally not included in the resection codes. The controversy thus lies in how to code for this additional procedure as currently a code for this procedure does not exist.

1. The use of 61618–61619

    These skull base codes are used for a secondary repair of the dura. The 2 scenarios are (1) no longer a common occurrence, a plastic surgeon performs the dural repair at the same operative session as the tumor is removed by the otolaryngologist and/or neurosurgeon, or (2) a return to the operating room is necessary to close a cerebrospinal fluid (CSF) leak by the otolaryngologist or neurosurgeon.

    Codes 61618–61619 are used when the original skull base procedure performed was reported using a skull base surgery code (61580–61616). If repair of a CSF leak occurs after a procedure where a skull base surgery code (61580–61616) was not used, then use another appropriate code such as 62100 or 31290.

2. The use of 15750

    CPT states the following about 15750: "This code includes not only skin but also a functional motor or sensory nerve(s). The flap serves to reinnervate a damaged portion of the body dependent on touch or movement (eg, thumb)." Therefore, it does not have application for skull base surgery procedures.

3. Unlisted code

    There are surgeons using an unlisted code to code for a nasoseptal flap. Because an unlisted code is being used for the endoscopic skull base approach and resection portions of the procedure, including the nasoseptal reconstruction in the unlisted code likely makes the most sense from a coding standpoint. The unlisted code will only be billed once, and the comparison code(s) can include those elements that would have been done had this been an open case. The neurosurgeon should code for their portion of the case with the unlisted nervous system code, 64999. Each surgeon should only include comparison codes for those aspects of the surgery that they performed.

Unlisted Skull Base Procedure Note

Attention Medical Review Department:
RE: [patient name, DOB, policy number]

On [date], Dr [neurosurgeon's name] and I performed a neuroendoscopic resection of a large olfactory groove meningioma on the above-mentioned patient. There is no specific CPT code for neuroendoscopic approach to the anterior cranial fossa, intradural; therefore, I am submitting the unlisted procedure code 31299 (*Unlisted procedure, accessory sinus*) for my work performing the approach.

The surgical approach performed on [patient name] may be reasonably compared to existing CPT code 61583 *Craniofacial approach to anterior cranial fossa; intradural, including unilateral or bifrontal craniotomy, elevation or resection of frontal lobe, osteotomy of base of anterior cranial fossa* in terms of physician work and practice expense. The endoscopic approach to the anterior cranial fossa for resection of tumors of the anterior cranial fossa requires extensive training and expertise of both an endoscopic skull base surgeon and a neurosurgeon with endoscopic training. The approach includes opening all of the paranasal sinuses (maxillary, frontal, ethmoid, and sphenoid) bilaterally and obtaining a vascularized nasoseptal flap for later reconstruction. After a superior septectomy, the cribriform plate and anterior skull base is drilled bilaterally from the limits of the posterior frontal sinus wall to the planum sphenoidale.

The use of angled instruments, multiple-angled endoscopes, and high-speed drills is necessary for the 2 surgeons to work via a binostril, 4-hand approach. After completion of bony resection and obtaining vascular control of the anterior and posterior ethmoid arteries bilaterally, a dural resection is performed to have direct access to the tumor without brain retraction. This endoscopic approach is significantly more complicated and more difficult that the CPT code described above but affords the surgeons much higher and direct access to the tumor with reduced morbidity to the patient.

Endoscopic repair requires more experienced training and instrumentation than open repair and offers advantages such as a superior close-up view of the relevant anatomy and an enlarged working angle provided with an increased panoramic view and excellent visualization of the skull base, orbit, optic nerve, or carotid artery. These procedures are less invasive because they bypass potentially extensive face-disfiguring surgical approaches that require large cranial opening and brain retraction. These procedures reduce hospital stay by eliminating extensive bone resection or skin incisions.

My usual charge for 61583 is $ [customary fee]. Therefore, I am requesting reimbursement of $ [customary fee] for my work involved as the surgeon who performed the neuroendoscopic approach.

Attached, please find a detailed copy of my operative report/office notes and a claim on the above-mentioned patient.

Sincerely,

Note, the letter can be expanded to include 61601-80 (or 82 in an academic center) if the otolaryngologist was involved in assisting the neurosurgeon with the intradural resection of the tumor.

Reference

1. Lee JT, Kingdom TT, Smith TL, Setzen M, Brown S, Batra PS. Practice patterns in endoscopic skull base surgery: survey of the American Rhinologic Society. *Int Forum Allergy Rhinol.* 2014 Feb;4(2):124–131.

CHAPTER 31

Robotic Surgery

Jason G. Newman, Bert W. O'Malley Jr., and Gregory S. Weinstein

Introduction

This chapter will cover codes used during robotic surgery. In otolaryngology, the most common indication for robotic surgery is the management of tumors of the oropharynx. However, other non-tumor indications including sleep surgery will also be discussed. The field of transoral robotic surgery (TORS) was first developed at the University of Pennsylvania in 2004 and is now over a decade old. With several thousand cases done annually in the United States, the discussion of coding is timely.

Key Points

Robotic approaches in the head and neck most resemble their open-surgical counterparts. Therefore, open surgical codes are the most appropriate codes to use in the performance of these cases. This is not endoscopic surgery. It adheres to the principles and techniques of en bloc classic open surgery. The robotic system enhances the surgeon's ability to achieve en bloc resection, and endoscopic approaches are typically piecemeal resections.

When performing surgeries with robotic assistance, there are no additional codes used for the professional component of the surgical procedures. In other words, the use of the robot does not itself generate additional coding or payment.

Often, during the surgical management of patients with oropharyngeal cancers, reconstruc-tive procedures are necessary. The appropriate flap codes are used in these cases, as they would be under nonrobotic circumstances. Codes such as 15732, 15756, 15757, and 15758 are often used for the reconstructive procedures. The coding for reconstruction follows the same principles as classic open en bloc resections and should be individualized for a given patient. In addition, many patients also undergo staged or concomitant neck surgery, necessitating the use of appropriate neck dissection codes. Coding for reconstruction and neck dissection are discussed elsewhere in this book.

Background and Practical Considerations

In December 2009, transoral robotic surgery using the Intuitive Surgical da Vinci robot was approved for use in a limited setting. The Food and Drug Administration (FDA) clarified that it was approved for "transoral otolaryngology surgical procedures restricted to benign and malignant tumors classified as T1 and T2," in the adult population only. Since that time, additional safety and efficacy studies have been performed. In February 2014 the FDA added "benign base of tongue resection procedures" to the list of approved use of the robot. They did not specify obstructive sleep apnea, as they commented in the decision that "the safety and effectiveness of this device for the use in the treatment of obstructive sleep apnea have not been established." However, base of tongue resection is often done for the indication of obstructive sleep apnea.

The adoption of robotic techniques in the field of otolaryngology may follow one of several pathways. Within the context of head and neck cancer surgery, the learning curve appears to flatten in the range of 20 procedures. Thus, practitioners and centers that do not see moderate to high volumes of head and neck cancers may not significantly benefit from the adoption of these techniques. Alternatively, practitioners with a strong interest in obstructive sleep apnea and a high surgical volume of patients undergoing tongue base resection for benign hypertrophy may find themselves using the robot more frequently for this indication. Given the high capital costs, need for specialized training by the operating room staff, and the learning curve of the procedure, a careful utilization analysis should be performed prior to investing in robotic technology.

Intuitive Surgical Inc. has been proactive in the patient safety arena and at the time of FDA clearance in 2009 worked with key thought leaders including the chapter authors (GSW, BWO) to create a training protocol for TORS. Completion of the training protocol then results in certification by the company for the individual surgeon. This is typically required by hospitals for the surgeon to obtain privileges to use the da Vinci system. The training protocol includes (1) online training on the Intuitive Surgical website; (2) inanimate computerized exercises on the robotic console taught by an Intuitive Surgical representative; (3) live pig lab learning robotic skills for a full day taught by an Intuitive Surgical representative; (4) surgeon-led cadaver training of basic procedures; and (5) proctoring of first cases by experienced TORS surgeon, arranged by Intuitive Surgical, Inc. Since FDA clearance, over 250 surgeons have been trained in the robotics lab at the University of Pennsylvania. Surgeons who have an interest in training can contact the senior author (GWW) or the Intuitive Surgical Inc. sales representative at their institution.

Key Procedures

31307 Laryngectomy, subtotal supraglottic, without radical neck dissection
wRVU 30.57; Global 90

31599 Unlisted procedure, larynx
wRVU 0; Global YYY

41120 Glossectomy; less than one-half tongue
wRVU 11.14; Global 90

41130 Glossectomy; hemiglossectomy
wRVU 15.74; Global 90

42120 Resection of palate or extensive resection of lesion
wRVU 11.86; Global 90

42842 Radical resection of tonsil, tonsil pillars, and/or retromolar trigone; without closure
wRVU 12.23; Global 90

42844 closure with local flap (eg, tongue, buccal)
wRVU 17.78; Global 90

42870 Excision or destruction lingual tonsil, any method (separate procedure)
wRVU 5.52; Global 90

42890 Limited pharyngectomy
wRVU 19.13; Global 90

42892 Resection of lateral pharyngeal wall or pyriform sinus, direct closure by advancement of lateral and posterior pharyngeal walls
wRVU 26.03; Global 90

42894 Resection of pharyngeal wall requiring closure with myocutaneous or fasciocutaneous flap or free muscle, skin, or fascial flap with microvascular anastomosis
wRVU 33.92; Global 90

Key HCPCS Level II Code

S2900 Surgical techniques requiring use of robotic surgical system (list separately in addition to code for primary procedure)
wRVU 0.00; Global XXX

Clearly the robot poses an additional cost to the facility in which the surgery is performed. However, on the physician surgical side, there is no additional *Current Procedural Terminology* (CPT) code used to indicate that robotic assistance is being used. There is, however, code S2900, a Healthcare Common Procedure Coding System (HCPCS) Level II code, to indicate that the procedure was performed robotically. This code may be added to the physician claim; however, unfortunately, most payers do not provide additional reimbursement for this code or use of the robot.

Key ICD-9-CM/ICD-10-CM Codes

146.0/C09.9 Malignant neoplasm; of tonsil, unspecified

141.6/C02.4 of lingual tonsil

145.6/C06.2 of retromolar area

147.1/C11.1 of posterior wall of nasopharynx

148.1/C12 of pyriform sinus

161.1/C32.1 of supraglottis

327.23/G47.33 Obstructive sleep apnea (adult) (pediatric)

474.11/J35.1 Hypertrophy of tonsils

Definition of Codes

31367 Laryngectomy; subtotal supraglottic, without radical neck dissection

Indicated for the management of select cancers of the supraglottic larynx. In practice, many surgeons are using this code to perform this surgery. However, as is often the nature with new surgical approaches to previously coded procedures, this procedure code, as currently listed, does not fully reflect the procedure as it performed robotically. The unlisted code, 31599, is an appropriate alternative for use in this situation. It may, however, require extra documentation, may prolong the payment process, and is associated with variable reimbursement patterns. Future robotic specific codes will be necessary to clarify this situation.

41130 Glossectomy; hemiglossectomy

Indicated for select cases of oropharyngeal cancers that involve the base of the tongue. In keeping with a subunit approach to surgery, patients with cancers involving the base of tongue undergo resection to the midline. This code is also appropriate for use in tongue base resections for sleep apnea. Although most insurance companies accept this code, some reject it. In those cases, 42870 (lingual tonsillectomy) can be used if indeed a lingual tonsillectomy was performed. This may make approval for an overnight stay problematic, so it is not preferable.

42842 Radical resection of tonsil, tonsil pillars, and/or retromolar trigone; without closure

Indicated for selected tonsil or retromolar trigone cancers. If the resection requires closure of the primary site, without the need for pharyngoplasty or free tissue transfer, consider: 42844 Radical resection of tonsil, tonsil pillar and/or retromolar trigone; closure with local flap (eg, tongue, buccal)

42892 Resection of lateral pharyngeal wall or pyriform sinus, direct closure by advancement of lateral and posterior pharyngeal walls

Indicated for limited tumors of the lateral pharyngeal wall or pyriform sinus.

Also indicated for cases of sleep apnea, where extensive tonsil tissue tracks along the lateral hypopharyngeal wall.

42894 Resection of pharyngeal wall requiring closure with myocutaneous or fasciocutaneous flap or free muscle, skin, or fascial flap with microvascular anastomosis

Indicated for extensive resection of tumor involving the lateral or posterior pharyngeal wall.

42999 Unlisted procedure, pharynx, adenoids, or tonsils

When a procedure is being performed for which no CPT code exists, this unlisted code should be used. When reporting an unlisted code to describe a procedure or service, it will be necessary to submit supporting documentation (eg, procedure report) along with the claim to provide an adequate description of the nature, extent, need for the procedure, and the time, effort, and equipment necessary to provide the service. At the present time, there are appropriate codes for each of the procedures in the head and neck approved for robotic use by the FDA. Therefore, this code may become more relevant in the future as the indications for robotic surgery expand.

Controversial Areas

In the modern health care arena, cost containment and "value"-based decision making play prominent roles in the delivery of surgical health care. By definition, this places robotic surgery at the forefront of procedures for which the question of cost/benefit comes up. In other subspecialties, like urology and gynecology, the role of the robot in several procedures has been under significant scrutiny. What is worth noting in otolaryngology is that the procedures performed commonly with the robot, transoral resection of base of tongue and tonsil cancers, were not generally done surgically prior to the use of this tool. That is to say, an adequate procedure to achieve negative margins for most tongue base or tonsil cancers required either a mandibulotomy, tracheostomy, percutaneous endoscopic gastrostomy (PEG) tube, or all 3. Only a select few centers performed nonrobotic versions (transoral laser microsurgery, or TLM) of the same procedures that are being done robotically. TLM preceded the use of the robot, but was not adopted widely, due in large part to the difficulty of the surgery itself. So, in essence, the use of the robot has allowed a surgery to be performed that was not widely being done previously. Many of the patients diagnosed with base of tongue and tonsil cancers were being treated with primary nonsurgical techniques. Thus, it is hard to compare raw "cost" of 2 surgeries, 1 with, and 1 without the robot. In the small studies that have been done to date comparing the "cost" of

treating patients with oropharynx cancer, using TORS or primary nonsurgical therapy, the cost of the robotic procedure is actually less than the nonsurgical therapy.

When it comes to benign base of tongue hypertrophy, the cost/benefit is even harder to judge. As of the time of the writing of this chapter, adequate financial data have not been accrued to easily answer this question. What can be said, however, is that, much like in cancer surgery, the robot has allowed us to perform a procedure that was not previously being routinely performed. Resection of a portion of the base of tongue, safely and adequately, was not easily achievable without the use of robotic assistance.

The Future

In the scheme of surgical medicine, robotic surgery is in its infancy. The relatively large arms, rigid shafts, and lack of haptic feedback will continue to improve. In fact, the next generation of robotic platforms is already FDA approved (despite not yet being available for clinical use). Single port systems with fully wristed instruments, snake-like movement of microinstruments, surgical navigation, and other technologic advancements are on the horizon. In addition, augmented-reality platforms that give surgeons additional information about the surgical field are already on the market. These technologies allow surgeons to see tumor vasculature, avoid underlying vessels and nerves, and navigate toward defined targets. This additional information will help make surgery safer, more efficient, and more effective. Otolaryngology represents a field in which access to multiple deep anatomic regions, through the nose, the mouth, and the ears, makes robotic surgery an obvious target. Some of the obstacles we currently face in the performance of our surgeries will be overcome as technology continues to evolve.

CHAPTER 32

Operative Pediatric Otolaryngology

Lawrence M. Simon

Introduction

This chapter will address the proper coding for surgical procedures in pediatric otolaryngology. Many of the codes in this chapter are performed primarily in the operating theater. However, several can also be performed in the office, and the site of service (facility vs nonfacility) will impact the associated relative value units (RVUs) and reimbursement from many payers. As already discussed in previous chapters, RVUs often change yearly and can be found in numerous places, including, among others, the Centers for Medicare and Medicaid Services (CMS) Medicare Physician Fee Schedule Final Rule, American Medical Association (AMA) publications, and the INGENIX Coding Companion. When performed on the same date as an evaluation and management (E/M) service, documentation must clearly establish the procedure as a separate service, and an appropriate modifier should be appended to the E/M service. Additionally, all operative procedures typically include a written and/or dictated note that details the indications, discussion of risks/benefits, anesthesia, detailed description of the procedure including technique, key equipment findings, and any complications encountered.

Key Points

- Most endoscopic codes have 0-day global periods per CMS guidelines.

- *Current Procedural Terminology* (CPT) makes a clear distinction between endoscopic and open procedures. Open procedural codes *cannot* be used when the procedure is performed endoscopically.
- Most otologic codes are unilateral and can be billed bilaterally, with modifier 50.
- All tonsillectomy codes include removal of both tonsils.
- All tonsillectomy and adenoid codes specify an age range.
- Certain codes contain descriptors that specify either with or without general anesthesia.
- Certain codes specify which approach is used (such as transoral vs external approach).

Key Procedure Codes

Foreign Body

For instance, removal of an earring backing embedded in the ear.

10120 Incision and removal of foreign body, subcutaneous tissues; simple
wRVU 1.22; Global 10

    10121 complicated
wRVU 2.74; Global 10

Nasal

Note. For epistaxis in children, typically 30901 or the endoscopic code 31238 will be used. The other epistaxis codes are included for completeness sake, but are rarely used in the pediatric population.

21315 Closed treatment of nasal bone fracture; without stabilization
wRVU 1.83; Global 10

> **21320** with stabilization
> *wRVU 1.88; Global 10*

30310 Removal foreign body, intranasal; requiring general anesthesia
wRVU 2.01; Global 10

30540 Repair choanal atresia; intranasal
wRVU 7.92; Global 90

> **30545** transpalatine
> *wRVU 11.62; Global 90*

30901 Control nasal hemorrhage, anterior, simple (limited cautery and/or packing) any method
wRVU 1.10; Global 0

30903 Control nasal hemorrhage, anterior, complex (extensive cautery and/or packing) any method
wRVU 1.54; Global 0

30905 Control nasal hemorrhage, posterior, with posterior nasal packs and/or cautery, any method; initial
wRVU 1.97; Global 0

> **30906** subsequent
> *wRVU 2.45; Global 0*

31238 Nasal/sinus endoscopy, surgical; with control of nasal hemorrhage
wRVU 2.74; Global 0

Neck

10140 Incision and drainage of hematoma, seroma or fluid collection
wRVU 1.38, Global 10

21501 Incision and drainage, deep abscess or hematoma, soft tissues of neck or thorax;
wRVU 3.98; Global 90

38510 Biopsy or excision of lymph node(s); open, deep cervical node(s)
wRVU 6.74; Global 10

42810 Excision branchial cleft cyst or vestige, confined to skin and subcutaneous tissues
wRVU 3.38; Global 90

42815 Excision branchial cleft cyst, vestige, or fistula, extending beneath subcutaneous tissues and/or into pharynx
wRVU 7.31; Global 90

Larynx

Most laryngeal surgery in children requires the use of the microscope and/or telescope. Both the nonmagnified codes and the codes with magnification are included in this section. If a procedure is done that is not listed, the unlisted code, 31599 should be used. This would include procedures such as endoscopic anterior cricoid split, supraglottoplasty, endoscopic posterior cricoid split, endoscopic scar division without dilation, and endoscopic cordectomy.

31520 Laryngoscopy direct, with or without tracheoscopy; diagnostic, newborn
wRVU 2.56; Global 0

> **31525** diagnostic, except newborn
> *wRVU 2.63; Global 0*

> **31526** diagnostic, with operating microscope or telescope
> *wRVU 2.57; Global 0*

> **31528** with dilation, initial
> *wRVU 2.37; Global 0*

> **31529** with dilation, subsequent
> *wRVU 2.68; Global 0*

31530 Laryngoscopy, direct, operative, with foreign body removal;
wRVU 3.30, Global 0

31531 with operating microscope or
telescope
wRVU 3.58; Global 0

31535 Laryngoscopy, direct, operative, with
biopsy;
wRVU 3.16; Global 0

31536 with operating microscope or
telescope
wRVU 3.55; Global 0

31540 Laryngoscopy, direct, operative, with
excision of tumor and/or stripping of
vocal cords or epiglottis;
wRVU 4.12; Global 0

31541 with operating microscope or
telescope
wRVU 4.52; Global 0

31561 Laryngoscopy, direct, operative, with
arytenoidectomy; with operating
microscope or telescope
wRVU 5.99; Global 0

31570 Laryngoscopy, direct, with injection into
vocal cord(s), therapeutic;
wRVU 3.86; Global 0

31571 with operating microscope or
telescope
wRVU 4.26; Global 0

31575 Laryngoscopy, flexible fiberoptic;
diagnostic
wRVU 1.10; Global 0

31580 Laryngoplasty; for laryngeal web,
2-stage, with keel insertion and removal
wRVU 14.66; Global 90

31582 for laryngeal stenosis, with
graft or core mold, including
tracheotomy
wRVU 23.22; Global 90

31587 Laryngoplasty, cricoid split
wRVU 15.27; Global 90

31588 Laryngoplasty, not otherwise specified
(eg, for burns, reconstruction after partial
laryngectomy)
wRVU 14.99, Global 90

31599 Unlisted procedure, larynx
wRVU 0.00; Global YYY

Trachea and Bronchoscopy

31600 Tracheostomy, planned (separate
procedure);
wRVU 7.17; Global 0

31601 younger than 2 years
wRVU 4.44; Global 0

31615 Tracheobronchoscopy through
established tracheostomy incision
wRVU 2.09; Global 0

31622 Bronchoscopy, rigid or flexible, including
fluoroscopic guidance, when performed;
diagnostic, with cell washing, when
performed (separate procedure)
wRVU 2.78; Global 0

31624 with bronchial alveolar lavage
wRVU 2.88; Global 0

31625 with bronchial or endobronchial
biopsy(s), single or multiple sites
wRVU 3.36; Global 0

31635 with removal of foreign body
wRVU 3.67; Global 0

31640 with excision of tumor
wRVU 4.93; Global 0

31641 with destruction of tumor or
relief of stenosis by any method
other than excision (eg, laser
therapy, cryotherapy)
wRVU 5.02; Global 0

31750 Tracheoplasty; cervical
wRVU 15.39; Global 90

31760 intrathoracic
wRVU 23.48; Global 90

31770 Bronchoplasty; graft repair
wRVU 23.54; Global 90

31775 excision stenosis and
anastomosis
wRVU 24.59; Global 90

31780   Excision tracheal stenosis and anastomosis; cervical
wRVU 19.84; Global 90

    31781   cervicothoracic
wRVU 24.85; Global 90

31785   Excision of tracheal tumor or carcinoma; cervical
wRVU 18.35; Global 90

    31786   thoracic
wRVU 25.42; Global 90

31800   Suture of tracheal wound or injury; cervical
wRVU 8.18; Global 90

    31805   intrathoracic
wRVU 13.42; Global 90

31820   Surgical closure tracheostomy or fistula; without plastic repair
wRVU 4.64; Global 90

    31825   with plastic repair
wRVU 7.07; Global 90

31830   Revision of tracheostomy scar
wRVU 4.62; Global 90

Oral Cavity

40810   Excision of lesion of mucosa and submucosa, vestibule of mouth; without repair
wRVU 1.36; Global 10

    40812   with simple repair
wRVU 2.37; Global 10

    40814   with complex repair
wRVU 3.52; Global 90

    40816   complex, with excision of underlying muscle
wRVU 3.77; Global 90

40818   Excision of mucosa of vestibule of mouth as donor graft
wRVU 2.83; Global 90

40819   Excision of frenum, labial or buccal (frenumectomy, frenulectomy, frenectomy)
wRVU 2.51; Global 90

41010   Incision of lingual frenum (frenotomy)
wRVU 1.11; Global 10

41115   Excision of lingual frenum (frenectomy)
wRVU 1.79; Global 10

41116   Excision, lesion of floor of mouth
wRVU 2.52; Global 90

41520   Frenoplasty (surgical revision of frenum, eg, with Z-plasty)
wRVU 2.83; Global 90

Pharynx

42700   Incision and drainage of abscess; peritonsillar
wRVU 1.67; Global 10

    42720   retropharyngeal or parapharyngeal, intraoral approach
wRVU 6.31; Global 10

    42725   retropharyngeal or parapharyngeal, external approach
wRVU 12.41; Global 90

42809   Removal of foreign body from pharynx
wRVU 1.86; Global 10

42820   Tonsillectomy and adenoidectomy; younger than age 12
wRVU 4.22; Global 90

    42821   age 12 or over
wRVU 4.36; Global 90

42825   Tonsillectomy, primary or secondary; younger than age 12
wRVU 3.51; Global 90

    42826   age 12 or over
wRVU 3.45; Global 90

42830   Adenoidectomy, primary; younger than age 12
wRVU 2.65; Global 90

    42831   age 12 or over
wRVU 2.81; Global 90

42835   Adenoidectomy, secondary; younger than age 12
wRVU 2.38; Global 90

42836   age 12 or over
wRVU 3.26; Global 90

42960   Control oropharyngeal hemorrhage, primary or secondary (eg, post-tonsillectomy); simple
wRVU 2.38; Global 10

> **42961**   complicated, requiring hospitalization
> *wRVU 5.77; Global 90*

> **42962**   with secondary surgical intervention
> *wRVU 7.40; Global 90*

60000   Incision and drainage of thyroglossal duct cyst, infected
wRVU 1.81; Global 10

60280   Excision of thyroglossal duct cyst or sinus;
wRVU 6.16; Global 90

> **60281**   recurrent
> *wRVU 8.82; Global 90*

64611   Chemodenervation of parotid and submandibular salivary glands, bilateral
wRVU 1.03; Global 10

67700   Blepharotomy, drainage of abscess, eyelid
wRVU 1.40; Global 10

Otology

69205   Removal foreign body from external auditory canal; with general anesthesia
wRVU 1.21; Global 10

69421   Myringotomy including aspiration and/or eustachian tube inflation requiring general anesthesia
wRVU 1.78; Global 10

69424   Ventilating tube removal requiring general anesthesia
wRVU 0.85; Global 0

69436   Tympanostomy (requiring insertion of ventilating tube), general anesthesia
wRVU 2.01; Global 10

69610   Tympanic membrane repair, with or without site preparation of perforation for closure, with or without patch
wRVU 4.47; Global 10

69620   Myringoplasty (surgery confined to drumhead and donor area)
wRVU 6.03; Global 90

Other

76942   Ultrasonic guidance for needle placement (eg, biopsy, aspiration, injection, localization device), imaging supervision and interpretation
wRVU (26) 0.67 (TC) 0.00; Global XXX

92502   Otolaryngologic exam under general anesthesia
wRVU 1.51; Global 0

CPT convention distinguishes "eg" from "ie" in code descriptors. When used, "eg" means "for example" and is followed by examples of the use of the code. In contrast, "ie" translates to "in other words" and is followed by an all-inclusive list that applies to the specified code.

Key Modifiers

24   Unrelated Evaluation and Management Service by the Same Physician or Other Qualified Health Care Professional During a Postoperative Period
This is used when seeing a patient during a postoperative global period when the reason for the visit is not related to the global period surgery.

52   Reduced Services
This is appended to a CPT code when a provider performs only part of a specified service, and a more appropriate code is not available.

57   Decision for Surgery
This is appended to the E/M code when a *separately identifiable* major procedure (defined as a procedure with a 90-day global period) is performed

on the same day. This modifier communicates to the coder that the *decision to perform surgery* was made at the specified E/M encounter as opposed to an earlier encounter.

59 Distinct Procedural Service

Modifier 59 is used when procedures that are not typically reported together are performed at the same operative session or same date of service. An example is reporting a direct laryngoscopy (31525) and bronchoscopy (31622) when using separate scopes for different indications and where both procedures were performed in their entirety. Modifier 59 is appended to the lower service to show it was indeed a separate procedure. CMS instituted, effective January 1, 2015, the "X modifiers" to replace modifier 59 because it was under a good deal of scrutiny. Therefore, CMS added modifiers XE, XS, XP, and XU to replace modifier 59 when clinically appropriate. CMS states modifier XE ("Separate Encounter") is used when the procedures are being separately reported because they occurred in separate encounters on the same date of service. XS ("Separate Structure") is used when the procedures are being separately reported because they were performed on separate structures on the same date of service. XP ("Separate Practitioner") is used when the procedures are being separately reported because they were performed by different practitioners on the same patient on the same date of service. XU ("Unusual Non-Overlapping Service") is used when the procedures are being separately reported because the smaller service does not overlap the usual components of the main service. CMS has not fully implemented the X modifiers at the time of this publication.

63 Procedure Performed on Infants Less Than 4 kg

This is appended to the CPT code anytime the procedure is performed on an infant with a mass less than 4 kg. This modifier may only be appended to codes 20005–69990, and it may not be used with E/M, anesthesia, radiology, pathology/laboratory, or medicine codes. Refer to Appendix F in CPT for the codes that are exempt from the use of modifier 63.

Key ICD-9-CM/ICD-10-CM Codes

Comment: Many of the *International Classification of Diseases, Ninth Revision, Clinical Modification* (ICD-9-CM) codes will cross-walk to one specific *International Classification of Diseases, Tenth Revision, Clinical Modification* (ICD-10-CM) code. Otitis media (OM) is a notable exception with multiple variations of OM being classified under ICD-10-CM code H65. For many codes, ICD-10-CM will also require the specification of right, left, or bilateral.

Airway

212.1/D14.1   Benign neoplasm of larynx

228.09/D18.09   Hemangioma of other sites

464.00/J04.0   Acute laryngitis

464.01/J05.0   Acute obstructive laryngitis [croup]

464.10/J04.10   Acute tracheitis without obstruction

464.11/J04.11   Acute tracheitis with obstruction

464.20/J04.2   Acute laryngotracheitis

464.21/J05.0   Acute obstructive laryngitis [croup]

464.30/J05.10   Acute epiglottitis without obstruction

464.31/J05.11   Acute epiglottitis with obstruction

464.4/J05.0   Acute obstructive laryngitis [croup]

476.0/J37.0   Chronic laryngitis

476.1/J37.1   Chronic laryngotracheitis

478.31/J38.01   Paralysis of vocal cords and larynx, unilateral (previously partial)

478.32/J38.01   Paralysis of vocal cords and larynx, unilateral (previously complete)

478.33/J38.02   Paralysis of vocal cords and larynx, bilateral (previously partial)

478.34/J38.02   Paralysis of vocal cords and larynx, bilateral (previously complete)

478.4/J38.1   Polyp of vocal cord and larynx

478.5/J38.3   Other diseases of vocal cords

478.74/J38.6   Stenosis of larynx

518.81/J96.00   Acute respiratory failure, unspecified whether with hypoxia or hypercapnia

518.81/J96.90   Respiratory failure, unspecified, unspecified whether with hypoxia or hypercapnia

518.83/J96.10   Chronic respiratory failure, unspecified whether with hypoxia or hypercapnia

518.84/J96.20   Acute and chronic respiratory failure, unspecified whether with hypoxia or hypercapnia

519.00/J95.00   Unspecified tracheostomy complication

519.02/J95.03   Malfunction of tracheostomy stoma

519.09/J95.01   Hemorrhage from tracheostomy stoma

519.09/J95.03   Malfunction of tracheostomy stoma

519.09/J95.04   Tracheo-esophageal fistula following tracheostomy

519.09/J95.09   Other tracheostomy complication

519.19/J39.8   Other specified diseases of upper respiratory tract

519.19/J98.09   Other diseases of bronchus, not elsewhere classified

748.2/Q31.0   Web of larynx

748.3/Q31.1   Congenital subglottic stenosis

748.3/Q31.3   Laryngocele

748.3/Q31.8   Other congenital malformations of larynx

748.3/Q32.1   Other congenital malformations of trachea

748.3/Q32.4   Other congenital malformations of bronchus

786.1/R06.1   Stridor

786.2/R05   Cough

V55.0/Z43.0   Encounter for attention to tracheostomy

Congenital Abnormalities/Syndromes

228.1/D18.1   Lymphangioma, any site

279.11/D82.1   Di George's syndrome

343.0/G80.1   Spastic diplegic cerebral palsy

744.41/Q18.0   Sinus, fistula and cyst of branchial cleft

744.42/Q18.0   Sinus, fistula and cyst of branchial cleft

744.46/Q18.1   Preauricular sinus and cyst

744.47/Q18.1   Preauricular sinus and cyst

744.49/Q18.2   Other branchial cleft malformations

748.0/Q30.0   Choanal atresia

750.29/Q38.8   Other congenital malformations of pharynx

758.0/Q90.9   Down syndrome, unspecified

758.32/Q93.81   Velo-cardio-facial syndrome

759.2/Q89.2   Congenital malformations of other endocrine glands

759.89/E78.71   Barth syndrome

759.89/E78.72   Smith-Lemli-Opitz syndrome

759.89/Q87.2   Congenital malformation syndromes predominantly involving limbs

759.89/Q87.3   Congenital malformation syndromes involving early overgrowth

759.89/Q87.5   Other congenital malformation syndromes with other skeletal changes

759.89/Q87.81   Alport syndrome

759.89/Q87.89   Other specified congenital malformation syndromes, not elsewhere classified

Swallowing and Vocal Disorders

315.31/F80.1   Expressive language disorder

527.7/K11.7   Disturbances of salivary secretion

527.7/R68.2   Dry mouth, unspecified

784.42/R49.0   Dysphonia

784.49/R49.8   Other voice and resonance disorders

787.20/R13.0   Aphagia

787.20/R13.10   Dysphagia, unspecified (can be further classified by phase)

Ear

One of the most commonly used codes in pediatric otolaryngology is otitis media. In ICD-10-CM, there is increased specificity for otitis media. H65 describes nonsuppurative otitis media. The next digit(s) defines the type, and the final digit describes laterality (left, right, bilateral, or unspecified). The following numbers replace the x and are defined as follows H65.x:

0   acute serous
1   other acute nonsuppurative
2   chronic serous
3   chronic mucoid
4   other chronic nonsuppurative
9   unspecified nonsuppurative

380.31/H61.129   Hematoma of pinna, unspecified ear

380.50/H61.309   Acquired stenosis of external ear canal, unspecified, unspecified ear

380.50/H61.599   Other acquired stenosis of external ear canal, unspecified ear

385.19/H74.19   Adhesive middle ear disease, unspecified ear

744.02/Q16.1   Congenital absence, atresia and stricture of auditory canal (external)

744.1/Q17.0   Accessory auricle

744.23/Q17.2   Microtia

744.43/Q18.2   Other branchial cleft malformations

V72.11/Z01.110   Encounter for hearing examination following failed hearing screening

Oropharynx/Retropharynx

462/J02.9   Acute pharyngitis, unspecified

463/J03.90   Acute tonsillitis, unspecified

474.00/J35.01   Chronic tonsillitis

474.01/J35.02   Chronic adenoiditis

474.02/J35.03   Chronic tonsillitis and adenoiditis

474.10/J35.3   Hypertrophy of tonsils with hypertrophy of adenoids

474.11/J35.1   Hypertrophy of tonsils

474.12/J35.2   Hypertrophy of adenoids

475/J36   Peritonsillar abscess

478.22/J39.0   Retropharyngeal and parapharyngeal abscess

478.24/J39.0   Retropharyngeal and parapharyngeal abscess

998.11/J95.830   Postprocedural hemorrhage and hematoma of a respiratory system organ or structure following a respiratory system procedure

Others

For most of the foreign body codes there is increased specificity. In addition to the side when relevant, the type of foreign body is significant (eg, unspecified, gastric contents, food, or other). A representative sample is given below. Please consult a coding book for the complete list.

215.0/D21.0   Benign neoplasm of connective and other soft tissue of head, face and neck

327.23/G47.33   Obstructive sleep apnea (adult) (pediatric)

373.13/H00.039   Abscess of eyelid unspecified eye, unspecified eyelid

527.6/K11.6   Mucocele of salivary gland

682.1/L03.221   Cellulitis of neck

682.1/L03.222   Acute lymphangitis of neck

750.0/Q38.1   Ankyloglossia

786.09/R06.00   Dyspnea, unspecified

786.09/R06.09   Other forms of dyspnea

786.09/R06.3   Periodic breathing

786.09/R06.83   Snoring

786.09/R06.89   Other abnormalities of breathing

786.30/R04.2   Hemoptysis

786.30/R04.9   Hemorrhage from respiratory passages, unspecified

919.6/T07   Unspecified multiple injuries

931/T16.XXXA   Foreign body in ear, initial encounter

932/T17.0XXA   Foreign body in nasal sinus, initial encounter

932/T17.1XXA   Foreign body in nostril, initial encounter

933.0/T17.200A   Unspecified foreign body in pharynx causing asphyxiation, initial encounter

933.0/T17.208A   Unspecified foreign body in pharynx causing other injury, initial encounter

934.0/T17.400A   Unspecified foreign body in trachea causing asphyxiation, initial encounter

934.0/T17.408A   Unspecified foreign body in trachea causing other injury, initial encounter

935.1/T18.100A   Unspecified foreign body in esophagus causing compression of trachea, initial encounter

935.1/T18.108A   Unspecified foreign body in esophagus causing other injury, initial encounter

Definition of Codes

1. Procedures with specific anesthesia designations:
   a. Intranasal foreign body removal: 30300 (without) vs 30310 (with)
   b. External auditory canal foreign body removal: 69200 (without) vs 69205 (with)
   c. Myringotomy: 69420 (without) vs 69421 (with)
   d. Tympanostomy tube insertion: 69433 (without) vs 69436 (with)

2. Procedures with specified age range designations:
   a. Adenoid and tonsil codes: under 12 years vs 12 years and older:
      i. Adenotonsillectomy: 42820 vs 42821
      ii. Tonsillectomy: 42825 vs 42826
      iii. Adenoidectomy, primary: 42830 vs 42831
      iv. Adenoidectomy, secondary: 42835 vs 43836
   b. Newborn vs not-newborn (a newborn is defined as birth through 28 days):
      i. Direct laryngoscopy: 31520 vs 31525
   c. 2 years and older vs younger than 2 years:
      i. Tracheostomy: 31600 vs 31601

3. Direct laryngoscopy/bronchoscopy code set (31520–31571; 31622–31641)
   a. *Indications*—Assessment and management of various pediatric airway conditions, including but not limited to stridor, obstructive symptoms, tumors/growths, and other mass-like lesions and stenosis.
   b. *Definitions*—Note the age clarification: CPT 31520 refers to diagnostic endoscopy in newborns specifically, while 31525 is used for all other patients.

c. *Key points*—Billing direct laryngoscopy (31525) and bronchoscopy (31622): CMS bundles the two codes with 31525 being inclusive of 31622. However, this bundling assumes that the same scope (eg, a flexible bronchoscope) is used to perform both endoscopies. Technically, the larynx and bronchi are separate anatomic sites, and 31525 and 31622 *can* be reported together when they are performed using separate scopes and for separate indications as long as a true bronchoscopy is performed with evaluation past the carina into the bronchi. When this is done, *modifier 59 is appended to 31525.* To qualify for separate reporting, you *should*:

   i. Use independent ICD-9-CM/ICD-10-CM billing codes for each procedure (CPT) code.

   ii. Document use of *different scopes* for each endoscopy. You must use a different scope for the bronchoscopy than was used for the laryngoscopy.

   iii. Document a true bronchoscopy. CPT 31525 *includes a tracheoscopy.* Therefore, if you only look down to the carina, then only 31525 should be reported. In order to report 31622, and bronchoscopy must be indicated, performed, and documented as evaluation of the mainstem bronchus.

d. *Definition*—Dilation: 2 codes describe dilation of subglottic stenosis—31528 and 31529. CPT 31528 is used to report the initial dilation (independent of surgeon); 31529 is used to report all subsequent dilations *by any surgeon.*

e. *Definition*—CPT 31541: This is a versatile code used to report removal of supraglottic, glottis, and subglottic lesions. This may include cysts, granulomas, papillomas, abnormal/diseased/damaged mucosa, and so on. The code is reported once regardless of the number of lesions addressed or laterality.

f. *Definition*—CPT 31561: This code is specific to the arytenoid and requires a full arytenoidectomy. It cannot be used for removal

of the cuneiform cartilages or redundant arytenoid mucosa.

4. Lingual Frenulum Surgery (41010, 41115, 41520): These codes all describe various ways of treating and repairing ankyloglossia (ICD-9-CM 750.0/ ICD-10-CM Q38.1).

a. *Indications*—Frenulum surgery is usually undertaken when poor tongue movement causes impairment of speech and/or swallowing (ICD-9-CM 315.31/ICD-10-CM F80.1 and ICD-9-CM 787.2/ICD-10-CM R13.1, respectively).

b. *Definition*—CPT 41010 describes simple division of the frenulum, such as might be done with scissors or electrocautery, with no further work being done besides hemostasis. Simple bedside division of the frenulum performed in a neonate for failure to latch would be reported with this code.

c. *Definition*—CPT 41115: Similar to 41010, except that the frenulum is actually excised —meaning that tissue (ie, a specimen) is removed from the floor of mouth. The actual removal of the frenulum is what distinguishes this code from 41010. Some sort of floor of mouth closure might also be performed as part of this code, although it would not be necessary.

d. *Definition*—CPT 41520: This code describes a more involved procedure in which the frenulum is either incised or excised and then repaired or reconstructed in some fashion. This procedure will typically be reported in older children with severe ankyloglossia and speech impediment or in patients with recurrent ankyloglossia and a sessile tongue that requires more extensive work to accomplish a full tongue release. At minimum, this code includes repairing/ reconstructing the frenulum with a suture line along the tongue and floor of mouth. However, it may also include using local flaps (eg, Z-plasty) and or mucosal grafts to reconstruct the floor of mouth. If a graft (eg, buccal mucosa) is used, the harvesting of it through a separate incision would be reported separately. Surgeons should also note that 41520 has a 90-day global period, as opposed to 41010 and 41115, each of which have 10-day global periods.

5. Post-Tonsillectomy Hemorrhage (42960–42962): This family of codes describes the treatment of post-tonsillectomy bleeding.
    a. *Definition*—CPT 42960: Describes simple treatment of the bleeding. One example of such management would be treatment with silver nitrate in the emergency department. The 2 key components of the code are that the patient was neither admitted nor brought to the operating room.
    b. *Definition*—CPT 42961: Applicable to patients whose bleeding can be stopped outside of the operating room, but still require hospitalization for observation and further care (eg, treatment of dehydration or anemia).
    c. *Definition*—CPT 42962: Used when a patient requires a return to the operating room to obtain hemostasis.

6. Myringoplasty (69610, 69620)
    a. *Indications*—These 2 codes are typically used to report simple repairs of tympanic membrane perforations when performed in lieu of a formal tympanoplasty (eg, post-tympanostomy tube perforations in young children).
    b. *Definition*—CPT 69610: This code describes the simple act of directly closing the perforation either by freshening the edges of the perforation, placing a synthetic patch (eg, cigarette paper, Gelfilm, or EpiDisc) or both. Surgery is confined to the tympanic membrane, and no autograft is harvested.
    c. *Definition*—CPT 69620 is used when the perforation is repaired with some sort of autograft in a direct transcanal approach *without* elevating a tympanomeatal flap. Surgery is confined only to the tympanic membrane perforation (drumhead) and the graft donor site. The drumhead work rarely extends beyond freshening the edges of the perforation. A fat graft myringoplasty is a typical example of the use of

this code. The code *includes* the graft harvesting. As such, the graft harvest *is not* reported separately.

7. Salivary gland chemodenervation (64611)
    a. *Indications*—Most commonly performed for drooling (ICD-9-CM 527.7/ ICD-10-CM K11.7) with or without cerebral palsy (ICD-9-CM 343.0/ ICD-10-CM G80.1).
    b. *Definition*—Involves use of botulinum toxin to denervate the submandibular and parotid glands *bilaterally*. If fewer than 4 glands are treated, then modifier 52 (reduced services) must be used because *only a part* (ie, *less than 4 glands*) of the procedure was completed.
    c. *Key points*—If ultrasound guidance is used *by the surgeon* to identify the glands and confirm needle placement, then CPT Code 76942 (Ultrasonic guidance for needle placement (eg, biopsy, aspiration, injection, localization device), imaging supervision and interpretation) is also billed.
        i. In order for the surgeon to bill 76942, he or she must be the sole provider interpreting the ultrasound. This code cannot be billed by the surgeon if the image is also read by a radiologist.
        ii. If the surgeon is not billing for the technical component of this service (eg, if the procedure is performed in the operating room/in a facility which owns the ultrasound machine and employs the technologist), then append modifier 26 (Professional Component) to 76942. This modifier allows for the facility to bill for the technical component (eg, use of the machine) and for the surgeon to bill for the interpretation of the imaging study.

8. Removal of congenital cysts/sinuses/fistulas
    a. *Definition*—CPT 42810: This code describes removal of a congenital branchial remnant that is *confined to the skin and subcutaneous tissues*. One such example is removal of *accessory auricles* (ICD-9-CM 744.1/ ICD-10-CM Q17.0- pre-auricular skin and cartilage remnants) and cervical auricles

(ICD-9-CM 744.43/ICD-10-CM Q18.2-superficial skin and cartilage remnants on the neck). Essentially, if the remnant is confined to the skin and subcutaneous tissue, then this code is appropriate. However, if the lesion extends to any deeper underlying structure, then this code is not appropriate.

b. *Definition*—CPT 42815: This code describes removal of a branchial remnant that *extends beneath the subcutaneous tissues*. Examples include *pre-auricular sinuses* (ICD-9-CM 744.46/ICD-10-CM Q18.1), branchial sinuses/fistulas of the neck (ICD-9-CM 744.41/ICD-10-CM Q18.0), and branchial cleft cysts (ICD-9-CM 744.42/ICD-10-CM Q18.0).

c. *Key points*—With codes 42810 and 42815, if more than one lesion is removed in a setting (eg, bilateral lesions), report the code once for each removal and append modifier 59 to each subsequent use. The anatomic structure of skin does not have laterality; therefore, modifier 50 is not appropriate.

   i. Example: Patient with bilateral preauricular pits/sinus undergoes removal of both pits on the same day—bill 42815, 42815-59. Append each code to diagnosis code 744.46/Q18.1.

9. Thyroglossal duct cyst (TGDC) (60000, 60280, 60281)

a. *Definition*—CPT 60000: This code describes incision and drainage (I&D) of an infected or abscessed TGDC. A needle aspiration alone would not meet the criteria for this code.

b. *Definition*—CPT 60280: This code is for the classic Sistrunk procedure for removal of a TGDC.

c. *Definition*—CPT 60281: This code is for excision of a recurrent TGDC.

d. *Key points*—One thing to note about these codes is that they are diagnosis specific. In many cases, when we excise a midline neck cyst, we may not know exactly what the lesion is (eg, dermoid vs TGDC) until final pathology is determined. In such cases, it

is appropriate to wait until the exact etiology of the lesion is determined prior to submitting a claim for services rendered.

10. Treatment of head and neck abscesses

a. *Definition*—CPT 21501: Incision and drainage, deep abscess or hematoma, soft tissues of neck or thorax. This code describes the classic incision and drainage (I&D) of a neck abscess.

b. *Key points*—There are 5 abscess codes that are abscess specific (42700, 42720, 42725, 60000, and 67700) addressed below). Outside of these 5 specific instances, code 21501 is used for treatment of a *deep* abscess or hematoma of the neck. This code is not appropriate for treatment of a superficial skin abscess or an abscess confined to the subcutaneous tissue; rather use 10140 for these procedures.

c. *Definition*—CPT 42700: Drainage of peritonsillar abscess. This same code is used for both bedside drainage in the clinic or emergency department or for drainage in the operating room. It will most commonly be associated with ICD-9-CM 475/ICD-10-CM J36 for peritonsillar abscess. If a Quinsy tonsillectomy is performed to treat the abscess, the tonsillectomy code is used in lieu of the I&D code. Also, if only a unilateral tonsillectomy is performed, modifier 52 (reduced services) must be appended to the tonsillectomy code.

d. *Definition*—CPT 42720: This code is used for transoral drainage of either a retropharyngeal *or* parapharyngeal abscess. Again, the code applies regardless of place of service; the procedure may be performed in the office, emergency department, or operating room. It will most commonly be associated with ICD-9-CM 478.24/ICD-10-CM J39.0 for retropharyngeal abscess and ICD-9-CM 478.22/ICD-10-CM J39.0 for parapharyngeal abscess.

e. *Definition*—CPT 42725: This code is used for external (lateral/transcervical) drainage of either a retropharyngeal *or* parapharyngeal abscess. The code requires an external (neck) incision for the approach. Again, the code applies to both bedside clinic in the ED/Clinic and for drainage in the operating room. It will most commonly be associated with ICD-9-CM 478.24/ICD-10-CM J39.0 for retropharyngeal abscess and ICD-9-CM 478.22/ICD-10-CM J39.0 for parapharyngeal abscess.

f. *Definition*—CPT 60000: Infected/abscessed TGDC (see above).

g. *Definition*—CPT 67700: This code will likely not be used very much be otolaryngologists, but it applies to drainage of an abscess of the eyelid. The corresponding ICD-9-CM and ICD-10-CM codes for eyelid abscess are 373.13 and H00.03-, respectively.

Controversial Areas

1. Laryngoplasty codes (31580–31588): This family of codes describes *open* treatment of laryngeal pathology. They are not appropriate for endoscopic laryngeal procedures, which are reported with codes 31520–31571 and 31599.

   a. *Definition*—CPT 31580: This code describes the procedure of open division of a laryngeal web with keel placement, such as might be performed on a child with Di George's syndrome (22q11 deletion). It is important to note that direct laryngoscopy (eg, 31525) is included and should not be reported separately in most circumstances. Additionally, the code requires the removal of the keel at a later date as it is part of a 2-stage procedure. Modifier 58 is appended to a second use of 31580 to indicate that it is the second stage of a staged procedure.

   b. *Definition*—CPT 31582: This code is used for treatment of laryngeal/subglottic stenosis. It describes the classic "laryngotracheal reconstruction (LTR)" and can be used for "single-stage" or "two-stage" procedures. Tracheostomy and a direct laryngoscopy/bronchoscopy are included in the

code. Of note, a graft or core mold of some kind *must be used* to report this code. If the procedure does not include a graft or core mold of some, then this code should not be used.

c. *Definition*—CPT 31587: This code describes the classic anterior cricoid split that is typically performed on neonates. It does not include any kind of graft placement and is not appropriate to use if a graft is placed. Direct laryngoscopy is bundled into the code if performed.

d. *Definition*—CPT 31588: This is a versatile code that can be used for any open laryngoplasty not otherwise specified above. An *open* repair of a type III laryngeal cleft would be an example of a procedure for which one would use this code. Again, laryngoscopy (eg, 31525) is included in the code.

e. Considerable controversy still surrounds this code set. It is anticipated that there will be CPT revisions in the near future, so monitor coding changes closely if you perform these services

2. Supraglottoplasty
   a. *Indications*—Supraglottoplasty is an endoscopic procedure used to treat laryngomalacia (ICD-9-CM 748.3/ICD-10-CM Q31.5).
   b. *Key points*—There are several types of supraglottoplasty, all of which are endoscopic (not open). In some cases, the epiglottis is pexied to the tongue base. In others, the aryepiglottic folds are cut, and still in others redundant tissue is excised from the posterior/lateral surface of the arytenoid cartilages. At times, a combination of these procedures is performed.
   c. *Coding controversy*—There is no specified code for supraglottoplasty. The most appropriate method for coding supraglottoplasty is to use 31599—Unlisted procedure, larynx. If a code other than 31599 is used, be sure that the work directly matches the description of the selected CPT code, and be sure to check payers to see how they would like the procedure to be reported.

Special Circumstances

Ear ring back removal from ear lobe: this is a common problem faced in pediatric otolaryngology where the back of an earring will become lodged in a patient's ear lobe and require removal. This procedure can be reported with CPT code 10120 (Incision and removal of foreign body, subcutaneous tissues; simple) and ICD-9-CM 919.6/ ICD-10-CM S00.45. Like the branchial cleft cyst/sinus/fistula codes, CPT 10120 is not associated with laterality. Therefore, bilateral removals would be coded by reporting 10120 twice and appending modifier 59 to the second code.

CHAPTER 33

Operative Sleep Surgery

Fred Y. Lin

Introduction

This chapter describes the procedures and diagnoses coded by an otolaryngologist concerning operative procedures for sleep apnea and sleep-related disorders. Indications for procedures will vary dependent on insurance carriers and can change yearly. Relative value units (RVUs) and reimbursement also can change yearly and can be found through the Centers for Medicare and Medicaid Services (CMS) website (http://www.cms.gov).

Key Points

- Surgical procedures can often be performed in lieu of or prior to continuous positive airway pressure (CPAP) trials for patients with mild obstructive sleep apnea.
- Most insurers will not cover palatal pillars, laser-assisted uvulopalatoplasty (LAUP) and tongue suspension procedures.
- Snoring procedures are generally not considered medically necessary and typically are not covered under most insurance plans.
- When performing multiple-level surgery, each procedure can be reported separately; add the appropriate modifier when necessary.

Key Procedure Codes

Evaluation Procedures

31575   Laryngoscopy, flexible fiberoptic; diagnostic
wRVU 1.10; Global 0

92502   Otolaryngologic examination under general anesthesia
wRVU 1.51; Global 0

Tonsil and Adenoid Procedures

42820   Tonsillectomy and adenoidectomy; younger than age 12
wRVU 4.22; Global 90

    42821   age 12 or over
wRVU 4.36; Global 90

42825   Tonsillectomy, primary or secondary; younger than age 12
wRVU 3.51; Global 90

    42826   age 12 or over
wRVU 3.45; Global 90

Soft Palatal Procedures

42140   Uvulectomy, excision of uvula
wRVU 1.70; Global 90

42145 Palatopharyngoplasty (eg, uvulopalatopharyngoplasty, uvulopharyngoplasty)
wRVU 9.78; Global 90

42299 Unlisted procedure, palate, uvula
wRVU 0; Global YYY

Tongue Procedures

41120 Glossectomy; less than one-half tongue
wRVU 11.14; Global 90

41512 Tongue base suspension, permanent suture technique
wRVU 6.86; Global 90

41530 Submucosal ablation of the tongue base, radiofrequency, 1 or more sites, per session
wRVU 4.51; Global 10

Hyoid and Osteotomy Procedures

21141 Reconstruction midface, Lefort I; single piece, segment movement in any direction (eg, for Long Face Syndrome), without bone graft
wRVU 19.57; Global 90

   21145 single piece, segment movement in any direction, requiring bone grafts (includes obtaining autografts)
   wRVU 23.94; Global 90

21196 Reconstruction of mandibular rami and/or body, sagittal split; with internal rigid fixation
wRVU 20.83; Global 90

21199 Osteotomy, mandible, segmental; with genioglossus advancement
wRVU 16.73; Global 90

21685 Hyoid myotomy and suspension
wRVU 15.26; Global 90

Nasal Procedures

30140 Submucous resection of the inferior turbinates, partial or complete
wRVU 3.57; Global 90

30520 Septoplasty or submucous resection, with or without cartilage scoring
wRVU 7.01; Global 90

30465 Repair of nasal vestibular stenosis (eg, spreader grafting, lateral nasal wall reconstruction)
wRVU 12.36; Global 90

Key Modifiers

52   Reduced Services
This can be used when a procedure is done which is less work or time than standard. An example of this is placing it on code 92502 when performing a sleep medicine evaluation under general anesthesia.

Key ICD-9-CM/ICD-10-CM Codes

327.3/G47.33   Obstructive sleep apnea (adult) (pediatric)

780.51   Sleep apnea with insomnia

780.53   Sleep apnea with hypersomnia

780.57/G47.30   Sleep apnea, unspecified

780.50/G47.9   Sleep disorder, unspecified

524.03/M26.02   Maxillary hypoplasia

524.04/M26.74   Mandibular hypoplasia

524.06/M26.06   Microgenia

Definition of Codes

1. Sleep Endoscopy (31575, 92502-52)
   a. *Indications*—Endoscopic evaluation of the airway during drug-induced sedation is used in situations for surgical planning or evaluation of the nature of obstruction.
   b. *Definition*—This procedure is performed by pharmacologically sedating the patient in an operative setting and evaluating the airway with a fiberoptic laryngoscope. Maneuvers can be performed during the

procedure to simulate therapy with an oral appliance (jaw thrust).

c. *Key points*—This procedure can be performed as a stand-alone procedure or in combination with other treatments. If performed in combination with other treatments (eg, UPPP, partial glossectomy), then neither 31575 nor 92502-52 may be reported, per *Current Procedural Terminology* (CPT) guidelines. An examination under anesthesia (92502, EUA) as well as a diagnostic procedure are included in all definitive surgical CPT codes. CPT 92502-52 may be reported by itself for a visual exam of only the oral cavity (no exam of the ears or nose).

2. Tonsillectomy and Adenoidectomy (42820–42821; 42825–42826)

a. *Indications*—Pediatric patients with an AHI (apnea-hypopnea index) of 5 or an AHI of 1.5 with excessive daytime sleepiness, behavioral problems, or hyperactivity. Adult patients with significant tonsillar hypertrophy with or without adenoid hypertrophy, and without other areas of obstruction.

b. *Definition*—Surgical removal of the tonsils and adenoids.

c. *Key points*—This can be performed as a complete tonsillectomy or intracapsular tonsillectomy. Tonsillectomy may be performed by excision or coblation; the method is not relevant to the coding.

3. Uvulopalatopharyngoplasty (UPPP) (42145)

a. *Indications*—Generally, patients who have (1) mild sleep apnea with or without a CPAP trial and symptoms of daytime somnolence, impaired cognition, cardiac disease, or mood disorders and insomnia; and (2) moderate/severe sleep apnea with a failed CPAP trial are candidates for surgery.

b. *Definition*—Procedure that enlarges the airway by removing or shortening the uvula with removal of the tonsils (if present) and/or modifying the palate.

c. *Key points*—Indications and approval for surgery will often vary by insurance company. This procedure is not to be confused with LAUP. LAUP removes the uvula and stiffens the palate with a CO_2 laser and has not been shown to be a reliable treatment for sleep apnea. CPT 42145 does not include a tonsillectomy according to CPT guidelines (refer to the *CPT Assistant*, August 1997, page 18); therefore, the tonsillectomy may be separately reported. However, many payers do not allow separate payment for the tonsillectomy. It is often helpful to add modifier 51 when reporting a tonsillectomy along with UPPP. Insurance approval varies widely for these cases. Most payers will approve a UPPP if there is mild sleep apnea or the patient has failed CPAP, as mentioned in the indications. Many payers will require precertification, and almost all will require precertification if the patient is admitted postoperatively. A few payers will not approve the procedure in cases of severe sleep apnea unless it is part of multilevel surgery with a tongue procedure included.

4. Palatal Stiffening Procedures (42299)

a. *Indications*—These procedures are primarily used to stiffen the palate to treat snoring.

b. *Definition*—These procedures, which include radiofrequency treatment (Somnoplasty), injection of a sclerosing agent (injection snoreplasty) and palatal implants (Pillar), stiffen the palate through various measures.

c. *Key points*—Most insurance companies will not cover these procedures and deem them not medically necessary. Their use for obstructive sleep apnea is still considered investigational, and snoring treatment is considered a lifestyle problem rather than a functional disorder. When appropriate, use the unlisted code for the palate and uvula listed above.

5. Radiofrequency Treatment of the Tongue (41530)

a. *Indications*—Most insurers consider these treatments investigational. Radiofrequency treatment of the tongue is indicated for patients that have base of tongue hypertrophy and narrowing of the hypopharyngeal airway.

b. *Definition*—Radiofrequency treatment of the tongue produces thermal lesions through coagulative necrosis causing volumetric reduction of tissue.

c. *Key points*—Treatment will often require multiple sessions for improved effectiveness although there are techniques that allow for single treatments. CPT 41530 includes ablation at any number of sites at a single operative session. Combination of this procedure with other upper airway procedures is often useful; the other procedures on different anatomic structures may be separately reported.

6. Partial Glossectomy, removal of less than half of tongue (41120)

a. *Indications*—Removal of a portion of the base of tongue is indicated for patients who have base of tongue hypertrophy and narrowing of the hypopharyngeal airway. A significant number of moderate and severe sleep apnea patients will have a hypopharyngeal component contributing to their sleep apnea.

b. *Definition*—Removal of a portion of the base of tongue to improve the posterior airway space. This can be achieved with resection or ablation with modalities such as electrocautery, laser, and coblation. If this procedure is completed using transoral robotic surgery (TORS), the same code is used, as TORS is FDA approved for upper airway surgery, though not specifically for sleep apnea. Healthcare Common Procedure Coding System (HCPCS) Level I code, S2900 (Surgical techniques requiring use of robotic surgical system (list separately in addition to code for primary procedure)) may also be reported with 41120, though payers are not likely to recognize this code in terms of added reimbursement. For more information on this code, refer to Chapter 31, "Robotic Surgery."

7. Tongue Suspension (41512)

a. *Indications*—Suspension of the tongue base can be used to improve the posterior airway space. Many payers consider this technique investigational.

b. *Definition*—This procedure is generally accomplished with a permanent suture that is fixated to the mandible suspending the base of tongue.

c. *Key points*—The most common technique is using the Repose system.

8. Maxillomandibular Advancement (21141 and 21196)

a. *Indications*—Advancement of the mandible and maxilla can be performed in cases of obstructive sleep apnea with failed CPAP in addition to narrowed posterior airway space and mandibular and maxillary hypoplasia.

b. *Definition*—This procedure includes advancement of the maxilla with a Le Fort I osteotomy and advancement of the mandible with a sagittal split osteotomy. Both advancements are fixated with hardware.

c. *Key points*—This can be combined with a hyoid suspension or genioglossus advancement. Lateral cephalometry showing a narrowed posterior airway space and/or maxillary or mandibular deficiency is generally needed for approval of this procedure. These codes are inherently bilateral procedures and should not be reported with modifier 50 (bilateral procedure).

9. Genioglossus Advancement (21199)

a. *Indications*—Advancement of the genioglossus muscle is indicated in patients with significant hypopharyngeal narrowing at the base of tongue. Posterior airway space narrowing can be seen on exam and lateral cephalometry.

b. *Definition*—A segmental osteotomy of the geniotubercle with advancement of that segment and its attachment to the genioglossus. This segment is then fixated with hardware.

c. *Key points*—This procedure is often included in multilevel surgeries that include the palatal/lateral pharyngeal airway and hypopharyngeal airway.

10. Hyoid Suspension (21685)

a. *Indications*—Advancement or suspension of the hyoid is used to treat narrowing of the posterior airway and hypopharyngeal space. This is often combined with other procedures to perform multilevel airway surgery.

b. *Definition*—This procedure involves advancement or suspension of the hyoid bone with fixation to the mandible or attachment to the thyroid cartilage.

c. *Key points*—This procedure is often included in multilevel surgery.

11. Nasal Procedures (30140, 30520, 30465)

a. *Indications*—Nasal procedures to improve nasal breathing are generally used to improve quality of life and CPAP tolerance. Having improved nasal airways generally allows for decreased CPAP pressure, and in some patients, decreased mouth breathing during sleep. Turbinate reductions in the office can be performed easily with radiofrequency or coblation. For insurance purposes, septoplasty and nasal procedures in the operating room are not indicated for sleep apnea but can be performed if documented nasal obstruction, rhinitis, septal deviation, and valve collapse with failure of conservative measures are noted and used for insurance approval.

b. *Definition*—These procedures involve improving the nasal airway and decreasing nasal obstruction via turbinate reduction, improving upon a septal deviation or nasal valve collapse.

c. *Key points*—Nasal procedures will generally improve a patient's quality of life, and some patients will report an improvement in snoring, mouth breathing, and possible CPAP tolerance. As mentioned above, it is important to specify that these procedures are being performed for nasal obstruction and not for sleep apnea when seeking insurance approval. CPT 30465 includes necessary osteotomies for valve repair; it is an inherently bilateral procedure so modifier 50 is not applicable. A septoplasty

(30520) is also an inherently bilateral procedure where modifier 50 should not be used. However, the submucous resection of inferior turbinates (30140) may be reported with modifier 50 when appropriate.

Controversial Areas

CPAP Versus Dental Appliance Versus Surgery

In most cases, insurance carriers will require a CPAP trial as initial therapy for moderate and severe sleep apnea patients. If the CPAP trial fails, the carrier will usually cover a dental appliance or surgery. For mild OSA, all 3 treatment modalities are options and up to patient preference. Dental appliances are covered by most medical insurance carriers (not Medicaid).

Postoperative Admission

One area of significant controversy is admission or 23-hour observation after sleep apnea surgery. Traditionally, almost all patients were admitted postsurgically due to the concern for perioperative airway issues. However, recent data in conjunction with the increased scrutiny toward costs of hospital stays have begun to change the philosophies of many sleep surgeons. There are no universal guidelines, although most surgeons will admit patients with a history of significant cardiac issues or those patients who have significant swelling in the operative areas. Documentation in the operative note and admission note is important with specific mention of the concern for airway obstruction and need for airway monitoring, parenteral corticosteroids, and intravenous pain control. Generally, 23-hour admissions are easily approved and do not require precertification in most cases.

Index

Note: Page numbers in **bold** reference non-text material.

A

AAO-HNS. *See* American Academy of Otolaryngology-Head and Neck Surgery
AAPC. *See* American Academy of Professional Coders
AASM. *See* American Academy of Sleep Medicine
ABN. *See* Advanced Beneficiary Notice
ABN modifiers, 176
Abscess drainage codes
   for office setting, 122, 126, 158–159, 196, 208
   for surgical setting, 265, 270, 271, 354, 356, 364–365
ACA. *See* Affordable Care Act
Accounts receivable, 42
Accounts receivable report, 42–43, **42**
Acoustic immittance testing, 167, 172
Acoustic neuroma, 268, 336
Acute maxillary sinusitis, 124
Acute respiratory failure, 359
Acute sinusitis, 245–246
Adaptation Test (ADT), 171
Add-on Category I codes (CPT), **9**
Adenoidectomy, 107, 353, 356, 367, 369
Adenoiditis, 210, 360
Adenotonsillectomy, 361
ADI. *See* Advanced diagnostic imaging
Adjacent tissue transfer
   office-based facial plastic surgery, 182–183, 187–188
   surgical setting, 282, 293–294, 321, 325
Adjustments report, 43
ADT. *See* Adaptation Test
Advanced Beneficiary Notice (ABN), 175–176
Advanced diagnostic imaging (ADI), 230
Advanced practice registered nurses (APRNs), 63
Affordable Care Act (ACA), 28, 34
AHIMA. *See* American Health Information Management Association
Airway surgery, pediatric, 356–359
Allergen immunotherapy, 130, 133
Allergy care, 129–134
   controversial areas, 133–134
   ICD-9-CM/ICD-10-CM codes, 131 132
   immunotherapy, 130, 133

   modifiers, 131
   procedure codes, 129–131
   sublingual immunotherapy, 134
   supervision, 134
   testing, 129–130, 132–133
Allergy testing, 129–130, 132–133
Allografts, 327
Alphabetic modifiers, 93, 113–115
Alternative payment models (APMs), 25
Alveolar ridge, fracture, 286, 299
Alveolectomy, 306
Ambulatory surgical center, 252
American Academy of Nurse Practitioners, 63–64
American Academy of Otolaryngology-Head and Neck Surgery (AAO-HNS), 24–28, 48, 50, 122, 164, 223
American Academy of Professional Coders (AAPC), 4
American Academy of Sleep Medicine (AASM), 215, 219
American Health Information Management Association (AHIMA), 4
American Medical Association (AMA)
   CPT® book, 3, 7, 24
   Relative Value Scale Update Committee (RUC), 26–27
   resources for coding, 5, 12, 28
American Nurses Credentialing Center, 64
American Rhinologic Society, 344
Anesthesia, 361
Ankyloglossia, 211, 361, 362
Anterior cranial fossa codes, 336–337, 338
Anterior epistaxis, 126
Anterior thorax, 308
Anti-Kickback Statute, 54
Antigen vials, 130, 133
Antrostomies, **102**
Antrotomy, 273
Aphagia, 258–259, 360
Aphasia, 149
Aphonia, 259
Apicectomy, 273–274
APMs. *See* Alternative payment models

Fenestration, 268, 276
Fine needle aspiration (FNA), 193, 200, 207
Flaps
    forehead flap, 328
    free flaps, 328–329, 333
    intranasal flaps, 344
    neurovascular pedicle flap, 340
    office-based facial plastic surgery, 183, 189
    osseous flaps, 329
    regional flaps, 328, 333
    soft tissue flaps, 329
    surgical settings
        reconstructive head and neck surgery, 328–329, 333
        skull base surgery, 340
Flexible bronchoscopy, 138, 143
Flexible fiberoptic endoscopic evaluation (FEES), 148
Flexible fiberoptic endoscopic evaluation of swallowing and sensory testing (FEESST), 149
Flexible laryngoscopy, 137, 143, 367
FNA. *See* Fine needle aspiration
Forehead flap, 328
Foreign body removal
    office-based procedures, 158, 159, 208
    operative procedures, 265, 271, 272, 353, 354, 357, 360–361
FPL. *See* Federal poverty level
Fractures
    alveolar ridge, 286, 299
    cranial fracture, 286
    mandibular, 286–287, 299 300
    nasal fracture, 183, 185, 189–190, 208, 284–285, 290, 298–299, 354
    neck fracture, 260
    orbital, 286, 299
    sinus fracture, 285, 299
Franklin, Benjamin, 43
Fraud
    Benefit Integrity Unity (BIU), 59
    compliance program audits, 56–57
    Recovery Audit Contractor (RAC), 3, 58, 60, **61**
    restitution, 61–62
    Zone Program Integrity Contractor (ZPIC), 59–60, **61**
Free fascia graft, 296
Free flaps, 328–329, 333
Free grafts, 326–327
Frenectomy, 209, 356
Frenotomy, 356
Frenulectomy, 213, 356
Frenulum surgery, 362–363
Front desk staff, 31–34
Front-end processes, 29–30, 31–36, **32**, 47–48

Frontal sinus, surgical treatment, 285, 299
Frontal sinus procedures, endoscopic, 250
Frontal sinusotomy, 243-244, 248, **248**, 250
Full-thickness skin grafts, 183, 189, 326–327

G

G-codes, 150–151
Genioglossus advancement, 370
Geographic practice cost index (GPCI), 25
Global period modifiers, **94**, 107–109
Global surgical package, 85, 98, 238
Global surgical periods, 4
Glomus tumors, 267, 274, 340
Glossectomy, 303, 306, 314, 350, 351, 368, 370
Goiter, 199
GPCI. *See* Geographic practice cost index
Grafts
    allografts, 327
    free grafts, 326–327
    office-based facial plastic surgery, 183, 189
    skin substitute graft, 287, 300, 327
    surgical setting
        bone, 325, 326
        ear cartilage, 276
        facial plastic surgery, 282–283, 284, 287, 300–301
        harvest, 321
        harvesting, 265, 300
        otology, 269, 276
        reconstructive head and neck surgery, 321, 325, 326–327
        skull base setting, 339–340
        skull base surgery, 339–340

H

HCPCS Level I modifiers, 93, **94**
HCPCS Level II codes, 3, 24, 94, 137, 155, 162, 168, 257–258, 350–351
HCPCS Level II modifiers, 93, 94, 113–115, 135, 137
Head and neck surgery
    office-based, 193–205
        controversial areas, 204–205
        definition of procedure codes, 200–204
        E/M code based on time, 203–204
        ICD-9-CM/ICD-10-CM codes, 197–199
        modifiers, 196–197
        procedure codes, 194–196
        surveillance visits, 204
        telephone encounters, 203
    practice management, 203–204
    surgical setting, 303–333
        controversial areas, 318–320

Excludes notes, 15–16
laterality, 16, 169, 184–185
transition to, 13
IDT. *See* Intradermal dilutional testing
Imaging
in ambulatory surgical center, 252
office-based, 194–195, 225–231
controversial areas, 229
CT accreditation, 229, 231
IAC accreditation, 230
ICD-9-CM/ICD-10-CM codes, 228
MIPPA, 229–230
modifiers, 228
procedure codes, 226–228
submission requirements, 230–231
stereotactic computer-assisted navigation (SCAN),
241, 244, 251–252, **252**, 309, 341
Immunotherapy
allergy, 130, 133
sublingual (SLIT), 134
Impacted cerumen, 159–160, 163, 270, 272
Implants, otological, 268
Improper Payments Information Act (2002), 3
In-office otolaryngology. *See* Office-based
otolaryngology
"Incident to," 175
Incident-to billing, nonphysician practitioners (NPPs),
65
Incision codes
for office setting
pediatric otolaryngology, 208
rhinology, 122
for surgical setting, otology, 273, 276, 364
Injection
botulinum toxin (Botox), 134, 136, 137, 141–142, 143,
144, 191
facial plastic surgery, 191
HCPCS Level II codes, 155
intratympanic steroid injection, **153**
Injection material, codes for, 263
Injury, Poisoning, and Certain Other Consequences of
External Causes, ICD-10-CM coding, 20–21
Inner ear, 157, 268, 276
Inpatient consultations, 89, **89**
Inpatient status, 86, **97**
Insomnia, 217–218
Insurance eligibility, 31, 34
Insurance fraud. *See* Fraud
Intermediate wound repair
office-based facial plastic surgery, 181–182, 187
surgical setting
facial plastic surgery, 281–282
reconstructive head and neck surgery, 322–323

Internal auditory canal/CPA, 337
*International Classification of Diseases, Ninth Revision,
Clinical Modification. See* ICD-9-CM
*International Classification of Diseases, Tenth Revision,
Clinical Modification. See* ICD-10-CM
Intersocietal Accreditation Commission (IAC), 229,
230
Intradermal dilutional testing (IDT), 129
Intranasal biopsy, 122
Intranasal flaps, 344
Intraoperative nerve monitoring (IONM), 304,
318–319, 341
Intraoperative ultrasonography, 317
Intrathoracic tracheoplasty, 355
Intratympanic steroid injection, **153**
Intratympanic therapy, 162
Intuitive Surgical da Vinci robot, 349
Intuitive Surgical Inc., 349, 350
InVitro allergy testing, 132–133
IONM. *See* Intraoperative nerve monitoring

K

Kickbacks, 53, 54

L

L codes, 168
Labyrinthectomy, 276
Labyrinthine dysfunction, 157
Labyrinthine fistula, 270
Labyrinthotomy, 268, 276
Lagophthalmos, 190–191, 284, 289, 298
Laryngeal disorders, 259
Laryngeal function studies, 148
Laryngeal sensory testing, 137–138, 142
Laryngeal surgery, 260–261
Laryngectomy, 255, 260, 303, 305, 313–314, 350, 351
Laryngitis, 358
Laryngocele, 259, 359
Laryngology
office-based, 135–144
controversial areas, 143–144
definition of codes, 140–143
ICD-9-CM/ICD-10-CM codes, 139–140
modifiers, 138–139
procedure codes, 136–138
operative, 255–263
controversial areas, 262–263
definition of codes, 260–262
ICD-9-CM/ICD-10-CM codes, 258–260
modifiers, 258
procedure codes, 255–258

(modifier 52), 93, **94**, 106–107, 113, **115**, 139, 148, 150, 169, 217, 222, 258, 357, 368
(modifier 53), **94**, 104, **115**, 288
(modifier 57), 83, 86, 94, **94**, 98–99, **98**, **116**, 357–358
(modifier 58), **94**, 107–108, **107**, **116**, 179, 184, 258, 288, 329, 342, 365
(modifier 59), 49, 94, **94**, 103–104, **103**, **104**, **116**, 150, 169, 184, 197, 245, 258, 269, 288, 303, 309–310, 319, 329–330, 358
(modifier 62), 93, **94**, 109–111, **111**, **116**, 321, 330, 336, 341, 342
(modifier 63), **94**, 104–105, **116**, 210, 358
(modifier 66), **94**, 111–112, **116**
(modifier 76), 93, **94**, 105, **116**, 124, 288
(modifier 77), 93, **94**, 105, **116**
(modifier 78), **94**, 108–109, **108**, **116**, 258, 342
(modifier 79), **94**, 109, **109**, **116**, 124, 155, 184, 197, 258, 288
(modifier 80), 93, **94**, 112, **116**, 321, 330, 342
(modifier 81), **94**, 112, **116**
(modifier 82), 69, 93, **94**, 113, **116**, 321, 330, 342
Motor Control Test (MCT), 171
Mouth. *See* Oral cavity
MPPF. *See* Multiple procedure payment formula
MRI. *See* Magnetic resonance imaging
MRND. *See* Modified radical neck dissection
MSLT. *See* Multiple Sleep Latency Test
Mucocele, 361
Multiple procedure payment formula (MPPF), 102
Multiple Sleep Latency Test (MSLT), 219–220
MWT. *See* Maintenance of Wakefulness Test
Myotomy, 262
Myringoplasty, 162, 274, 357, 363
Myringotomy, 161, 266, 273, 357

N

Narcolepsy, 218
Nasal airway surgery, 279–280, 288, 290–292, 371
Nasal biopsy, 122
Nasal deformities, 280, 292
Nasal disorders, 245
Nasal endoscopy, 194, 341
Nasal fracture
    office-based facial plastic surgery, 183, 185, 189–190, 208
    surgical repair, 284–285, 290, 298–299, 354
Nasal polyp excision, 127
Nasal septal perforation, 302
Nasal vestibular stenosis, 292, 302
Naso-orbito-ethmoid (NOE) complex, 285, 299
Nasomaxillary complex fracture, 285, 299
Nasopharyngoscopy, 147, 162–163, 194
Nasopharynx, 158, 271, 331–332

National Correct Coding Initiative (NCCI or CCI) Policy Manual, 5, 27, 31, 82
National Correct Coding Initiative (NCCI or CCI) edits, 175
National coverage determinations (NCDs), 27, 54
National Medicare Physician Fee Schedule Database, 4, 83, 99, 110
National Outcomes Measurement System (NOMS), 151
National provider identifier (NPI) number, 64, 65, 165
NCCI. *See* National Correct Coding Initiative (NCCI or CCI) Policy Manual
NCCI edits. *See* National Correct Coding Initiative (NCCI or CCI) edits
NCDs. *See* National coverage determinations
Neck
    dissection, 303, 305, 306, 312–313, 316, 319–320
    pediatric otolaryngology, 209, 354
    See also Head and neck surgery; Reconstructive head and neck surgery
Neck fracture, 260
Needle biopsy, 200
Needle electromyography, 136, 137, 142, 309
Neoplasms, 16–17, 198, 199, 259, 270, 280–281, 288–289, 292–293, 304, 308, 310–311, 330, 331, 332, 351, 352, 361
Nerve graft, 284, 296
Nerve repair, surgical, 324–325
Net collections percentage, 42
Neuroendoscopy, 308
Neurovascular pedicle flap, 340
New patients
    E/M coding, 73, 74–75, **81**
    preregistration, 34
No-show patients, 33
NOE complex. *See* Naso-orbito-ethmoid (NOE) complex
NOMS. *See* National Outcomes Measurement System
Nonendoscopic codes, rhinology, 122, 127
Nonphysician practitioners (NPPs)
    billing, 63–66, **66**, 67–68, **67**, **70**, 71
        direct billing, 64
        incident-to billing, 65
        split/shared billing, 65–66
    resources, 70–71
Nose
    deformities, 280
    office-based pediatric otolaryngology, 208
    surgical procedures
        pediatric otolaryngology, 354
        reconstructive head and neck surgery, 330–331
        trauma repair, 284–285
    See also under Nasal
NPI. *See* National provider identifier number

Radioguided parathyroidectomy, 317

Radiology CPT codes, 10

Ranula, 307

RBRVS study. *See* Resource-Based Relative Value Scale (RBRVS) study

Reasonable and necessary services, 53

Reconstructive head and neck surgery, 321–333

  controversial areas, 333

  definition of procedure codes, 333

  ICD-9-CM/ICD-10-CM codes, 330–332

  modifiers, 329–330

  procedure codes, 322–329

  skull base surgery, 339–341

Recovery Audit Contractors (RAC), 3, 58, 60, **61**

Recurrent laryngeal nerve, 319

Referrals, 31, 34

  defined, 55

  self-referrals, 53, 55

Regional flaps, 328, 333

Relative Value Scale Update Committee (RUC), 26–27

Relative Value Units (RVUs), 24–26, 121

Resection, skull base surgery, 338–339

Resident physicians, 70

Resource-Based Relative Value Scale (RBRVS) study, 24–25, 26, 28

Respiratory failure, 359

Respiratory system diseases, 17–18

Respiratory system surgery, 305

Restitution, 61–62

Retropharyngeal abscess, 360, 364

Review of systems (ROS), 77

Rhinology

  office-based, 121–128

    ICD-9-CM/ICD-10-CM codes, 124–125

    modifiers, 123–124

    procedure codes, 122–123

  operative, 241–253

    controversial areas, 252–253

    definition of codes, 246–252

    ICD-9-CM/ICD-10-CM codes, 245–246

    modifiers, 244–245

    procedure codes, 242–244

Rhinoplasty, 279, 288, 290–292, 301–302

Rhytidectomy, 284, 297

RND. *See* Radical neck dissection

Robotic surgery, 262, 349–352, 370

ROS. *See* Review of systems

Ross Information Processing Assessment, 149

Rotary chair, 171

Round window fistula, 268, 275

RUC. *See* Relative Value Scale Update Committee

RVUs. *See* Relative Value Units

S

S codes, 168

Salivary duct, 201

Salivary glands

  chemodenervation, 363

  ICD-9-CM to ICD-10-CM mappings for, **19**

  neoplasm, 198

  procedures, 195, 201

  reconstructive head and neck surgery, 332

  surgical procedures, 307, 363

Same-day service modifiers, **94**, 99–105

SCAN. *See* Stereotactic computer-assisted navigation

Scar revision, 295

Second-level appeals, 52

Secondary dural repair, 339

Self-referrals, 53, 55

Semicircular canal dehiscence, 277

Semont maneuver, 163

Sensorineural hearing loss, 169

Sensory Organization Test (SOT), 171

Septal fracture, 189–190, 284, 285

Septoplasty

  billing for, 35

  coding for, 99, 101, **247**, 302, 368

  global period, 4

  surgical, 237, 242, 292

Sequestrectomy, 306

Severity modifiers, 150–151, **151**

SGR formula. *See* Sustainable growth rate (SGR) formula

Sialadenitis, 210

Sialoadenitis, 199

Sialodochoplasty, 195, 201

Sialoendoscopy, 193, 204

Sialolithiasis, 199, 204

Sialolithotomy, 195, 201

Simple grafts, 326

Simple wound repair

  office-based facial plastic surgery, 181, 187

  in surgical setting

    facial plastic surgery, 281

    reconstructive head and neck surgery, 322

Sinography, 229

Sinonasal lesions, 246

Sinus endoscopy, 194, 242–243, 248, **248**, 249, 250, 252

Sinus fracture, 285, 299

Sinus implantation, 252–253

Sinus ostial dilation, 127, 128

Sinus surgery, 241

  endoscopic, 242–243, 248, **248**, 252

  reconstructive, 330–331

Sinusitis, 124, 245–246

Sinusotomy, 248
Sistrunk procedure, 364
Skin
  office-based otolaryngology
    facial plastic surgery, 179–192
    pediatric otolaryngology, 208
  reconstructive head and neck surgery, 322–324
Skin and subcutaneous tissue diseases, ICD-10-CM coding, 19
Skin grafts, 326–327. *See also* Grafts
Skin lesions, 179–180, 280–281, 292–293
Skin substitute graft, 287, 300, 327
Skin tags, 208
Skin tests, for allergies, 129–130, 133
Skull base surgery, 268, 304, 308–309, 317–318, 335–346
  controversial areas, 343–345
  ICD-9-CM/ICD-10-CM codes, 343
  modifiers, 342
  procedure codes, 336–342
  procedure note, **346**
Sleep apnea, 215, 218, 361, 368, 371
Sleep endoscopy, 368–369
Sleep medicine
  office-based, 215–223
    controversial areas, 222–223
    definition of codes, 219–222
    ICD-9-CM/ICD-10-CM codes, 217–218
    modifiers, 217
    procedure codes, 216–217
  operative, 367–371
    controversial areas, 371
    definition of codes, 368–371
    ICD-9-CM/ICD-10-CM codes, 368
    modifiers, 368
    procedure codes, 367–368
Sleep studies, 216
SLIT. *See* Sublingual immunotherapy
SLPs. *See* Speech-language pathologists
SMAS. *See* Superficial muscular aponeurotic system
Smell testing, 127–128
Smith-Lemli-Opitz syndrome, 359
Snoring, 211, 218, 222, 361, 367
Social history, documentation, 77
Social Security Act, 54
Soft tissue flaps, 329
SOT. *See* Sensory Organization Test
Speech-generating devices, 148
Speech-language pathologists (SLPs), 147
Speech pathology, 147–153
  definition of codes, 150–152
  modifiers, 149–150
  office-based, ICD-9-CM/ICD-10-CM codes, 150
  procedure codes, 147–149

Speech studies, 148
Sphenoidotomy, 237
Sphenopalatine ligation, 236, 249
Spine, skull base surgery, 338
Split/shared billing, 65–66
Split-thickness grafts, 326, 339
Spontaneous nystagmus, 166
Squamous cell carcinoma, 289, 311, 330
Staff
  billing staff, 30, 38–40, **41**, 42–43, **42**
  educating and empowering, 43–44
  front desk staff, 31–33
  training, 43
Stand-alone Category I codes (CPT), **9**
Stapedectomy, 267, 275
Stapedotomy, 267, 275
Stapes, 267
Stapes mobilization, 275
Stark laws, 55, 223
State and local law, physician practices, 54–56
State law, practice management, 56
Stent placement, office-based, 123
Stereotactic computer-assisted navigation (SCAN), 241, 251–252, **252**, 309, 341
Stridor, 211
Stroboscopy, 137, 147
Subglottic stenosis, 359
Sublingual immunotherapy (SLIT), 134
Sublingual salivary gland, 198, 307, 332
Submandibular gland stone, 201
Submandibular salivary gland, 332, 357
Submaxillary salivary gland, 307
Substernal thyroidectomy, 316
Subtotal supraglottic laryngectomy, 313
Subtotal thyroid lobectomy, 315
Superficial muscular aponeurotic system (SMAS), 297
Supraglottoplasty, 365
Suprahyoid lymphadenectomy, 306
Suprahyoid neck dissection, 313
Surgeon role modifiers, **94**, 109–113
Surgery
  robotic surgery, 262, 349–352, 370
  teaching setting rules, 69, **70**
  See also Surgical code modifiers; Surgical coding; Surgical otolaryngology
Surgical assistance services, 64, 69–70, **70**
Surgical code modifiers, 99–113, 237
  complexity modifiers, **94**, 105–107
    (modifier 22), **94**, 105–106, **115**, 149–150, 168–169, 209, 244, 258, 287, 303, 309, 329, 342
    (modifier 52), 93, **94**, 106–107, 113, 115, 139, 148, 150, 169, 217, 222, 258, 357, 368
  diagnostic code modifiers, 113

Surgical code modifiers *(continued)*
  global period modifiers, **94**, 107–109
    (modifier 58), **94**, 107–108, **107**, **116**, 179, 184, 258, 288, 329, 342, 365
    (modifier 76), 93, **94**, 105, **116**, 124, 288
    (modifier 77), 93, **94**, 105, **116**
    (modifier 78), **94**, 108–109, **108**, **116**, 258, 342
    (modifier 79), **94**, 109, **109**, **116**, 124, 155, 184, 197, 258, 288
  same-day service modifiers, **94**, 99–105
    (modifier 50), 93, **94**, 100, **101**, 102, **102**, 114, **115**, 123, 136, 139, 155, 210, 244, 258, 269, 309, 353
    (modifier 51), **94**, 101–102, **102**, **115**, 184, 197, 210, 244, 258, 287
    (modifier 53), **94**, 104, **115**, 288
    (modifier 59), 49, 94, **94**, 103–104, **103**, **104**, **116**, 150, 169, 184, 197, 245, 258, 269, 288, 303, 309–310, 319, 329–330, 358
    (modifier 63), **94**, 104–105, **116**, 210, 358
    (modifier 76), 93, **94**, 105, **116**, 124, 288
    (modifier 77), 93, **94**, 105, **116**
  surgeon role modifiers, **94**, 109–113
    (modifier 62), **94**, 109–111, **111**, 321, 330, 336, 341, 342
    (modifier 66), **94**, 111–112, **116**
    (modifier 80), 93, **94**, 112, **116**, 321, 330, 342
    (modifier 81), **94**, 112
    (modifier 82), 69, 93, **94**, 113, **116**, 321, 330, 342
Surgical coding, 235–239
  ambulatory surgical center, 252
  controversial areas, 239
  CPT codes, 10, 50–51
  global surgical package, 85, 98, 238
  medical necessity, 57, 235, 236–237
  modifiers. *See* Surgical code modifiers
  multiple procedures, 237
  new technology, 236
  operative note, 235–236, 239
  selecting a code, 236–237
  unbundling, 237–238
  unlisted codes, 238–239, 249
  See also Postoperative global period; Surgical code modifiers; Surgical otolaryngology
Surgical endoscopy, 125–126
Surgical otolaryngology, 235–371
  coding basics, 235–239
  facial plastic surgery, 279–302
  head and neck surgery, 303–320
  laryngology, 255–263
  otology, 265–277
  pediatric otolaryngology, 353–366
  reconstructive head and neck surgery, 321–322
  rhinology, 241–253
  robotic surgery, 252, 349–352

  skull base surgery, 268, 304, 308–309, 317–318, 335–346
  sleep surgery, 367–371
  See also Surgical code modifiers; Surgical coding
Surgical wound preparation, office-based facial plastic surgery, 183, 188–189
Suspension microlaryngoscopy, 255
Sustainable growth rate (SGR) formula, 25
Swallowing disorders, 150, 151, 259–260, 360
Swallowing tests, 137–138, 142, 148
Symptoms, Signs, and Abnormal Clinical and Laboratory Findings, ICD-10-CM coding, 19–20

T

"T" codes (CP), **9**
Teaching physicians, billing by, 68–70, **70**
Teaching setting
  defined, 68
  surgical assistance in, 69–70
  surgical procedures in, 69
Telephone encounters, 203
Temporalis fascia graft, 276
Tendon graft, 326
TGDC. *See* Thyroglossal duct cyst
Therapeutic office-based procedures, 140–141
Therapeutic vocal fold injection, 136
Thermocauterization, 284
Thymectomy, 308
Thyroglossal duct cyst (TGDC), 357, 364
Thyroid glands, surgical procedures, 307–308
Thyroid nodule, 199, 227
Thyroidectomy, 303, 315–316, *315*
Thyroplasty, 260
Thyrotoxicosis, 199, 311
Time-based codes, 152
Tinnitus, 157, 168, 169, 173
Tissue grafts, 300, 339–340
Titration skin tests, for allergies, 129–130
TLM. *See* Transoral laser microsurgery
Tongue, 209, 213, 306, 352
  glossectomy, 303, 306, 314, 350, 351, 368, 370
  radiofrequency treatment, 369–370
  suspension, 367, 368, 370
Tonsillectomy, 106–107, 353, 356, 361, 363, 367, 369
Tonsillitis, 210, 360
Tonsils, 210, 306, 350, 351, 361
TORS. *See* Robotic surgery
Total glossectomy, 314
Total laryngectomy, 313
Total thyroidectomy, 315
Tracheal disorders, 259
Tracheitis, 358
Tracheo-esophageal fistula, 359